ELECTRONIC

MEDICAL

RECORDS

For a catalogue of publications available from ACP–ASIM, contact:

Customer Service Center
American College of Physicians–American Society of Internal Medicine
190 N. Independence Mall West
Philadelphia, PA 19106-1572
215-351-2600
800-523-1546, ext. 2600

Visit our Web site at www.acponline.org

ELECTRONIC MEDICAL RECORDS

A Guide for Clinicians and Administrators

JEROME H. CARTER, MD, FACP

A|C|P

AMERICAN COLLEGE OF PHYSICIANS
PHILADELPHIA, PENNSYLVANIA

Clinical Consultant: David R. Goldmann, MD
Manager, Book Publishing: David Myers
Production Supervisor: Allan S. Kleinberg
Acquisitions Editor: Mary K. Ruff
Editorial Coordinator: Alicia Dillihay
Interior and Cover Design: Kate Nichols
Indexer: Nelle Garrecht

Printed in the United States of America
Composition by Fulcrum Data Services, Inc.
Printing/binding by McNaughton & Gunn, Inc.

American College of Physicians (ACP) became an imprint of the American College of Physicians–American Society of Internal Medicine in July 1998.

Publisher's Note—Although a number of EMR vendors and products are mentioned within the text of this book and some chapter authors are formally affiliated with an EMR vendor, this in no way implies an endorsement of the products or vendors by the editor or the American College of Physicians—American Society of Internal Medicine.

Library of Congress Cataloging-in-Publication Data

American College of Physicians–American Society of Internal Medicine.
    Electronic medical records: a guide for clinicians and administrators / [edited by]
Jerome H. Carter.–1st ed.
        p. ; cm.
    Includes bibliographical references and index.
    Contents: Part 1. Electronic medical records for clinicians and administrators –
Part 2. EMR implementation (workbook).
    ISBN 1-930513-01-1
    1. Medical records--Data processing. I. Carter, Jerome, H., 1955-
[DNLM: 1. Medical Records Systems, Computerized. WX 173 E383 2000]
R864.A42 2000
651.5´04261´0285–dc21   00-049594

01 02 03 04 05 / 9 8 7 6 5 4 3 2 1

CONTRIBUTORS

Jeroan J. Allison, MD, MS
Associate Professor of Medicine
Division of General Internal Medicine
Department of Medicine
University of Alabama–Birmingham
    School of Medicine;
Director, UAB Pittmam General Clinical
    Research Center Informatics Core
Director, UAB Center for Outcomes and
    Effectiveness Research
Education Data Management Unit
Birmingham, Alabama

Bryan Bergeron, MD
Director, Medical Informatics
    Laboratory
Department of Anesthesia and
    Critical Care
Massachusetts General Hospital
Brookline, MA

Lyle L. Berkowitz, MD
Medical Director
Proxicom, Inc.;
Attending Physician
Northwestern Memorial Hospital;
Instructor in Clinical Medicine
Northwestern University Medical
    School
Chicago, Illinois

Stephen E. Brossette, MD, PhD
Chief Technology Officer
MedMind, Inc.
Birmingham, Alabama

Jerome H. Carter, MD, FACP
Director of Informatics
1917 Research Clinic
Division of Infectious Diseases
Department of Medicine
University of Alabama–Birmingham
Birmingham, Alabama;
Adjunct Assistant Professor
Health Informatics Program
Dept. of Health Services Administration
School of Health-Related Professions
University of Alabama–Birmingham;
Chair, Medical Informatics Subcommittee,
    1997-2001
American College of Physicians–
    American Society of Internal Medicine
Philadelphia, Pennsylvania

Sarah T. Corley, MD, FACP
Associate Professor
Department of Health Care Sciences
George Washington University School of
    Medicine;
Medical Director
Internal Medicine Associates
Arlington, Virginia

Daniel C. Davis, Jr., MD, FACP
Medical Director, Clinical Informatics
The Queen's Medical Center;
Chief, Division of Medical Informatics
Department of Medicine
John A. Burns School of Medicine
University of Hawaii
Honolulu, Hawaii

Erica L. Drazen, ScD
Vice President
First Consulting Group
Lexington, MA

Patricia L. Hale, PhD, MD
Private Practice, Internal Medicine
Gansevoort, NY;
Member, Medical Informatics
    Subcommittee
American College of Physicians–
    American Society of Internal Medicine
Philadelphia, Pennsylvania

J. Michael Hardin, PhD
Professor, Health Informatics and
    Biostatistics
Deparrtment of Health Services
    Administration
School of Health-Related Professions
University of Alabama-Birmingham
Birmingham, AL

John J. Janas III, MD
Attending Internist and Pediatrician
Family Care of Concord;
Medical Director, Physician Information
    Services
Capital Region Healthcare
Concord, NH

Merida L. Johns, PhD, RRA
Director, Master of Science Program in
    Information Systems Management
Information Systems and Operations
    Management Department
School of Business Administration
Loyola University
Chicago, Illinois

Terri Thompson Mallett, MBA, JD
General Counsel
Greater Southeast Healthcare System
Washington, DC

Daniel R. Masys, MD, FACP
Director of Biomedical Informatics and
    Associate Clinical Professor of
    Medicine
University of California - San Diego
    School of Medicine
La Jolla, California

**Blackford Middleton, MD, MPH, MSc,
FACP**
Chief Medical Officer
Medscape, Inc.;
Associate Professor (Adjunct) of Medical
    Informatics and Outcomes Research
Department of Medical Informatics and
    Outcomes Research
Oregon Health Sciences University
Hillsboro, Oregon

**Matthew W. Morgan, MD, MSc,
FRCP(C)**
Director of Healthcare Informatics
Per-Se Technologies;
Practicing General Internist;
Assistant Professor
Department of Medicine
University of Toronto
Toronto, Ontario, Canada

Bruce Slater, MD, MPH, FACP
Assistant Professor of Health Care Sciences
    and Medicine
George Washington University Medical
    Center
Washington, DC

The contributions of **Steven Spadt and
Linda Sundberg** of the American
College of Physicians–American
Society of Internal Medicine to
Appendix A are much appreciated.

PREFACE

The inspiration for this book came from the many clinicians whom I have encountered over the past four years who found themselves in the frustrating position of wanting to implement an electronic medical record (EMR) system and having no idea where to start the process. Invariably, their first words to me after the usual pleasantries were "Which system should I buy?" My response always began with "That depends..." and the ensuing brief discussion was rarely sufficient to answer their query.

This book is an attempt to answer the many questions that arise when implementing an EMR system. As an aid to the reader, the book is divided into two parts. In Part One the reader will find in-depth discussions of technologies, issues, and processes. When applicable, references for further reading are provided. However, this should in no way be understood to imply that Part One is an academic work with little practical value. It offers the background information required to understand the important EMR issues that arise as one journeys from initial curiosity to final implementation. Think of Part One as providing the "what" and "why" of EMR-related technologies and issues.

Part Two has a completely different approach. It is designed as a Workbook. Here the goal is to offer practical advice on the actual steps involved in implementing an EMR system. The information provided in its chapters is thoroughly infused with the "hands-on" experience of the authors. Though Part Two offers useful advice for readers in all practice environments, it should be particularly useful to those in a solo practice or small group and to others who cannot afford to retain the services of major consulting firms or do not have access to a good deal of on-site technical expertise. Part Two covers the everyday issues of negotiating a contract, evaluating products, understanding practice needs, and planning.

How To Use This Book

Electronic Medical Records for Clinicians and Administrators contains a good deal of information, much of it quite technical—all of it necessary to achieve a working knowledge of the important issues faced when moving from paper to an EMR. It is expected that readers will come to this work with quite different backgrounds, and to that end the following suggestions are offered based upon the knowledge of the reader and the type of resources that are at his or her disposal. The following groups should encompass the majority of readers.

Clinician/Administrator with Little Technical Knowledge and Access to Limited Resources

Often in small groups or solo practices the clinician or administrator has little technical knowledge and access to limited resources. A major consulting firm is out of the question, and the technical person involved may be the retailer who sold you the practice management system (or possibly a relative who "knows a lot about computers"). The cost of failure will be high in terms of dollars and morale. If you fall into this group, caution is the keyword. Take time to read Chapters 1–3, 5–7, 10–12, and all of the Workbook (Part Two). These chapters offer insight into the issues most pressing for those in your situation. Once you have become familiar with the concepts and issues that they discuss, then go back and finish the remaining chapters. Do not take lightly the admonitions offered in the Workbook. Most of all, do not allow your desire to do "something" make you do something that you come to regret.

Clinicians/Administrators who are Members of "Selection Committees"

Usually a selection committee implies a fair-sized practice or a more diverse setting (e.g., hospital, multi-specialty group). In such cases technical personnel and consultants are often available, both of whom can be very helpful during product selection and implementation. If you are a member of this group, you will likely have little direct say over the most important issues. Your role becomes that of protecting the interests of those you represent (unless of course you are the committee chairman!). Your understanding of the key issues is extremely important. If you have a fairly good grasp of technical matters, then issues related to work-flow, practice environment, and general operations should guide your reading. Chapters 6–12 will probably be most helpful initially, with Chapters 1–5 acting as an occasional reference. The Workbook will be useful in helping you prepare your colleagues for the changes that lie ahead.

Medical Directors

The implementation of an EMR system may be either a godsend or the worse thing that has ever happened in your professional life. As the spokesman for the medical staff your opinion counts tremendously and therefore should be well-informed. Very likely you have access to technical staff and consultants. Unfortunately, they may have a vested interested in influencing your opinion. Part One has the information you need to understand the terms and concepts that will be discussed repeatedly in your meetings, demonstrations, and site visits. If quality improvement is a major reason for the implementation (e.g., order entry, guidelines), Chapters 6–10 and 16 should be given particular scrutiny. If a clinical data repository is being considered, Chapter 4 should be added to the must-read list.

CEO/CIO and Other High Level Administrators

All of the issues covered in the book are important to you. However, because many jobs will be delegated to those with appropriate expertise, the information that you require is likely to be at a fairly high conceptual level. Consequently, Chapters 8–12 will probably be most useful. In addition, the chapters in the Workbook that discuss Requests for Proposals and contracts might provide a few useful insights (see especially Chapter 18).

Technical Personnel with Little EMR Knowledge

Few health care sites have installed an EMR system, and there is no shortage of horror stories of failed implementations. Many of the failures are caused by nontechnical issues (e.g., poor planning, inadequate training). However, often the problem is a poor understanding of the technical issues associated with EMR software. For example, response times under full load, file importation, database structure, clinical vocabulary, and system integration are technical matters that can delay or doom an EMR installation. Those who may be best able to understand the potential pitfalls at an early stage are knowledgeable technical personnel. Chapters 1–5 and 16 should be of particular value to technical personnel involved in EMR projects.

Final Remarks

If you find that you do not fit into any of these groups, reading the book from beginning to end also works quite well. But do not read this book in a vacuum. Many vendors offer fully functioning demonstration programs, at little or no cost, that may be used to aid in understanding EMR features and issues. Supplement your reading with other materials; there are a number of helpful Web sites and magazines (see Appendix B). One result of the diligent reading of this book will be the mastery of the concepts and jargon associated with EMR systems. You will be surprised at how quickly once-incomprehensible technical articles and discussions begin to make perfectly good sense.

Acknowledgements

I would like to thank all those who have made this book possible. The Editorial Staff members of ACP-ASIM—Mary Ruff, David Myers, and Alicia Dillihay—have been very understanding, supportive, and patient. Former staff members of the College's Medical Informatics Department—Bob Spena, Jerry Osherhoff, Linda Sundberg, Chris Dwyer, and Steve Spadt—provided very helpful comments and suggestions.

Michael Saag, Jim Raper, Betty McCulloch, Michael Kilby, Tracey Reid, and the staff of the 1917 Research Clinic at the University of Alabama–Birmingham demonstrated exceptional patience and understanding during my many months of endless questions, interviews, meetings, and report writing. Having gone through a full-scale systems-and-requirements analysis for our home-grown EMR project, they remain cheerful and eager to continue. Thank you for your support and good humor.

Doing a book of this scope would have required more time than I alone could possibly have dedicated to such an important task. Also, the quality would not have been nearly as high without the valuable contributions of my fellow authors. I am honored to be in such good company.

Finally, I would like to thank all those who have attended my talks and seminars over the years for helping me to focus the content of the book and to understand what the important issues really are.

Jerome H. Carter, MD, FACP
February 2001

CONTENTS

PART ONE

Electronic Medical Records for Clinicians and Administrators

SECTION I

Infrastructure

1 / What is an Electronic Medical Record?

Jerome H. Carter

R eports of the use of computers to support clinical data management activities date back to the late 1950s. Over the years computer systems have been designed that support most major activities related to health care business practices and clinical processes. The most common types of systems are listed in Table 1-1.

Until recently, hospitals led the way in the development of clinical information systems. This was owing, in part, to several factors: 1) the cost of these systems (including personnel) made information technology too expensive for smaller entities, and 2) hospitals had greater needs of meeting regulatory and financial requirements. Hospital Information Systems (HIS) usually have, as their central component, an Admission, Discharge, and Transfer (ADT) system that manages census and patient demographic information. Billing and accounting packages are also frequently included as core components. In many community hospitals, financial and ADT systems along with Laboratory Information Systems (LIS) comprised the complete HIS package until recently. In the last ten years most hospitals, regardless of size, have created fairly complete Information Systems (IS) solutions via integration of departmental systems with the core HIS.

Departmental systems, especially those for Pharmacy, Radiology, and Laboratory, have evolved from a focus on administrative tasks (scheduling, order-entry, billing) to more clinically oriented functions. For example, modern pharmacy systems commonly provide drug interactions, allergy alerts, and drug monographs as part of their standard functions. When looking at the evolution of clinical information systems, it is instructive to consider how the end-user has changed over the years. Departmental systems were designed primarily for use by workers within those departments, not health care providers. Thus drug-interaction information was available

Table 1-1   Common Health Care Computer Systems.

System Type	Function
Master Patient Index	Registration and assignment of unique identifier
Pharmacy Information System	Medication dispensing, inventory, billing, drug information and interactions
Radiology Information System	Scheduling, billing, results reporting
Picture Archiving System	Storage and presentation of radiologic images
Nursing Information System	Storage and collection of nursing documentation, care planning, administrative information
Hospital Information System	Core system manages hospital census (admission, discharge, transfer) and billing; most often linked to departmental systems (pharmacy, laboratory, etc.)
Chart Management/Medical Records Systems	Assist in the management of paper records and required statistical reporting; used by Medical Records Personnel
Practice Management System	Outpatient system for managing business-related information; may contain some clinical information (CPT, ICD)
Laboratory Information System	Ordering of laboratory tests, results reporting; covers blood bank, pathology, microbiology, etc.

only to pharmacists and their staffs, not directly to doctors and nurses. Clinical information systems were labeled as such because they were utilized in areas that supported clinical activities, not because they were intended for use primarily by clinicians.

Of all the systems that fall under the rubric of clinical information systems, only a few are designed primarily for use by health care providers: Intensive Care Unit (ICU) systems, Picture Archiving (PAC) systems, and Electronic Medical Record (EMR) systems. ICU systems monitor a number of physiologic variables and thereby aid in decision making; PAC systems provide access to radiologic images at locations throughout the enterprise. Both have well-defined domains and may work quite well without close integration with other departmental systems. EMRs are quite another story. The EMR is intended to integrate information from all departmental systems and deliver that information to health care providers at or close to the point-of-care. This is no small task.

The Electronic Medical Record Concept

Aside from having health care providers as primary users, EMRs have a another trait that sets them apart from other clinical information systems; they are designed to capture and re-present data that accurately capture the clinical state of the patient. Symptoms, physical examination findings, and treatment plans find their home in EMRs. The EMR, as a concept, is a tool that helps the clinician manage all aspects of patient care. The data-capture functions help to ensure that all pertinent patient data are accurately entered, appropriate for the stated diagnoses, and legible. However, it is the presentation functions that drive the EMR concept. Here reside the means to look at data in new ways, whether they be trends in serum glucose values, medication history, or a list of patients who have not received recommended preventive health interventions. Unlike the paper chart, the EMR is capable of presenting previously stored data in novel ways. Trends may be reviewed for one patient or an entire group. The potential impact on decision making is almost unlimited.

Origins

Early efforts at building what are now referred to as EMRs began in the 1960s with the COSTAR system, developed by Barnett at the Laboratory of Computer Science at Massachusetts General Hospital (1). Subsequent efforts at Duke University (2) and the Regenstrief Institute at Indiana University Medical Center (3) have given rise to robust EMR systems that contain data for thousands of patients. Commercial versions of EMRs are available from over 200 companies. However, despite these successes, EMR technology is not widespread. It has been estimated that only 3% to 5% of doctors have access to or use EMRs on a regular basis (4). Given the nearly forty years of development activity, it is difficult to understand why EMRs are not a more commonly used clinical tool. The answer may lie in the complexity of the issues that surround the design and implementation of these systems.

EMR and CPR Defined

In 1991 the Institute of Medicine (IOM) published a landmark report, "The Computer-Based Patient Record: An Essential Technology for Health Care" (5). This document served to focus attention on the issues surrounding EMR design and implementation. Perhaps one of its more valuable contributions is in the area of terminology.

When perusing publications concerned with EMRs and associated technologies, one is quickly struck by the number of terms used to describe what are often represented as the same entity. *Electronic medical record, electronic patient record, electronic health record, computer-stored patient record, ambulatory medical record,* and *computer-based medical record* are at varying times applied to the same type of system. Are they the same thing? The IOM report suggests very useful definitions, and these will be used for these terms throughout this book. It defines the CPR (Computer-based Patient Record) as an

> electronic patient record that resides in a system designed to support users through availability of complete and accurate data, practitioner reminders and alerts, clinical decision support systems, links to bodies of medical knowledge and other aids.

The report goes on to define a CPR system as

> the set of components that form the mechanism by which patient records are created, used, stored, and retrieved... It includes people, data, rules, procedures, processing and storage devices, and communications and support procedures.

Further amplification was later provided by one of the report's editors, Richard Dick, who states (6):

> The CPR is a representation of all of a patient's data that one would find in...the paper-based record, but in a coded and structured, machine-readable form. It incorporates a messaging standard for common representation of all pertinent patient data. Clinical documentation is completed via computer and is coded within the patient's CPR. Stored data are indexed with sufficient detail to support retrieval for patient care delivery, management and analysis.

He then proceeds to discuss the features of EMRs and EPRs:

The EMR and EPR, which are, in fact reasonably synonymous, are electronic, machine-readable versions of much of the data found in paper-based records, comprising both structured and unstructured patient data from disparate, computerized ancillary systems and document imaging systems. Clinical documentation may originate in either paper records or computerized data; however, the data are not comprehensively coded. One might consider the EMR or EPR as transitional between the paper-based record and the CPR.

The perspective offered by Dick relates the CPR, EMR, and EPR along a continuum based upon, among other factors, the level of granularity of stored data. A true CPR requires that every data item be uniquely coded and individually searchable; an EMR/EPR does not. EMR systems only require that the data be in electronic form. An example may make this point clearer. This chapter is being written using a word processor. Therefore it is in electronic form. However, there is no index to this document that would permit one to answer questions such as how many lines contain the word *almost*. A clinical example might be: "Retrieve all records for patients who have an S3 recorded for their most recent physical exam." In both examples, an indexed database of terms is required to perform an efficient query. Of course, to ensure that all retrieved records actually relate to the same phenomenon and that all records of patients with an S3 are in fact found, some means has to be in place to find records that do not explicitly contain the term S3. Records that have a "third heart sound" or a "summation gallop" recorded as findings would be overlooked. A controlled vocabulary, as well as a mechanism for creating searchable terms, is required. A CPR requires both of these features along with many others. Commercially available systems are EMRs. In fact, the author is unaware of any true CPR system, commercial or otherwise. The EMR, while not the ultimate patient record system, is still a very complex technology.

An Introduction to Electronic Medical Record Systems

The availability of a standard definition for EMR helps when discussing products and concepts but does little to aid in the evaluation of systems. One reason for this is that an EMR may be a stand-alone product or a virtual system created via integration of existing systems. Two levels of integration are possible: presentation and data level.

At the presentation level, users will be able to view data from all connected systems through a common interface. The user may access a single terminal to review patient information. Laboratory work may be reviewed, medications ordered, and so on. Systems like this are quite useful but very limited when users wish to do more than simple data retrieval. These systems only *seem* to be one coherent system because a single interface is utilized to interact with all of its components. Much of the enthusiasm for the Intranets and Web browsers are due to their ability to support, with relative ease, presentation-level system integration.

Data-level integration is much more desirable and considerably more difficult. Data-level integration requires that all system components use a consistent scheme for labeling (coding) data elements and that a mechanism be present for movement of data between systems (from components to the central system). In the case of a hospital system, the central system may be a database on the mainframe or a server with connections to all component systems. Data integration in a mainframe-dominant environment is rarely seen unless all departmental systems are provided by the same IS vendor. Clinical data repositories (databases which accept data from a number of departmental systems and combine them into a centrally, searchable form) provide another mechanism for data-level integration (see Chapter 4).

In the setting of a single hospital or integrated delivery system, system integration is difficult and seldom completely accomplished. Most successful systems achieve only presentation-level integration. The downside to presentation-level integration is the lack of query capability across all systems. For example, it would not be possible to issue a command such as "Find all patients with a diagnosis of congestive heart failure who are not taking an ACE inhibitor" because the patient problem list and medication record reside on two different computer systems. The billing system may hold the problem list and the pharmacy system the medication profile. For a system to qualify as an EMR some degree of data-level integration should exist. All references to EMRs in this text will assume the existence of data-level integration (a feature found in all commercially available packages).

Information systems in hospitals or Integrated Delivery Systems (IDS) represent a special problem for EMR implementation due to the presence of "legacy" systems (older systems currently in place). These older systems often cannot be easily replaced and so must become part of newer systems. In many instances presentation-level integration is all that is possible. Another issue for hospitals and IDS is that few stand-alone EMR packages exist for larger enterprises. Even so, "enterprise" EMR packages bring their own integration headaches and may create as many problems as they solve.

The EMR is one instance in which ambulatory practice sites are in a much better position to implement new technologies than their often wealthier inpatient cousins. First, ambulatory care sites tend to be simpler. ICU and nursing systems are not an issue. Laboratory information system requirements often are not present (however, obtaining data in electronic form from outside labs can be problematic). Pharmacy function requirements are usually limited to those required by health care providers (prescription writing, drug interactions, etc.). Second, stand-alone systems that support most major EMR functions are available from many vendors.

EMR Building Blocks

Databases

From the preceding discussion it should be clear that databases are the foundation of any EMR system. A database is a software program that permits the storage and retrieval of information. Databases can store data in large blocks (documents or images) or as discrete items (numbers or single words). Modern database systems may hold billions of data items. Finding anything quickly would be very difficult if not for the presence of indexes. Indexes are ordered files (alphabetical, numeric, or a combination) that indicate exactly where each stored data item may be found.

A database may reside on a single computer (the server) or multiple computers. Data repositories are special types of database programs. All EMRs contain a database of some type. In a stand-alone EMR, the database contains all chart notes, laboratory values, medication lists, problem lists, etc. This is the situation with most commercial systems aimed at outpatient practices. Database management systems are software programs that provide all the functions required to manipulate the information stored in databases. In addition, they provide development tools for creating specialized applications such as EMRs. A few such programs dominate the market: Oracle, SQL Server, and Sybase provide the underlying database system for most currently available EMRs.

Data Input Technologies

Data entry is a major EMR implementation issue. The traditional means of interacting with computers, the keyboard, is not feasible for many EMR users. Other data entry methods are being investigated as adjuncts or substitutes for keyboards. The two that have received the most attention are pen and voice-based input.

Pen-based input relies on a pointing device that may operate much like a mouse or it may be used to write actual characters. In the latter case, the computer must learn to decipher what has been written (handwriting recognition) prior to storing it in the database. Success with handwriting recognition has been limited when large amounts of data are entered. As the technology improves, however, this may become a more viable data entry option. Pen-based input (mouse type) is available with many EMR systems and may for some providers be a workable answer to data entry needs (7).

Voice recognition technology has progressed significantly over the last few years. Second-generation voice recognition systems are available that can handle continuos speech (no unnatural pauses between words) with relatively few errors. They are also much more affordable. Voice recognition has yet to be widely adopted as an EMR data-entry mechanism. However, the technology is sufficiently mature to warrant an evaluation (8).

Networking

Even in the setting of a solo practice networking is required to reap the full benefits of an EMR. Until the appearance of the Internet, *networking* referred to the practice of wiring computers directly together in order to permit communication and sharing of resources. Local Area Networking (LAN) is the name given to this practice. LAN technology makes computing more affordable because it permits a build-it-as-you-need-it approach to purchasing and installing hardware and software. The main computer in LAN is referred to as the *server*. Depending upon the amount of computing power required, a server may be a fast personal computer with extra memory or a special computer designed just for this purpose. In either case a server for a small office can be purchased for less than $3000. LANs are constructed by physically connecting computers and other devices using some type of wiring. Wiring an office requires time and a good deal of planning; every time the computers are moved the wiring has to be adjusted accordingly. All things considered, however, LANs are very cost-effective solutions for implementing EMRs.

Internet technologies also provide a means for networking that is very cost-effective and in many cases superior to other ways of sharing information and resources. One important benefit of using the Internet as the networking technology is that it is relatively platform independent. The essential piece of software required for accessing the Internet is referred to as a *browser* (e.g., NetScape Navigator and Microsoft Internet Explorer). Any software written to obey the communications and display protocols that govern the Internet will be able to send and receive information from any browser. A server connected to the Internet may be used by any other computer that can establish a connection to the server. Since Internet protocols can be used over standard telephone lines, a virtual network can be established simply by attaching a server to the Internet and making that address known to those with whom you wish to share information. If you wish to limit access to a group of computers or people, it can be accomplished quite easily with an Intranet (a system that uses Internet rules but has access restricted to a specific site or group). A growing number of vendors are offering Internet and Intranet EMR applications, and these may prove to be very attractive to smaller practice sites.

Wireless computer capability is also changing the networking equation. Wireless networks rely on radio frequency transmissions to communicate. One great feature of using wireless technology is that users are not tied to one location. No more worrying about wiring schemes and which rooms should have terminals. The cost of wireless technology is decreasing in cost while becoming more powerful. It is worthy of consideration when planning your networking strategy.

Biometrics

Maintaining the security of the information stored in an EMR is of the utmost importance. The standard mechanism in most EMRs for restricting access to sensitive information is passwords. Passwords can be quite effective if guarded properly. However, they can be easily forgotten or stolen. A newer approach to identifying users is via the use of biologic markers (9). Fingerprint and iris scanning technologies are already enjoying fairly widespread use in a number of fields. In fact, iris scanning is reputed to have an error rate of only 1 per 1.2 million scans. Voice and face recognition systems are also available. Biometric identification is superior to passwords in two ways: they cannot be forgotten or stolen. The role of biometric identification for EMR security has yet to be fully determined. Practice sites with many employees may find that biometrics offers a more manageable solution to data security than do traditional passwords.

Storing Clinical Information

EMRs exist to store clinical information. The exact means used to accomplish this task, however, is anything but straightforward. Two fundamental data-related issues must be addressed when implementing an EMR: movement of information between systems and the format to be used for ultimately storing the data. A number of solutions are possible for each task, some sufficiently widespread that it is possible to grant them the status of a "real world" standard. (A number of officially defined standards exist; however, they are not widely used).

Messaging

Perhaps the most widely accepted standard for messaging between systems in the United States is Health Level 7 (10). HL-7 was initiated in 1986 as a cooperative effort between health care providers and technology vendors. HL-7 is the messaging standard for moving clinical and other types of data (orders, referrals, test results, administrative information, etc.) between computer systems. It supports a range of data types and even includes provisions for handling structured text notes. HL-7 is supported by most commercial EMR and clinical information systems vendors. It is a "must have" for any system under consideration.

Like HL-7, DICOM (Digital Imaging and Communications in Medicine) is another widely used standard (11). It addresses issues related to the processing of imaging data. DICOM is a joint product of the American College of Radiology and the National Electrical Manufacturers Association. All major types of radiologic images are covered in the standard. Due to the massive nature of imaging files and their storage requirements, specialized computer systems, Picture Archiving and Communications Systems (PACS), are used. PACS, which are usually found in larger health care facilities, are an important component of any EMR implementation.

The American Society for Testing and Materials (ASTM) also has a major role in defining standards for health care data exchange (12). This organization collaborates with the developers of both HL-7 and DICOM. ASTM Committee E-31 is responsible for health care related standards and has sponsored many publications.

Codes and Classifications

Once received from another system or via data entry, data must be stored in a manner that permits their use for clinical and research purposes. There are a number of competing "standards" in this area; here they will be considered by area of application.

The EMR is an application aimed primarily at caregivers. Aside from the problem of getting data into the system, the matter of ensuring that when retrieved the data are properly interpreted is a very important issue. The problem list is an essential component of any medical record. A notation of "ESRD" in a patient's progress note would be taken by most internists to mean "end-stage renal disease" but could have another meaning or not be recognized at all by someone from a different medical specialty. Coding systems help to reduce ambiguity by offering a common notation for clinical concepts. The codes are chosen by the provider and have standard definitions and representations. The ICD (International Classification of Diseases) offers a standard set of codes for capturing diagnostic information and concepts (13). The ICD code set is published by the World Health Organization and is the accepted standard for diagnostic coding in the United States. Of course, this only partially addresses the problem of ambiguity. After all, codes are selected by the clinician. If an incorrect code is entered, the data in the system will be incorrect and may cause harm to the patient. Incorrect codes may result from oversight or errors in clinical judgement. For example, a patient who presents with 2+ pitting edema may be given a code for congestive heart failure when the real problem is peripheral vascular disease. Thus a coding standard does not necessarily mean accurate patient information.

Current Procedural Terminology (14) is a coding system for diagnostic and therapeutic procedures used primarily for billing purposes. The CPT code set is published by the American Medical Association. Most EMR systems utilize CPT and ICD codes as the only means of storing patient data (aside from free-text).

A third coding system commonly found in EMR systems is SNOMED (Systemized Nomenclature of Medicine), a product of the College of American Pathologists (15). SNOMED is a somewhat more complex coding system than either CPT or ICD. Whereas ICD terms are meant to be used as single entities, SNOMED terms may be combined to form more complex concepts. The downside to this expressive freedom is that there are multiple ways to encode the same clinical concept, which may lead to ambiguity.

Aside from the possibility of erroneous entries, the aforementioned coding systems offer only the barest indication of the actual clinical state of the patient. That information is usually found in an uncoded portion of the record—the progress note. The development of a coding scheme for data contained in the progress note is a major area of inquiry. (Most EMR systems make no provision for this.) However, two viable systems do exist.

The Read Clinical Classification codes (16) were developed in the early 1980s by a British physician. They were later adopted by the British National Health Service. The Read codes have the very ambitious goal of providing a term for all concepts that clinicians might enter into a patient's chart. The second system, developed by a private vendor in the United States, is MEDCIN (17), which directly addresses the problem of encoding the progress note. MEDCIN consists of 75,000+ findings that represent clinically valid terms. Neither of these systems is commonly found in commercial systems within the United States, although MEDCIN is licensed by a few major American-based EMR vendors.

The remaining classification systems are usually buried within the EMR out of sight of clinicians, but they are valuable tools for managing clinical data. Laboratory test and clinical observation coding is the aim of LOINC (Logical Observations Identifiers Names and Codes) (18). It has been adopted by a number of major laboratory systems vendors and major medical centers. NDC (the National Drug Code), a system for classifying pharmaceuticals (19), is widely used within the pharmaceutical industry and may play a key role in future EMR implementations.

The significance of these systems to those planning to implement an EMR system is, for the present, dependent upon the anticipated practice environment. Large sites (hospitals, IPAs, etc.) will likely have a number of clinical systems that must be integrated. In such cases, the use of standard coding systems may lower the cost of system implementation and maintenance. HL-7 capability is a must in larger environments and may be quite helpful to those in much smaller practices where transmission of laboratory data is desired. ICD and CPT codes are a feature of all systems due to their role in billing and administrative activities. The role of clinical nomenclatures such as MEDCIN has yet to be defined. However, as it becomes more important to capture granular patient information for use by clinicians and other EMR components (i.e., decision support subsystems), the interest in and use of such systems is sure to increase.

Summary

Over the last 40 to 50 years clinical systems have undergone significant evolution. The Computer-Based Patient Record is the ultimate goal of those who see the value of information systems in the care of patients. The Electronic Medical Record, in its current incarnation, is a valuable tool and a significant step toward the CPR. However, much remains to be done in the areas of data coding, data entry, user interfaces, database design, and security before CPR becomes a reality.

REFERENCES

1. **Grossman JH, Barnett GO, Koespell TD.** An automated medical record system. JAMA. 1973;263:1114-20.

2. **Stead WW, Hammond WE.** Computer-based medical records: the centerpiece of TMR. MD Computing. 1988;5:48-62.

3. **McDonald CJ, Blevins L, Tierney WM, Martin DK.** The Regenstrief medical records. MD Computing. 1988;5:34-47.

4. **McCormack J.** Wooing physicians to embrace electronic records. Health Data Management. 1999;7:56-68.

5. **Dick RS, Steen EB, Detmer DE.** The computer-based patient record: an essential technology for health care. The Institute of Medicine, 1991.

6. **Andrew W, Dick R.** Venturing off the beaten path: it's time to blaze new CPR trails. Healthcare Informatics. 1997;14:36-42.

7. **Lussier YA, Maksud M, Desruisseaux B, et al.** PureMD: a Computerized Patient Record software for direct data entry by physicians using a keyboard-free pen-based portable computer. In: Proceedings of the Annual Symposium on Computer Applications in Medical Care. Institute of Electrical and Electronics Engineers. Piscataway, NJ; 1992:261-4.

8. **Gillespie G.** For physicians talk is cheap. Health Data Management. 1999;7:92-6.

9. http://www.zdnet.com/pcweek/reviews/1027/27bioapp.html

10. www.HL7.org

11. www.nema.org

12. www.astm.org

13. www.vaccines.ch/whosis/icd10/index.html

14. www.ama-assn.org/med-sci/cpt/cpt.htm

15. www.snomed.org/

16. www.schin.ncl.ac.uk/mig/terms.htm

17. www.medicomp.com

18. www.regenstrief.org/loinc/loinc_information.html

19. www.fda.gov/cder/ndc/

2 / Computer Hardware and Enabling Technologies

Daniel C. Davis, Jr.

Introductory Concepts

Nowhere is the phrase "form follows function" more important than in the selection of computer hardware for the clinical practice. Hardware selection (form) is determined by software and workflow (function). In the office computer system, the physical components of the system should be determined by the functions of the system. The physical components of the office system include the equipment (the hardware), how the hardware is linked together (the network), and the locations of the equipment within the office. An understanding of fundamental computing concepts and the basic parts of a computer will help determine how well different hardware components will support workflow functions in the office.

Fundamental Computer Concepts

Computers are nothing more than sophisticated calculating machines that perform mathematical operations using a binary number system. Understanding basic concepts about computers will help in planning the medical office computer system.

The computer has four fundamental parts:

1. *Input*, the data fed to the computer.
2. The *computer itself*, which is often called the *processor*.
3. A *program* that tells the computer how to mathematically manipulate the input.
4. *Output*, the data presented to the user or another computer program.

Input

Data can be fed to the computer from many sources and in many forms. The input data, whether words or numbers, are translated by the computer into a machine code that the computers can understand. This code is actually a binary mathematics system consisting of just "1's" and "0's" that can represent a vast array of numbers, letters, words, and concepts. A string of input data might look like "00000001" and "00000010", which are binary codes for the numbers 1 and 2.

Processor

The processor receives the binary input data and performs mathematical operations on the input data under the direction of a set of instructions called a *program*. For example, a program might instruct the processor to add "00000001" to "00000010" to get "00000011", the binary equivalent of $1 + 2 = 3$.

Program

The computer program is a set of instructions, or rules, that dictate what the processor should do with the input data.

Output

Once the processor has manipulated the input data according to the program instructions, the processor spits out the result data, which is called *output*. This output comes from the processor in the form of binary code. In our trivial example of "Add 1 + 2", the output is "00000011". The binary output is then translated into a format useable by humans, by another program, or by another computer. In our example, "00000011" translates to the numeral 3.

To summarize, in the fundamental computer, input is fed to the processor, which follows the program's instructions to produce output.

Parts of the Basic Computer

The computer system in the medical office consists of one or more personal computers (PCs) connected by a network. The basic computer in this network contains six components:

1. Central Processing Unit (CPU)
2. Random Access Memory (RAM)

3. Storage memory
4. Input devices
5. Output devices
6. Connectivity devices

Central Processing Unit

The processor in modern computers is often called the *Central Processing Unit* (CPU) to distinguish it from other processors in the computer box, such as video and audio processors. The CPU is a computer chip that can be identified as a flat black square or rectangle, about an inch on a side, attached to the big green plastic motherboard inside the computer case. CPUs have evolved rapidly over the past fifty years, shrinking in size and growing in power by many orders of magnitude.

CPUs are classified by families and by speed. The large chip manufacturers use names and numbers to identify families of chips; some examples include Intel 386 and Intel 486; Pentium, Pentium II, Pentium III, and Pentium IV; and Motorola's 68000 and PowerPC chips. Each new generation of chips gets faster. The chips are rated by the speed of the processor, which depends in part on how fast a tiny quartz crystal in the chip vibrates. This quartz crystal, called the *clock*, acts as a timer for the CPU. These timers vibrate several million times per second. One million vibrations per second is one megahertz. The number of megahertz at which the quartz crystal vibrates is called the *clock speed*. The faster the quartz crystal oscillates, the faster the chip can process instructions. In addition to clock speed, the speed of the CPU depends on how many transistors are embedded in the chip. More transistors allow the CPU to process more instructions simultaneously. Every six months or so new generations of chips are released, each new generation having more transistors and faster clock speeds. The combination of more transistors and faster clock speed in successive generations of CPUs has allowed a tremendous increase in the computing power that can be purchased for each dollar.

Random Access Memory

Random Access Memory (RAM) is one of two types of memory in the computer. (The other type of memory is *storage memory*; see next section.) RAM is located in special computer chips that can be identified as rectangular dull black chips often lined up side by side either on the motherboard or on a green card sticking up from the motherboard. Within the RAM chip are thousands of microscopic transistors that act as tiny electrical switches that are either "on" or "off". If a transistor is in the "on" state, it is said to have a value of "1"; if the transistor is in the "off" state, it is said to have a value of "0".

How these microscopic transistors work is very interesting. A memory chip consists of a silicon sandwich that contains crisscrossing wires that are only a few molecules thick. One wire carries a current of electrons, but the current cannot flow along the wire because the wire is interrupted periodically by tiny breaks in the wire. The wire on one side of the break (called the *source* because it is the source of electrons) provides electrons that are trying to jump across the break in the wire. On the downstream side of the break, the wire is called the *drain*. Electrons would like to jump across the break in the wire but cannot do so because there is a special kind of insulating silicon that fills the gap between the source end and the drain end of the wire. When no current flows across this gap, the transistor is said to be "off" and have a value of "0". Running perpendicular across the gap is another wire. If a positive current is applied to this second wire, negatively charged electrons are attracted by the positive current into the gap between the source and the drain causing the gap filling silicon to become a conductor rather than an insulator. This allows a current of electrons to flow from the source to the drain, thus turning the transistor "on". The "on" transistor is said to have a value of "1". Thus a transistor's "on" or "off" state can represent one digit of a binary number, either "1" or "0". The value of the transistor is either "on" or "off", "1" or "0".

This binary limitation of the transistor explains why machine code uses binary mathematics. The value of a transistor is called a *bit*. Eight "bits", that is eight transistors, comprise a "byte" of information. A series of transistors can represent a series of binary numbers, which can be translated into a standard Arabic number, a letter of the alphabet, and even logical values of "true" and "false". Many thousands of transistors in the memory chip can store information that represents input data, output data, programs, and Boolean logic.

Computer chips are engineered to work with maximum length binary numbers or words. Thus, the earlier chips were "8-bit chips", meaning that the largest binary number the chip could handle was eight digits long. The largest 8-bit binary number is "11111111", which translates into the numeral 65,536. Newer and larger chips can handle binary numbers up to 32 bits, representing the numeral 4,294,967,296. Sixty-four bit chips are on the way and will produce huge gains in computing power.

A group of transistors in RAM memory can be assigned an "address", much like a street address. Specific information is stored at specific addresses within RAM so that the computer can find this information quickly.

RAM is an important determinant of how fast your computer works. When the CPU needs input data, that data must often come from storage memory (e.g., a disk drive). When the CPU gives output data, that data must be sent somewhere (e.g., a disk drive). Sending data to and from storage memory is one of the slowest tasks performed by the computer. Sending data to and from RAM is much faster than using a disk drive. RAM allows the computer to store input data, output data, and program instructions in a place that can be accessed much faster than the disk drives. More RAM, with faster clock speeds and larger number lengths, results in a much faster computer.

RAM is measured in size as "megabytes", meaning millions of bytes of memory. Current consumer and business computers are shipping with progressively larger amounts of RAM, typically 32 to 64 megabytes. Even small medical groups are buying server computers with 256 or more megabytes of RAM. RAM is characterized as word size (32-bit or 64-bit words), speed, and amount supplied in the computer.

An important characteristic of RAM is that it is volatile, meaning that when the computer is turned off, the contents of the memory disappear. Because RAM does not store data after the computer is turned off, the computer needs another means of storing data permanently. Memory that stores information permanently is called *storage memory*.

Storage Memory

The second type of computer memory is storage memory. Because RAM memory is volatile (i.e., the information in RAM disappears when the power is turned off), the computer must have a place to store information permanently. Information stored in storage memory is often the type of information that is used repeatedly, such as computer programs, input data files, and output data files. There are many forms of storage memory. The three most common are floppy disks, hard disks, and CD-ROM disks. Less common types of storage memory include compact disks, magnetic tape, DVD disks, optical disks, memory PCMCIA cards, and memory sticks. All but the hard disks are removable media (i.e., the storage memory can be removed from the computer either for safekeeping or for transfer to another computer).

Floppy disks are thin plastic disks enclosed in a protective plastic case. The older 8-inch-diameter and $5^1/_4$-inch-diameter floppy disks had protective cases that were thin and pliable, hence the name *floppy disk*. The thin plastic disk inside the floppy is coated with a very thin film of iron particles. Each tiny spot on the disk can be magnetized or unmagnetized, representing a binary "1" or "0". The floppy disk is placed into a floppy drive. The drive spins the floppy disk, much like a record on a turntable, but much faster at several thousand revolutions per second. The disk drive pivots a "read-write" arm over the disk, much like the tone arm of a record player. At the end of the read-write arm is a tiny coil of wire, called a *head*, that "reads" whether each location on the floppy is magnetized or not and translates the sequential magnetic information into binary "1's" and "0's" that are used by the computer. The read-write head can also write to the floppy. When sequential pulses of current travel through the coil of wire in the head, a tiny magnetic field is generated. The magnetic field of the read-write head can then magnetize the iron particles at discrete spots on the floppy, thus recording "1's" and "0's" in the form of magnetic spots onto the floppy disk. Most floppy disks are now $3^1/_2$ inches in diameter and hold much more information (1.44 megabytes) than did the old 8 or $5^1/_4$ inch varieties. Smaller floppies with larger capacity are being introduced.

The terms *hard disk* and *hard drive* are used interchangeably because unlike the floppy disk, which can be removed from the floppy drive, the hard disk is fixed permanently inside the hard drive and is never removed. Hard disks are called *fixed media*, and other storage media are called *removable media*. Hard disks work on the same principle as the floppy disk, using read-write heads and tiny magnetic fields to store and retrieve information on the drive. However, hard drives use rigid rather than floppy platters and use several platters and several read-write heads simultaneously. The magnetic spots on hard disks are more densely packed. These techniques allow the hard disks to store much more information than floppies. Hard disks that are currently shipping with business PCs often hold more than 10 gigabytes of information. One gigabyte equals 1 billion bytes of information.

Input Devices

The computer gets data from the user through various input devices. The basic input devices are the keyboard and the mouse.

THE KEYBOARD Basic input from the user comes from the *keyboard*. When the user presses a key on the computer keyboard, a tiny voltage change is generated from the mechanical action. This voltage change is translated into a unique code for the key press or combination of presses. This digital code is then sent to the computer and used as input to a program. The keys on a basic keyboard are arranged like a standard typewriter. Most keyboards also have a numeric keypad placed on the right end of the keyboard. There also are special keys that are assigned commands by individual programs or by the user. These keys are called *function keys* and are usually labeled F1 to F12. The function keys are typically located in a line across the top of the keyboard. Another group of keys, called *program keys*, are used alone or in combination with the standard keys to send program commands to the computer. Some of these program keys are the "Control" key, the "Alt" key, the "Escape" key, the "Print screen" key, and the "Break" key. Different programs may assign slightly different functions to the program and function keys. There are many variations on the basic keyboard design. Some of these useful variations are discussed in the Peripheral Devices section.

THE MOUSE The other basic input device is the *mouse*. The mouse is the most common pointing device. A *pointing device* is a tool that allows the user to move the cursor to any place on the monitor screen and "point" to an area for input or to select a function displayed on the screen. The *cursor* is a blinking symbol that draws the user's attention to the area on the monitor screen where input or output is being manipulated by the user. Older computer programs used a character and line-based method of display that limited the cursor to the end of a typed line, just like an old typewriter. Modern programs use a graphical user interface, called for short a *GUI* and pronounced "gooey", that allows the user to move the cursor anywhere on the computer screen by manipulating a pointing device. When the user moves a pointing device, like a mouse, in a given direction, speed, and distance, the cursor on the computer screen moves in the same direction, speed, and distance across the screen. The *keypad mouse* is called that because it is about the size of a large mouse and has a wire sticking out of one side that looks like a mouse's tail. There are many other kinds of pointing devices but they all do principally the same thing—move the cursor about the screen. (Other pointing devices are described in the Peripheral Devices section below.)

Output Devices
The computer program manipulates the input data, thereby producing new output data. The output data can be presented to the user or can be sent to another program or to a second computer. The devices that manage output data are called *output devices*. The output devices of the basic computer are the monitor and the printer.

THE MONITOR *Monitors* come in a variety of sizes, shapes, and image quality. Monitors are also called *displays, display terminals, CRTs (cathode ray tubes)*, and *VDTs (video display terminals)*. The most familiar computer monitor looks like a television. These monitors use cathode ray tubes similar to television tubes. Size of the monitor is measured by the diagonal length of the screen, measured from upper corner to the opposite lower corner. These monitors range in size from about 12 inches diagonally to 21 inches diagonally. Larger and smaller sizes are not practicable for the office. The standard office monitor is 15 inches. A significant disadvantage of the standard CRT monitor is its overall size. As screen size increases, so does the front-to-back length of the CRT. A 15-inch CRT monitor may be entirely too big for a small desk in the typical examining room or at a nurse station. Monitors also are manufactured as flat panel displays like those seen in laptop computers. Most flat panel displays use LCD (liquid crystal display) technology rather than CRT technology. The flat panel displays save desktop space but are currently three or four times more expensive than the standard CRT monitors.

The quality of the image displayed by the monitor is determined by the resolution of the monitor. Generally, higher resolution is better. Resolution is determined by the number of pixels the monitor can display, by the dot pitch of the screen, and by the number of colors the monitor can display. Occasionally one may find use for a monochrome monitor, but most modern software takes advantage of color to improve the user interface.

Pixel is a word coined from the term *picture element*, which refers to the dots of light the monitor screen displays. The number of pixels that can be displayed along the horizontal axis and along the vertical axis of the screen are stated in an expression of resolution such as "640 × 480" on the low end or "1024 × 768" on the high end. Higher and lower resolutions are rarely used in the office setting. A physical characteristic of monitors is dot pitch. *Dot pitch* refers to the size of the individual points of light displayed by the monitor. The smaller the dot pitch, the finer is the quality of the image displayed. Currently standard office monitors are manufactured with a dot pitch of 0.28. Also, monitors can display a variable number of colors. The more colors the monitor displays, the higher the image quality. Image quality depends not only on the physical characteristics of the monitor but also on special image software and hardware in the computer. Dot pitch and maximum resolution are physical characteristics of the monitor. Within the hardware and software limitations of the computer, one can select the number of pixels and colors displayed by the monitor. The hardware limitations are determined by the monitor itself and by the video card capabilities. The video card connects the monitor to the computer motherboard. The software limitations of the display are determined by software called a *video driver*.

Which monitors one chooses for the office setting depend on which functions are important to the users. For example, if the receptionist uses a scheduling program that requires only large print on the screen, the monitor can be a low-resolution monochrome model. If the receptionist's work area has a lot of desk space, a standard 15-inch CRT monitor might be adequate. A low-resolution 15-inch CRT would be a relatively inexpensive option for the receptionist. On the other hand, if the physician is using a computer in a small exam room for an electronic medical record (EMR) program or for patient education with an anatomy program, then a high-resolution 14-inch flat panel display would be a better investment.

THE PRINTER *Printers* are important output devices that are often overlooked. Despite the attraction of the "paperless office", few medical offices are truly paperless. The function of paper, its generation, flow, and disposition in the office must be understood. As with all other hardware choices, form follows function. The printer that is optimal for printing prescriptions at the nursing station is not likely to be the best printer for producing hundreds or thousands of multi-part billing statements. Printers are characterized by print technology, whether they handle multi-part forms, whether they feed paper by tractor or by single sheet, and how easily they handle envelopes. One must also consider printer resolution, color versus black and white, speed, cost per page, noise, and size.

Three common printer technologies are in use in the medical office:

1. Dot matrix printers
2. Laser printers
3. Ink jet printers

Dot matrix printers are the old workhorses of the medical office. The dot matrix printer consists of a print head that contains a collection of small wires that spring from the print head and strike an inked printer ribbon to deposit onto the paper a tiny bit of ink, much like the key-and-ribbon action of a typewriter. Dot matrix printers tend to be faster than other printer types, last longer, and cost less per page printed but are noisier and produce lower print quality. They are excellent for printing large amounts of paper and for printing multi-part forms such as statements and insurance claim forms. Dot matrix printers are usually found in the business office and are less suited for a quiet reception area or exam room.

Laser printers are popular because they can produce excellent print quality, are quiet, and are easy to operate. Laser printers tend to be slower than dot matrix printers and cannot handle multi-part forms such as billing statements or insurance claim forms. They are excellent for printing a few on-demand charge slips in the reception area because they are quiet and because on-demand printing of charge slips is usually a low-volume function. For similar reasons, laser printers are a good choice for the exam room. Compared with dot matrix printers of equal speed, laser printers cost more to purchase. Because the costly print mechanism must be replaced when the laser printer runs out of ink, laser printers cost more per printed page.

Ink jet printers are less expensive to purchase and have an intermediate cost per printed page. They tend to be slower and are a little nosier than laser printers. Ink jet printers are manufactured in very small and portable sizes. They are attractive in environments where small size is more important than speed or quiet operation. Ink jet printers cannot handle multi-part forms. Ink jets use single-sheet paper rather than continuous-feed paper.

The paper type required by a clinical function often influences the type of printer. For example, correspondence requires high-quality twenty-pound 8.5 by 11 inch cut sheet paper. A laser printer works well for correspondence. Similar heavy, expensive paper is not desirable for generating high volume chart notes, charge tickets, or appointment schedules. Inexpensive, lightweight, continuous-feed tractor drive paper is a more cost-effective choice for these latter uses. Printing prescriptions with the computer presents special problems. Prescriptions are traditionally written on small 4 by 5 inch pads, a unique paper size that is used in few other office functions. One can either dedicate printers to print prescriptions only or one can print prescriptions on standard 8.5 by 11 inch paper. Printing prescriptions for controlled substances is a problem because many states require sending duplicate prescriptions to the pharmacy. Multi-part statements must be printed on heavy-duty dot-matrix printers; laser and ink-jet printers cannot print on multi-part forms. Envelope and label printing present additional challenges.

Printer speed is another consideration. The difference in speed of printers, typically measured in number of pages per minute, may not seem significant until one considers office workflow. Color printing, although attractive, is slow and more costly. The three minutes it takes to print a pretty color patient handout may be too costly to the nurse when multiplied by 20 or 30 patients per day. In contrast, the 15 seconds it takes to print a black and white patient education form on a fast laser printer may generate critical time savings in the patient-flow process.

Other factors that influence printer choice are the physical size of the printer relative to work space, the flow of foot traffic, noise generated by the printers, and paper dust.

Summary

There are many choices to be made in selecting basic computer hardware for the medical office. These choices should be determined primarily by a careful analysis of the workflow and function of the persons using the computers in the office. The hardware configurations required by the front-office receptionist or by the back-office clerk are likely to be different from the physician who is using the computer in the exam room. Again, form follows function.

Hardware Technologies and Applications

Types of Computer Systems

Computer systems can be classified by their complexity and size. Recent computer technology has blurred the lines between microcomputers, mini-computers, mainframes, client-server systems, and Web-based systems.

Microcomputers are single CPU computers that are used by one user at a time. They may be stand-alone machines or they may be linked into a network.

Minicomputers are designed for use by more than one user at a time, typically 5 to 100 users. Minicomputers may have more than one CPU. The term *minicomputer* was used more commonly a decade ago to distinguish the smaller minicomputers, which are slightly bigger than the standard desktop PC, from large and very expensive mainframe computers. Minicomputers functioned like mainframes but on a smaller scale. Like mainframes, they used dumb terminals rather than PC workstations. As PC-based networks have become more powerful, the minicomputer has become less popular as a small business solution.

Mainframe computers are very large computers that once occupied an entire room. New technologies have shrunk mainframes down to refrigerator size or smaller. Mainframes are typically run by large institutions such as hospitals and insurance companies that may have hundreds or thousands of simultaneous users. Mainframes have single or multiple CPUs and typically are very fast compared with PCs. As with the minicomputer, more powerful PC-based networks are taking over many of the functions of the older mainframes.

The *client-server computer system* is a newer type of computer architecture in which the end-user PCs share some of the processing functions and data with the larger central server computer. The central server computer is typically larger and faster than the client PC and can handle multiple users at one time. The server also stores data that are used in common by many of the users. The users typically connect to the server using their PC, which, in this configuration, is called a *client computer*. The client computer runs client software that is designed to work closely with the server software. The idea is that the central server provides services, such as sharing of data files, printers, programs, modems, and other external connections, to the client PCs. Because most PCs do not need all of these services at one time, the services can be shared among many PCs and provide economies of scales. The economies of client-server architecture often apply even to the small medical office.

The newest computer system architecture is based on Internet and Web technology. The thin client software has become the Web browser. In some Web-based clinical applications, the client PC may need no other software than the browser. The Web server sends data when requested by the browser. The user modifies the data and returns it to the central Web server where the data are stored. If the client browser needs additional programs, these can be downloaded to the client browser in the form of small program applications called *applets*. Web-based computer systems can be confined to the office—an Intranet—or can be connected to the public Internet outside the office. Also, the office Web-based system can be connected to other remote systems through a virtual private network. There are many problems to be solved before Web-technology becomes the principal clinical computing architecture. Many Web-based applications are too slow for the busy office practice. There are challenging security and privacy issues. The best office systems have not yet been restructured to take advantage of Web technology. However, these barriers are being overcome rapidly. Within a few years many medical offices will be served primarily by Web applications.

Office Workstation Choices

"Form follows function" also applies to the choice of computer workstations for the users in your office. There are several workstation types to choose from:

- Full-size PCs
- Laptops, notebooks, and subnotebooks
- Network PCs
- Hand-held computers

The choice of workstation will depend on several important factors:

1. Software Requirements
   - Does the software require specific workstation speed, RAM, and hard disk capacity?
   - What are the specific software functions that each person will use?
   - What is the optimum size and resolution of the monitor for the information to be displayed?

2. Space and Environmental Requirements
   - How much space is available for the user's workstation and printer?
   - Does the space required by the workstation leave enough desk or counter space for the user to work with other documents, books, or charts?
   - Is there sufficient desk space to use a mouse or should space-saving alternative pointing devices be used, such as track-balls, track pads, joy sticks, touch screens, or light pens?
   - Will the user be standing or sitting?
   - Will the heat generated by computer equipment be an issue for workers?
   - If voice recognition is to be used, will ambient noise interfere with accuracy?
   - Can the user's dictation be overheard by other patients?
   - Will multiple speakers be sharing the same computer? If so, will the time required to load each user's speech profile interfere with patient flow?

3. Electrical Power Issues
   - Are there enough power outlets to accommodate each workstation and printer?

- Is there enough power capacity to run the equipment on each power circuit?
- What is the quality of the electrical power? Are there surges, spikes, or brown-outs?

4. Portable Workstations
   - Are portable workstations preferred over fixed workstations?
   - How will the portable workstations connect to the network? By infrared wireless, radio wireless, or hardwire cables?
   - What will prevent portable workstations from being lost or stolen?
   - Does the portable have a keyboard with sufficient functions to allow the user to input data with optimum speed?
   - How long will the batteries last?
   - Where and how do the batteries get recharged?
   - If you rely on swapping out discharged batteries, where are the charged replacements stored?
   - Are data lost if the batteries are changed or run down?
   - Does the portable have "instant-on" capabilities so that the user can resume work at exactly the same place as when he or she turned the portable off? Or must the portable be rebooted every time it is turned on?

Full-Size Personal Computers

Full-size PCs tend to have more RAM, faster CPUs, and larger hard drives than other PCs. The former have larger cases, typically 18 to 24 inches in length and width and 6 to 8 inches in height. Some full-function models are designed to be placed on top of the user's desk and hence are called *desktop PCs*. The combination of a standard desktop case, 15 to 17 inch monitor, keyboard, and mouse consumes a large part of a standard size desk. A large desk in the physician's private office may accommodate full-size computer equipment, but these "space hogs" may overwhelm the small desks and counters used in the clinical areas. Other full-function PCs, called *tower models*, are designed to stand vertically. They fit nicely on the floor next to the desk, under the desk, or even hidden in a cabinet. Two advantages of the full-size PCs are price and flexibility. Full-size PCs tend to be less expensive than PCs that have been specially engineered for space saving because full-size PCs can accommodate generic hard drives, CD-ROMs, and modems. Another advantage of the full-size PCs is that they have more available expansion slots than the smaller PCs. These extra expansion slots allow the addition of upgrades and new functions such as extra modems, scanners, network interface cards, or video cameras. As computer components shrink in size the overall dimensions of full-function PCs shrink. Some new models of desktop PCs are one third the size of standard PCs of two years ago.

Laptops, Notebooks, and Subnotebooks

Laptop, notebook, and subnotebook PCs should be considered for office workstations where saving space or portability is important. Laptops are portable PCs that are designed to be used sitting on your lap. They are generally the bigger of the portables and weigh about 7 to10 pounds but usually come with many built-in features such as a full-size keyboard, floppy drive, hard drive, CD-ROM, modem, and pointing device. Notebook PCs are similar in design to the laptops but are somewhat smaller and lighter and may have a smaller keyboard. Subnotebook PCs are smaller yet: New models weigh less than three pounds. Subnotebook keyboards may be smaller than is comfortable for the average user. The screen size is smaller. To save size and weight, the sub-notebooks often use an external floppy drive and external CD-ROM. All of these portable devices run common PC software and standard operating systems. All of these can connect to the office network through network interface cards called *PCMCIA cards*, or *PC cards* for short. The PC cards slide into special slots on the side of the portable computer. The PC cards are credit-card size devices that provide the physical wiring connection to the network. PC cards can be designed for other functions such as radio network connection, modems, extra storage memory, CD-ROM, tape backups, video cameras, and digital cameras.

Network Personal Computers

Network PCs are designed to work only on a network rather than as standalone PCs. Network PCs rely on the concept of using the central network server to store and manage most of the data used by the network PC. Even programs may be stored on the central server rather than on the PC. The main advantage of the network PC architecture is the reduced cost of maintaining large numbers of PCs in big networks. This cost over the life of a PC connected to the network is called *total cost of ownership*. The total cost of ownership over the useful life of each standard PC on the network may be ten times the original purchase price of the PC. Network PCs are stripped-down versions of full-function PCs. The network PC has a CPU, relatively little RAM, a keyboard, a mouse, and a monitor. Storage memory for the network PC is located on the central server. The network PC may have a floppy drive. A network PC may not even have a hard drive or CD-ROM.

Network PCs are not in widespread use in medical offices. This is due to falling prices of full-function PCs, the fact that physicians are more familiar with standard PCs, and because networks in the typical medical office are small.

Another option for the office workstation is to use the thin client model, such as in the Citrix Winframe/Microsoft Metaframe architecture. A thin client is a very small piece of software that can run on a variety of inexpensive, stripped-down PCs or even hand-held WinCE devices. The Citrix client can run on many different types of computers, thus allowing a great deal of flexibility in the choice of workstations in the medical office. This is one way of accommodating both Apple MacIntosh and Windows PC users in the same office. When the user wants to run a program, he starts the Citrix client software. This software then attaches to the Citrix server, which then starts up a "virtual PC" on the server to be used by the one user. Multiple users can attach to the same server using multiple "virtual PCs" running on the same server. The virtual PCs running on the Citrix server can share hardware resources like RAM, hard drives, and modems. This configuration allows all of the processing and software maintenance to be done by the central server, allows the user to have a wide range of choices of cheap PCs, decreases cost of maintaining user equipment and software, and also allows for low bandwidth connectivity between client and server.

Hand-Held Computers

Though not designed as true workstations, very small hand-held computers are gaining popularity among clinicians, principally as personal information managers. These small computers can be held in one hand and usually fit into a shirt or coat pocket. Hand-held computers run on batteries and are designed for ultimate portability. Hand-held computers come in four principal forms: 1) full-function PCs, 2) Windows CE devices, 3) palm computers, and 4) DOS computers.

Full-function PCs are becoming progressively smaller. The smallest full-function PCs run Windows 98 and most popular Windows programs. Advantages of these little PCs are high portability, full compatibility with desktop PCs, no learning curve for the user of desktop PCs, the same wide range of software selection available for desktop PCs, and network connectivity through PCMCIA cards. These machines are often held with one hand while using the other hand to type. Their small size is also a disadvantage. The display screens are small and sometimes difficult to read depending on font size and lighting conditions. Keyboards are small, making touch-typing difficult. Battery life is often too short. In addition, most of these machines do not have an "instant-on" function but rather must go through a boot-up cycle every time they are turned on.

Another type of hand-held computer is the Windows CE (WinCE) computer. These computers use the Windows CE operating system, which provides functions familiar to Windows users. WinCE machines come in several sizes that range from true palm size with very small keyboards and screens to larger sizes with 10 to 12 inch screens and full-size keyboards. Some WinCE machines have touch-sensitive screens that aid in navigation. A popular WinCE function is the "instant-on" function. This function allows the user of a WinCE computer to resume work at exactly the same spot as when the machine was turned off without having to reboot. This instant-on function saves several minutes that would otherwise be consumed by a boot-up process. Because WinCE machines are often carried in a pocket throughout the office and hospital, they may be turned on and off 20 to 30 times per day. Without the instant-on function, the user would waste 30 to 60 minutes per day just waiting for the computer to boot up. The WinCE machines usually have built-in modems and can be connected to a network via PCMCIA cards. The screens are backlit, making viewing in low-light situations easy. However, most WinCE screens are difficult to read in full daylight. The short battery life requires charging stations, plug-in power sources, or replacement batteries to be readily available at the work site. The batteries are proprietary and are specially configured for each model. There are few medical programs available for WinCE computers, but the number is increasing. WinCE devices can be connected to a network and to the Internet. They can run regular Windows programs, including EMR software, if connected through Citrix Winframe or Windows Metaframe network architecture.

Palm computers have become very popular in the past few years. These devices are held in the palm of one hand. The other hand writes on the touch-sensitive screen to spell out input data. A hand-writing recognition program recognizes the pen strokes and translates them into computer text. The user must learn a special method of writing for the computer to translate effectively. Like the WinCE machines, the palm computers have built-in software that serves most personal information management needs. Though the built-in personal information management software can be useful to the individual physician, there are few medical software packages for palm computers. Electronic reference software is now available for palm computers, and EMR applications are being developed. The best known palm computer is 3Com's Palm Pilot series. The newer Palm Pilots have modem and wireless connectivity.

A fourth type of hand-held computer is the Hewlett-Packard LX 200. This computer runs the old DOS operating system, is simple to operate, and has a wide range of valuable medical applications. It is used primarily as a personal information and reference manager. Some clinicians use the built-in word processor or DOS-based commercial word processors to complete history and physical exams or consultations at the patient's bedside and then fax or print the medical document for the chart. These computers are not designed for network use or for a full-function EMR system. The LX200 runs on two generic AA batteries that may last a month or more. The keyboard is very small. Many users learn to "thumb type" because they cradle the LX 200 in the fingers of both hands leaving the thumbs above the keyboard for typing. The screen is not backlit and is difficult to see in low-light situations such as taking CME notes in a darkened auditorium. The screen is easier to see in bright daylight than are the screens of most WinCE computers.

Summary
Most offices will choose full-size PC workstations or laptops. Some clinics large enough to benefit from economies of scale may use WinCE devices running through WinFrame network architecture. Hand-held computers, while useful as personal information management tools, are not yet suitable as true workstations in the medical office network.

Peripheral Devices

Peripheral devices are equipment attached to the PC other than the basic monitor, keyboard, and mouse.

Other Input Devices
There are many variations on the basic keyboard and mouse, some of which might be of special use in the office computer system. These special input devices include wireless keyboards, track-balls, touch pads, and "joy sticks" that may be separate devices or may be integrated into the keyboard. Other input devices include light pens, touch-sensitive screens, and voice input.

The wireless keyboard with integrated track-ball is particularly attractive for use in the exam room. Wireless connection between the keyboard and PC occurs through either an infrared signal or a radio signal. The infrared connections tend to be limited by line of sight in contrast to the radio-linked keyboards that are multidirectional. A skillful clinician can place the wireless keyboard on his or her lap and input clinical notes while facing the patient and maintaining direct eye contact. With a trackball mounted on the keyboard, the clinician can avoid fiddling with a mouse on the desktop. If one needs to input sketches or draw on anatomy diagrams, drawing on a touch pad is more natural than trying to draw with a mouse or track-ball. Touch pads range from less than 2 inches wide to larger than a sheet of notebook paper.

CD-ROMs

CD-ROMs are a storage medium that uses laser technology to increase storage memory capacity. CD-ROM stands for "compact disk–read only memory". CD-ROMs work like music CDs but with a computer. CD-ROMs are platters that spin rapidly in a special CD drive. The CD platter contains a foil-like material sandwiched between two layers of plastic. Information is stored on the CD by a sharply focused laser beam that burns tiny pits into the foil. The presence or absence of a pit indicates a binary "1" or "0". Because the laser can be focused in a much smaller area than can the magnetic read-write head of a hard disk or floppy disk, the CD-ROM can store much more data in a given area. Until recently, CD-ROMs were "read only", meaning that the usual CD drive could not write to the CD. Writing to the CD required expensive writers that were beyond the resources of most small businesses. However, some PCs are now being shipped with inexpensive CD drives that are capable of both reading from and writing to special CDs. In addition to storing a large amount of data, CDs are also removable and can serve as back-up media. A disadvantage of CDs is that moving information between the CD and the computer is slower than with hard drives, although every few months faster and faster CD systems are being released. Besides the familiar single-user CD, CD drives can be purchased in a tower configuration containing multiple CD drives. Single- and multi-drive CD units can easily be placed on the office network.

Scanners

Even when using EMR, few offices can become truly paperless because the typical medical office receives paper communication from many sources, such as radiology reports and consultations. Scanners can convert these paper documents into electronic documents that are stored in the computer.

Three types of scanners are commonly used in the medical office. They are distinguished from each other by how the scan head moves relative to the document being scanned. In *flat-bed scanners*, the document is placed flat on a piece of glass and the scan head moves past the stationary document. In a *sheet-fed scanner*, the document is moved past the scan head by a set of rollers much like the rollers in a typewriter or printer. *Hand-held scanners* are drawn across a stationary document by the user's hand. Each scanner type has its own advantages. High-volume scanning operations use the sheet-fed scanner type. Though sheet-fed scanners cost more to purchase, they save on labor. Sheet-fed scanners can scan only flat documents and cannot scan books. Flat-bed scanners can scan books and other thick objects. Flat-bed scanners require an attendant to move the original page to and from the scan bed and are labor intensive. Sheet-fed scanners can be loaded with multiple documents and require less labor. Hand-held scanners are inexpensive, slower than the other types, and are suitable only for occasional use in the medical office.

Scanned documents can be stored either as document images or as text files. If documents are stored as images, the computer cannot search text content within the document. If the documents are to be stored as text files, then the documents must be scanned using an optical character recognition (OCR) program.

The advantages of scanning documents into electronic format are

- Less storage space required for paper records
- Fewer lost documents
- Viewing scanned documents from multiple places
- Neater office with less paper clutter
- Easier archive and retrieval

Disadvantages of scanning clinical documents are

- Scanned documents are more easily used if integrated into an EMR system.
- Scanning documents can be labor intensive.
- Indexing of documents for later retrieval can be a problem. By what data elements and key words should each document be indexed? Who will do the indexing? How accurate must the index be?
- If documents are scanned using OCR, additional issues arise. Because no OCR system is 100% accurate, who will be responsible for proofreading and editing the OCR documents? If the OCR

documents are not proofread, who will take responsibility for content errors in the scanned medical documents? Can the source document be destroyed if the clinicians using the information are not highly confident in the accuracy of the scanned copies?

- If image scanning is used, what benefits are lost by not being able to search on content that is not computer readable?

Modems

Many office computer systems will have a modem to connect the system to the outside world. Outside connectivity may allow for software maintenance over the telephone, access to medical records from the physician's home, or access to an Internet service provider. A modem is a device that connects the computer to a telephone line in order to connect the computer to remote computers by translating digital computer signals into analog telephone signals.

The word *modem* is a contraction of "modulator-demodulator". Modems modulate (change) the digital output of the computer into analog noises that can travel over standard telephone lines. The modem on the destination computer "demodulates" (changes) the analog noises into digital signals that the destination computer can understand. Modems are classified by the speed at which they work and by the type of telephone line over which they operate. Standard modems can transmit data over a standard telephone line at a maximum speed of 56 kilobaud per second. A baud is the unit of measure of modem speed; think of it as bits per second. Faster telephone lines include ISDN (Integrated Digital Subscriber Network) and ADSL (Asymmetric Digital Subscriber Line), plus several new variations of ASDL, as a class denoted xDSL. Each type of line requires a matching type of modem. Cable modems use the a cable TV system instead of telephone lines to connect computers at very high transmission speeds, up to 10 megabits per second.

Protecting Computer Equipment and Data

Another very important hardware consideration for the medical office is protecting computer equipment from electrical disasters. The quality of the electricity supplied by the outlets in the office is not as good as one might expect. The voltage drifts up and down. Occasional spikes of electrical current occur when the power is turned on or off in the building or during electrical storms. All of these unexpected electrical events can damage delicate computer equipment unless the equipment is protected. To guard against unexpected surges of electrical power, all office computer equipment and peripherals should be protected with surge and spike protectors. To guard against power failure, an uninterruptable power source (UPS) should power the server. The UPS can give the server a few minutes to shut itself down in an organized manner rather than crashing to a halt and damaging data or hardware when the power goes off. Higher priced UPSs can power the server for hours.

In addition to protecting hardware, software and data should be protected with regular backups. The backup process copies data from the computer's hard drive to removable media, usually magnetic tape or CDs. PC workstations should be backed up as well as the server. Backups of irreplaceable billing data and medical records should be made daily. It helps to automate the process. Not only should one plan for electrical events harming data, one must also worry about physical problems such as fire and flood. Whole servers have been stolen from offices. Though hardware can be replaced easily, replacing data is almost impossible. Backup tapes should be removed each day from the office premises and stored in a secure environment.

Novel Devices for the Office Computer System

Combinations of the aforementioned hardware comprise the basic office system. To make the office workflow more efficient, there are some special computer peripherals that might serve special needs in the medical office. Which peripheral devices are appropriate depends primarily on the workflow and the benefits expected from computerizing the office. Remember again, form follows function.

Pointing Devices
Several alternative pointing devices that may be useful in the medical office are track-balls, track-pads (touch-pads), joysticks, and touch-screens. The *track-ball* is a popular pointing device that works like a mouse turned upside down exposing the ball to the user. With the ball on the topside of the pointing device, the user's index finger or thumb rolls the ball to move the pointer on the screen. Track-balls can be separate from the keyboard or built into it. With the track-ball integrated with the keyboard, the doctor can hold the keyboard in his or her lap, enter clinical findings into the EMR, and talk to the patient simultaneously. With a little practice, the

computer can be integrated into the doctor-patient interaction in the exam room. Another popular input device is the *track-pad*, also called a *touch pad*. This is a touch-sensitive plastic pad over which one drags the finger to move the pointer on the screen. Touchpads come in several sizes, from only 1.5 inches square to 8.5 by 11 inches. Some very large touch pads can be used as drawing tablets, which allow digitization of anatomic drawings. The *joystick*, the third common pointing device, is a small stick that stands up from the keyboard. These sticks are covered with a soft material that resembles a pencil eraser, and many people refer to them as *eraser heads*. *Touchscreens* are migrating from the WinCE environment to the full PC environment. These screens allow the user to move the pointer on the screen by simply touching the screen and dragging the finger to the desired area.

Wireless Keyboards

Another nontraditional computer peripheral is the wireless keyboard. These keyboards attach to the PC not with a wire but with a wireless infrared light beam or a radio transmitter. Because these keyboards are not physically attached to the PC, they often have a built-in pointing device. This allows the physician more freedom in using the computer in the exam room.

Digital Cameras

Another useful input device is a digital camera. These cameras can be used to import photos into the electronic patient record. The photos can remind the staff of what a patient looks like so that the patient is recognized by sight when returning to the office after a long absence. Another use of the digital camera is to record the appearance of skin lesions for the patient's medical record or for e-mailing to a colleague.

Choreographing the Doctor-Patient-Computer Interaction

Successful implementation of a computer system in the doctor's office requires many skills. In addition to developing a business case for computerizing the medical office, one should analyze the flow of patients, personnel, and work through the office. Integrating the movement, spatial relationships, and timing of how people and computers interact in the office is similar to choreographing a dance. Where and when patients, personnel, and doctors walk, sit, stand, and talk are important factors. Consider who can view the information on the computer screen. One the one hand, sharing the screen information with a patient may be important when doing patient education in the privacy of the exam room. On the other hand, when scheduling a patient for a follow-up visit, the patient should not be able to see other patients' names and diagnoses on the screen.

The amount of physical space taken up by computer equipment is an important consideration. The desk space required by a desktop or tower PC, a 15-inch CRT monitor, and a printer may consume all the available desk area at the nurse station. Because space is often an issue, think about space-saving alternatives such as the new, smaller PCs. Consider placing PCs under the desk or on a sturdy bookshelf high off the desk. Think about sharing network printers in order to decrease computer clutter in the exam room. The new, flat panel monitors save a lot of desk space but are two or three times more expensive than standard monitors. Laptop, subnotebook, and small WinCE computers may save space.

When using a computer in the exam room, think carefully about the placement of the doctor, the patient, and the computer equipment. Avoid placing computer equipment between the doctor and the patient. If the patient is encouraged to view the computer screen, such as an anatomical diagram or a problem list, the display must be large enough and positioned so that both doctor and patient can see the image. This may require a triangular relationship between doctor, patient, and computer display.

Be wary of extraneous noises. Computer noise can distract from the doctor-patient conversation. Choose a quiet keyboard. Avoid keyboards that produce irritating mechanical key clicks. Some keyboards are programmed to generate key click sounds through the computer speaker. If possible, disable these computer-generated key clicks. Turn down the volume of alarms from the computer.

There must be an artful arrangement of patient flow, workflow, computer hardware, and geographic space in the medical office to implement a computer system successfully.

Emerging Technologies and Issues

Emerging technologies will increase the usefulness of computers in the medical office. These include voice recognition, biometrics, telemedicine and video conferencing, and wireless networks.

Voice Recognition

One of the most common computer fantasies of physicians is to bark out an order and have the computer respond instantly, with absolute accuracy, and with complete understanding, asking no questions.

> The doctor, speaking rapidly, says, "Computer, Mr. Smith needs a CBC, retic count, ferritin, and stools about a week after he gets the UGI. Next, Computer, begin Mr. Doe's note... This 45-year-old male complains of...."
> The computer, speaking not so robotically, says, "Yes, Master", orders the tests on Mr. Smith, and begins transcribing the doctor's dictation.

Though it will be many years before the office computer will do everything asked of it, computer speech recognition can be useful today in the right clinical setting. With the right equipment and commitment from the clinician, a speech recognition program can be a powerful adjunct to the office computing environment.

The short explanation of how speech recognition works is that the speaker's words are digitized by a sound system in the PC. The digitized speech is then compared by the speech recognition program to a previously recorded file of words and phonemes using a system of artificial intelligence rules that consider word frequency, order, associations, context, and the speaker's personal pronunciation patterns. The expert system then attempts to execute the tasks requested or to transcribe the speech into text that is displayed on the computer monitor. Faster processors, more RAM, and improved speech algorithms are making speech recognition sufficiently fast and accurate to be considered for the medical office.

There are some significant issues regarding speech recognition technology that may not be apparent to the inexperienced computing physician. Older speech recognition systems required the speaker to say each individual word discretely with a brief pause between words. This form of dictation, called *discrete speech*, is a slow and unnatural way to speak. The newer speech recognition systems allow the user to speak in a natural cadence without discrete pauses between words, the system being one of *continuous speech* recognition. Continuous speech recognition is a more natural way of dictating medical notes to the computer. Another differentiating factor among speech recognition systems is whether the system is limited to a single user or can accommodate multiple users. If the speech recognition system is able to accommodate multiple users, one needs to know how quickly the system can switch from one user to another. If a user's voice file takes several minutes to load before he or she can use the system, then it will be impractical for clinicians to switch between speech recognition computers in a busy office practice. Each clinician may require a dedicated voice recognition computer.

Another issue to consider regarding speech recognition is the difference between issuing verbal commands to the computer, the *command mode*, versus automated transcription of dictated speech, the *transcription mode*. Some inexpensive speech recognition programs are limited to a command mode of speech recognition and are not suitable for transcribing clinical notes.

Also to be considered is the relative value of structured data input versus free text input. Full speech recognition allows the physician to input long, rambling, unstructured free-text notes. Free-text notes cannot easily be searched by the computer. Structured clinical data are stored in a structured computer database that allows searching for specific elements such as medications. A searchable clinical database will facilitate management of a patient population (e.g., the ability to identify all patients who have been prescribed a recalled medication). However, physicians have difficulty inputting data into highly structured EMRs. Some speech recognition systems allow dictation directly into the data fields of the EMR. The advantages of such a system are that it provides the speed of dictation, the cost savings of speech recognition, plus the structured database of the EMR. Some speech recognition systems will not allow dictation directly into the EMR. Rather, these systems require the user to dictate into a special text box and then to manually cut and paste the transcribed text into an EMR field. Such a cut-and-paste requirement will slow the busy clinician.

Three related speech recognition issues are accuracy, proofreading, and editing. Speech recognition systems are often advertised as having accuracy rates of 95%. However, 95% accuracy means that one out of every twenty words will be an error. Because these errors contain correctly spelled but inappropriate words, finding these word errors by proofreading after the fact is more difficult than finding spelling errors. Catching the errors on the fly during the dictation-speech recognition process is difficult because the user must juggle three mental activities at the same time. First, the user must be thinking ahead about what he is going to say. Second, the user must say what needs to be said at that very moment. Third, because the speech recognition system delays typing on the screen by a few seconds, the user must also be mentally comparing what was previously said to what is being typed on the screen. Juggling several mental speech processes at once can be very disconcerting to the speaker and requires a great deal of practice. In addition, correcting errors can be cumbersome and time consuming.

Most speech recognition systems are very sensitive to background noise. Some do not function well when the speaker is hoarse. Another consideration is deciding when during the patient flow process to do the dictation. Will it be in front of patients in the exam room? Many physicians are uncomfortable dictating medical record entries in the presence of a patient. Will the clinician dictate between patients? If so, is the speech recognition computer easily accessible in the immediate vicinity of the exam rooms in which the clinician is working?

To maximize the benefit of speech recognition in the medical office, one should very carefully map out clinician workflow and commit to spending hours learning the speech recognition system, training other users, and purchasing a high-powered PC and the proper medical vocabularies.

Biometrics

Maintaining privacy of health information in the computer age is very important. One element of the privacy equation is knowing that the individual using the computer system is who he says he is. This requires authentication of users. Most systems are currently protected by passwords. Passwords can be stolen, shared inappropriately, or guessed. More sophisticated systems use digital certificates. A digital certificate is a specially encoded file issued to a specific computer by a certificate authority that uniquely identifies that specific computer. Digital certificates alone do not authenticate the user of that computer. The combination of passwords and digital certificates is better than either alone, but soon biomteric systems will be used to authenticate users and patients. Biometric authentication systems take a reading of a unique biologic parameter from the user and compare the parameter to a database of authenticated users. Biometric parameters that are now emerging include fingerprint recognition, iris scanning, retinal scanning, and voice-print recognition. It is quite likely that within the next few years users of EMR systems, whether in the office, hospital, or home, will be required to authenticate themselves to the computer using one of these biometric methods.

The section on Other Hardware Issues: Privacy and Portability further discusses the topic of privacy.

Telemedicine and Video Conferencing

Telemedicine is an emerging technology that may soon play a role in the medical office. Telemedicine has been eagerly awaited but has met with only limited success so far. Rapidly improving video technology, increasing bandwidth, and reimbursement of telemedicine services may cause telemedicine to become an important part of clinical care.

Room video conferencing, with large TV-like monitors in auditoriums or large conference rooms, is commonly used for CME activities and medical conferences. Good quality desktop video conferencing equipment, available for less than $1000 per PC, can allow the clinician to see colleagues or patients at the other end of the computer link. Medical images, such as radiographs, Gram stains, and digital pictures of skin lesions, can easily be attached to e-mail or shared with colleagues using communications software such as Microsoft NetMeeting. The largest barriers to wider use of telemedicine have been the lack of adequate bandwidth required for high-quality video, the cost of video conferencing equipment, and the cost of telemedicine peripheral scopes and cameras. As more bandwidth becomes available and the cost of equipment falls, clinicians and patients will find sufficient value in telemedicine to make it a part of daily practice.

Wireless Networks

Installing the wires that form the office network presents a signficant cost and a number of challenges. Various grades of computer cable must be matched to the computer system and to the distance of the devices from the server. Building codes require certain computer cable specifications. Even details such as avoiding electromagnetic interference from fluorescent lights and other electrical power sources must be considered. The new wireless network technology addresses many of these issues. Wireless networks connect devices to the computer system through radio links rather than standard computer cables. Wireless connectivity is typically accomplished by installing a wireless access point onto the wired network. This access point is a radio that transmits and receives information to and from other PCs, printers, or modems that contain small receiver-transmitters. The wireless network obviates the need for stringing cable and provides the ability to move devices frequently about the office. The cost of wireless networks has fallen and the reliability and ease of installation have improved considerably, making wireless local area networks a reasonable alternative or addition to the traditional wired office network.

Other Hardware Issues:
Privacy and Portability

Several hardware initiatives can enhance security and privacy of patient information in the medical office. Screen savers and passwords should be placed on all PCs and terminals that can be accessed by patients and non-medical staff such as cleaning people, building maintenance persons, and building security personnel. Screen savers are applications that cause the CRT image to be replaced by a blank screen or pattern. Requiring that a password be entered in order to recover the screen will help prevent inappropriate browsing of computer information.

All applications that contain confidential information should be password protected. Passwords should be unique to each user and should not be shared. A commonly overlooked risk for confidentiality breaches is the inappropriate management of paper output from the computer. Reports with patient-specific information should be discarded properly by shredding or burning or by cutting the patient identifier from the documents. Paper output should not be left in areas where patients may be tempted to read about other patients.

Back-up media, such as computer tapes, floppy disks, and CD-ROMs, should be closely guarded. Ideally, any media that leaves the office should have encrypted data files so that, if the disk or tape is lost, others cannot read confidential patient information.

Many physicians are beginning to carry laptops from the office to home or the hospital in order to have patient information at their fingertips. These laptops can be lost or stolen. Confidential information in the files on these mobile computers should be protected by password and should be encrypted.

Summary

A successful computer system for the medical office requires thoughtful business planning, a clear understanding of office functions and workflow, and reasonable knowledge about computer hardware and software. The hardware and network configuration chosen for the office is always defined by office functions, workflow, and software requirements. Form (the hardware) follows function (workflow and software).

An understanding of fundamental computer concepts and how basic hardware works will help with planning the office system and will allow appropriate adoption of new technologies. Different computer technologies have different strengths and weaknesses. Understanding these weaknesses can help avoid computer disasters such as lost data. Understanding the strengths of new technologies will help the clinician provide better care. Like choreographing a dance, thoughtful attention to space (the placement of hardware), timing (workflow process), and roles (office personnel, clinicians, and patients) will enhance the doctor-patient-computer interaction.

See Appendix B for additional sources of information concerning hardware and technology resources.

3 / Operating Systems and Programming Languages

Stephen E. Brossette

O perating systems and programming languages are two pillars on which the foundation of modern computing rests. Since the landscape of each field changes rapidly, however, a basic knowledge of each is essential so that new technologies can be understood and used. Without such a framework, modern computing becomes a poorly understood morass of buzzwords and catch-phrases. In this chapter, operating systems and programming languages are addressed in sufficient detail to afford the reader a basic understanding of each, and to facilitate further independent investigation where desired.

Operating Systems

An operating system is a program that makes a computer easier to use, more reliable, more efficient, and more flexible in application. Since it is difficult to define an operating system in less abstract terms, the best way to understand what an operating system is, is to understand what one does. In-depth treatments of operating systems principles can be found elsewhere (1, 2). This section highlights the important features of the modern OS and surveys of some of the more popular modern operating systems including UNIX, DOS, Microsoft Windows, the Macintosh OS, OS/2, and Novell NetWare.

Early Features

The first computers were very expensive and were capable of running only one program at a time. Each program was entered manually by flipping switches or loading cards and was responsible for controlling all of the computer's hardware including input/output (I/O) devices, the central processing unit (CPU), and memory. Programs that used the same I/O devices controlled the same low-level device-specific operations and therefore contained duplicate instructions. To reduce this redundancy, I/O subroutines or device drivers were created. A *device driver* is a program that controls an I/O device and provides an interface for other programs to communicate with that device.

Device drivers were the first mechanism of abstraction in shielding the programmer, or user, from hardware. In other words, device drivers control I/O devices so that programmers and users don't have to. As a result, programmers were freed from writing device-specific codes. A program written to run on one computer could now run on another with different devices with only small modifications to the program. Modern operating systems sometimes contain thousands of device drivers that control everything from printers, video cards, and hard disks, to network adapters and modems.

Since the first computers were so expensive, efforts were made to minimize the time that they were not actually computing—downtime. In the beginning, computer time was scheduled by sign-up sheets, and programmers had to be on-site at their scheduled time to load programs, run them, debug them, and collect the output. Because these programmers, usually scientists, were not very efficient at operating computers, dedicated operators were hired to minimize downtime. Programs were queued with the operator. If one finished early, sometimes by error, the program could be removed by the operator and another started, without the programmer having to be present. The programmer would interpret results or debug off-line and add the program back to the queue if needed. This improved efficiency but eliminated interaction between the programmer and the running program.

The human operator was soon replaced by the *resident monitor program* (RMP). Programs were loaded in memory, by this time from tape, and, when one finished, the next was loaded and started by the RMP. This worked more efficiently than the human operator but was still plagued with the same problems. Namely, if a program crashed or hung, human intervention was required. Additionally, there was still no interaction between the programmer and the executing program. The RMP was, however, the first example of process management (the loading and running of programs) by computer, and, together with device drivers, comprised the first-generation operating system.

Multitasking

The RMP scheduled and ran one program at a time. A single running program, however, inefficiently utilizes the CPU and I/O devices. This inefficiency is due to the discrepancy in speeds between I/O devices and the CPU. For example, in the time between the keystrokes of a fast typist at a keyboard (an I/O device), a modern CPU can perform millions of operations. Therefore, when a program needs data from an I/O device, even a hard disk, the CPU sits idle for relatively long periods of time until the I/O device returns data. On the other hand, if a single running program keeps the CPU busy, then the I/O devices stay idle. In either case, computers that run one program at a time underutilize valuable computing resources.

To solve this problem, the computer must be able to manage more than one program at a time and be able to switch between them so that when one program is waiting for I/O another can run on the CPU. This is called *multitasking* and requires two important operating system features: interrupts and context switching.

An *interrupt* is an asynchronous signal generated by an I/O device that alerts the CPU when the device has completed a request for service. For example, if a program needs input from the keyboard, it sends a request to the keyboard's device driver via a system call, then waits for that device to return data. Instead of the OS repeatedly polling the device to see if the user has typed anything, the device itself generates a hardware signal, an interrupt, to inform the OS that a key has been pressed. The OS recognizes the signal, gets the data, then continues running the program which made the request.

Context switching, the other necessary feature for multitasking, allows the operating system to change running programs so that a program waiting for I/O can be set aside while another program uses the CPU. In general, a program in a multitasking operating system can be in one of three states: running, blocked, or ready. A program changes states from running to blocked when it submits a request to a device driver, from blocked to ready when that request is complete (signaled by an interrupt from a device), and from ready to running when the scheduler makes it so. Specifically, when a program requests service from an I/O device, information about the current state of the program is saved, and the OS marks the program as *blocked* (awaiting I/O). In the meantime, the OS, through its *scheduler*, selects another program that is ready to run (i.e., not blocked) to use the CPU. When the *interrupt handler* (part of the OS) receives an interrupt for the blocked program, the blocked program becomes ready, and can run on the

CPU when the CPU becomes available.

Unless a program requests the service of an I/O device, and therefore blocks, it will not relinquish control of the CPU to allow another program to run. This scheme, in which the operating system depends on the behavior and cooperation of programs to voluntarily give up the CPU so that other programs can run, is appropriately named *cooperative multitasking*. In reality, however, programs are not so cooperative, and the performance of operating systems that depend on cooperative multitasking (e.g., Macintosh OS, Windows 3.1 and, to some extent, Windows 95) is unpredictable.

Multiple Users and Preemptive Multitasking

In order to have fast interaction response times between multiple users and programs on the same computer, timer interrupts are required. A *timer interrupt* is a fixed-rate (e.g., 60 per second), clock-driven signal that is recognized by the CPU. At each timer interrupt, the scheduler selects a program ready to run, saves the state of the running program, and makes a context switch. Since the time between timer interrupts, the *time slice*, is very short compared with the speed of human-computer interaction, the computer can run many programs over a short period of time which, to the user, makes it seem as if the computer is running the programs simultaneously. This scheme, where the OS interrupts a running program to start another, is called *preemptive multitasking*. In operating systems that support preemptive multitasking (e.g., UNIX, Linux, OS/2, Windows NT), the scheduler is clever in selecting the next program for execution. It does so based on how I/O intensive the program is, to keep the CPU and I/O devices busy, and how important the program is, to give important programs, or those owned by important users, higher priority. With multitasking and multiple users, however, the operating system has additional problems to address such as protection and security.

Protection and Security

Safeguards against programs corrupting other programs become necessary in multitasking environments. Without *protection*, any program could control a device or write to any location in memory, even if that memory contains another program or data for another program.

Since the OS is also a program, the hardware must allow for two distinct modes of operation to facilitate memory protection: user mode and protected mode. In *user mode*, instructions responsible for memory management and direct control of I/O are disabled. With no direct access to these resources, programs must request these services from the OS, which can switch the hardware to a *protected mode* where privileged instructions can be executed. Before giving control back to application programs though, the OS switches the hardware back to user mode. This gives the OS sole control over the direct manipulation of vital resources to coordinate their use and to protect one program from being inadvertently or maliciously interfered with by another. Larger computers have supported protected mode operation for some time because it is desirable for multitasking. Personal computers began offering protected mode operation with the introduction of the Intel 80386 microprocessor, although DOS and early versions of Windows do not use this feature.

Operating system *security* refers to the management of users, groups, and their access privileges. The goal of security is to prevent users from having unauthorized access to other users' or groups' files and programs. This is usually accomplished by log-in and password identification and file systems that keep file ownership and file access information.

Files and File Systems

A *file* is an abstraction for a program or data stored as bits on disk or tape. A *file system* is a logical structure for organizing files on one or more storage devices. Operating systems create and maintain file systems and provide functions that application programs can use to create and delete files, locate them, and transfer data to and from them. The operating system controls the details of file manipulation so that application programs don't have to. For example, if a program needs data stored in a particular file, it calls an OS function to open the file, then calls other OS functions to locate data and copy it into memory. The operating system locates the file, which may be stored in several pieces on the disk, and transfers the data from disk to memory—a process that is more involved than it appears.

File systems also determine the maximum length of a file name and how many files can be stored on a disk partition of a certain size. They can also provide data security by storing copies of files on other disks and keeping track of file ownership and access privileges. Each operating system fully supports at least one file system and may partially support several others.

Multithreading

A *thread* is a single pathway of instruction execution through a program.

Many programs have one thread. Sometimes, however, a program can be separated into distinct threads such that more than one can be executed simultaneously, thereby improving execution speed. Such a program is *multi-threaded* and usually consists of some primary thread that may, for example, handle user interaction, and one or more other threads that perform background tasks, such as rendering images on the screen.

In a multitasking operating system, each thread of a multithreaded program is handled separately so that the program can take advantage of multitasking. While one thread is running, others can be blocked or ready. This improves the performance of a single program by allowing the threads of the program more access to the CPU and I/O devices. UNIX, Linux, OS/2, Windows 95, and Windows NT support multithreaded programs.

Memory Management and Virtual Memory

Just as the OS manages files stored on external media, it also manages programs and data in memory. A secure operating system (e.g., UNIX, Linux, OS/2, and Windows NT) prevents a program from accessing memory that it does not own. This is accomplished by assigning each program its own address space that can be accessed by the program itself but by no other application or user program. Other memory management features of the OS include allocating memory for running programs, keeping track of data and programs scattered through memory, reclaiming unused memory so that it can be used again, and managing virtual memory.

Virtual memory exists not in memory but on disk. When a program requests memory from the OS, but none remains, the OS can use a piece of the hard disk as memory. To do this, it moves less frequently used chunks (pages) of bits from memory to disk so that the space cleared in memory can be used for the new request. When the bits stored on disk are needed again by a program, they are moved back to physical memory by swapping places with other pages. The extra overhead required for swapping pages in and out of memory makes this process slower than simply accessing bits in memory but gives application programs the illusion that there is more physical memory than actually exists.

User Interfaces

Operating systems allow the user to interface with the computer so that programs can be started, files can be deleted, etc. Common examples include text-based interfaces, such as the DOS command line or the UNIX bash shell, or graphical user interfaces (GUIs), such as X-Windows for UNIX and Linux or those with Macintosh OS, OS/2, and Microsoft Windows.

Multiprocessing

Multiprocessing refers to an operating system's ability to support more than one CPU so that more than one program or task can run simultaneously, one on each CPU. This is different from multitasking on a single-processor machine in which programs only appear to be running simultaneously. In fact, on multiprocessor machines, multiprocessing and multitasking are often used at the same time.

A number of schemes exist for dividing work between two or more processors, and some of the ways in which operating systems do this are complicated. The most complex, powerful, and reliable of these is *symmetric multiprocessing* (SMP) in which all processors are connected to a common memory, share the same I/O devices, and are capable of performing the same tasks. UNIX, Windows NT, and NetWare 5 support SMP.

Network Operating Systems

The network operating system is an operating system that provides services for connecting a computer to other computers to create a local area network (LAN). Within a LAN, some computers run programs that act primarily to serve information to different programs on other computers. The serving programs are called *servers*, and the receiving programs are called *clients*. This *client-server* paradigm is responsible for most of the data transferred on the Internet. (Client-server computing also describes two or more programs on a single multitasking machine that interact with each other in a client-server relationship.) By tradition, machines that run important server programs, like an HTML server for Web pages, are themselves called *servers*, whereas machines that run client programs, like a Web browser, are called *clients*.

The term *network operating system* is usually reserved for operating systems that only run on LAN servers. Network operating systems are not used on client machines. UNIX and Microsoft NT, for example, can run on servers, but they are also used on client machines. Novell NetWare, on the other hand, is found only on servers.

POSIX

Little can be read about modern operating systems without encountering the term POSIX. POSIX (Portable Operating Systems Interface in UNIX) is a set of standards maintained by IEEE that defines an interface between operating systems and application programs (3). It is a standard aimed to facilitate the construction of portable application programs. A program that uses POSIX system calls should be portable amongst POSIX-compliant operating systems. Today, many versions of UNIX, Linux, and Windows NT are POSIX compliant.

A Survey of Popular Modern Operating Systems

UNIX

UNIX is the legendary multiuser, multitasking, network-capable operating system first developed at AT&T in the late 1960s and early 1970s, and later at the University of California at Berkeley, that has become the most widely used operating system on computers other than PCs. Originally developed for computers in academic and government environments, UNIX can now be found on machines of all types, from supercomputers to PCs, and in all work environments, from major corporations to the home. UNIX is also the most widely used operating system on computers that provide content on the Internet (e.g., HTML servers) and on company computers that contain mission-critical transaction systems and important databases.

UNIX has many attractive features. It is secure and stable. It is multiuser, multitasking, and POSIX compliant. It can act as a network server and is available for virtually any hardware platform, including multiprocessor machines. Additionally, many distributions come with compilers and other useful software not found in other OS distributions, and many vendors and independent organizations offer training and certification. UNIX also supports file systems that can handle large hard disks and other external storage devices efficiently.

There are many versions of UNIX and many vendors. Sun, Silicon Graphics, HP, Compaq and IBM are but a few companies that sell versions of UNIX. Perhaps the most exciting development of late, however, has been the emergence and success of Linux, a very capable UNIX developed by Linus Torvalds and a small army of programmers in a decentralized, noncorporate effort that has come to exemplify the Open Source movement (4,

5). Linux was developed for the PC but is now available for the DEC Alpha and the PowerPC, with other ports underway.

Linux is free and comes with a variety of powerful application programs, including the Apache Web server. The operating system and application programs are often packaged in *distributions*, each from a different organization. Most can be downloaded for free. Alternatively, some can be purchased along with proprietary programs, such as word processors, from distributors for a nominal charge. Now companies such as Caldera (6) and Red Hat (7) not only maintain and sell Linux distributions but offer support, training, and certification in the way that other companies do for commercial operating systems.

Linux has become a popular, affordable, and capable alternative to more expensive and sometimes less capable commercial operating systems. As a result of Linux's growing popularity, third-party software manufacturers, including database makers Oracle and Sybase, are now porting industrial strength business software to run on Linux. Additionally, some PC manufacturers, such as Dell, now offer a choice of Linux or Microsoft Windows with a new PC or server (8).

In the past, UNIX has been considered an expert's operating system, and it is true that it is generally not as user-friendly as other operating systems that have sophisticated GUIs and self-configuring installation programs. With the growing popularity of Linux, however, UNIX is becoming friendlier to the nonexpert user as GUIs and other software that simplify installation and maintenance are being created.

Whereas a great deal of software exists for UNIX systems in general, not so much exists for PC versions of UNIX, such as Linux, as for other popular PC operating systems like Microsoft Windows. This too, however, is quickly improving as Linux gains market share, prompting software manufacturers to port programs to run on Linux platforms.

MS-DOS

MS-DOS (or simply DOS) was, for all practical purposes, the original operating system of the personal computer. Developed by Microsoft for the first IBM PC, MS-DOS version 1.0 was released in 1981. Since then, it has gone through many versions and gained features such as a hierarchical file system (v2.0), installable modular device drivers (v2.0), a background print spooler (v2.0), some networking capabilities (v3.0), the support of several communication ports (v3.3), the support of 1.44 MB floppy disks (v3.3), the support of 2GB hard disks (v4.0), and improved memory management (nearly all versions). The last version of MS-DOS, unofficially known as version 7, is the foundation for Microsoft's Windows 95 and Windows 98 operating systems. Though DOS has been eclipsed in many ways by more sophisticated operating systems, it maintains a strong presence in the PC world due to its tremendous popularity in the 1980s and the fact that many computers still run DOS and DOS-based applications.

DOS has served the personal computer well, but it has many limitations. It is 16 bit, single user, single tasking (vs. multitasking), has poor memory management, and does not support virtual memory. Perhaps the most notorious shortcoming of DOS, however, is its inability to run in protected mode, a capability of PC CPUs from the Intel 80386 forward. As a result, DOS cannot stop application programs from directly writing to memory or controlling I/O devices. This has been used to the advantage of some programmers (especially game programmers) to get direct control of hardware to maximize program speed. Ultimately, however, this feature makes DOS unsafe and unstable because without protected mode operation, any program can, intentionally or not, corrupt any other program in memory including DOS itself.

The inability of DOS to run in protected mode also restricts DOS programs to 1 MB of addressable memory, of which only 640 KB are available to application programs. (Data, but not programs, can be stored in memory beyond 1 MB with MS-DOS v4.0 and later versions.) This notorious 640 KB addressable memory ceiling is the remnant of the maximum addressable memory of the Intel 8088 and 8086, which were the 16-bit CPUs of the first IBM PCs.

Although Microsoft stopped development of MS-DOS in favor of its Windows line of operating systems, DOS programs are supported by Windows 3.1, Windows 95, Windows 98, and OS/2. Windows NT supports DOS programs through a DOS emulator, and DOS emulators exist for UNIX and the Macintosh OS. Additionally, Lineo distributes Dr-DOS, a version of DOS with some networking and multitasking features (9).

Microsoft Windows

Microsoft Windows (10) dominated the PC operating systems market in the 1990s. The successor to MS-DOS, Microsoft Windows (or just Windows) has evolved through many product generations including Windows 3.x (which includes Windows 3.0, 3.1, and 3.11), Windows 95, Windows 98, Windows NT, and Windows 2000. In addition to giving the PC a Macintosh-like graphical user interface (GUI), the Windows operating systems have provided a number of desirable OS features previously unavailable with DOS. These include memory access beyond 640 KB (Windows 3.0), virtual memory (Windows 3.0), a 32-bit architecture (Windows 95), built-in networking (Windows 95), plug-and-play hardware support (Windows 95), true preemptive multitasking (Windows NT), improved security and stability (Windows NT), POSIX compliance (Windows NT), symmetric multiprocessing (Windows NT), and server capabilities (Windows NT Server). With the exception of Windows NT Server, all are single-user operating systems.

Windows 3.x, 95, and 98 all depend to some extent on DOS version 7. Otherwise, Windows 3.x is significantly different from Windows 95 and Windows 98, which are very similar. In addition to the new GUI style, the notable difference between Windows 3.x and Windows 95/98 is that the latter have a 32-bit architecture whereas Windows 3.x has a 16-bit architecture. This means that with Windows 95/98, 32-bit application programs can utilize the ability of the Intel 80386 and newer CPUs to transfer information around the hardware in 32 bits at a time. Windows 3.x, on the other hand, has a 16-bit architecture designed to run on the Intel 80286 CPU. It does not support 32-bit software.

Multitasking improved from Windows 3.x to Windows 95/98. Whereas Windows 3.x has only cooperative multitasking capabilities, Windows 95/98 can preemptively multitask 32-bit Windows programs (though it must still cooperatively multitask 16-bit programs).

Windows 95/98 support the FAT32 file system, which allows more efficient data storage and supports larger hard disks than the FAT16 file system. The maximum hard- disk size supported by FAT16 is 2 GB. Anything bigger must be divided up (partitioned) into logical partitions, each no larger than 2 GB. FAT32, on the other hand, with 32-bit addressing, supports disks up to 2 terabytes on a single partition.

Windows 95 also supports *plug-and-play*, a hardware standard that allows the OS to determine the identification of plug-and-play I/O devices so that it automatically configures them and installs their device drivers. Windows 95 also provides built in networking with TCP/IP support (the data transfer protocols of the Internet) as well as support for other network communication protocols.

Whereas Windows 3.x, 95, and 98 are all based on DOS to some extent, Windows NT is not, making it the first in a new line of operating systems from Microsoft. Windows NT is an advanced 32-bit operating system available for the Intel x86 line of CPUs and the DEC Alpha. It contains many features that the DOS-based Windows systems do not, including preemptive multitasking for 16-bit and 32-bit programs, multithreading, symmetric multiprocessing, support for the NTFS file system, improved stability and security, and POSIX compliance. Windows NT comes in a client version (Windows NT Workstation) and a server version (Windows NT Server).

Windows NT supports the same GUI as Windows 95/98 but does not have plug-and-play capabilities. Windows 2000, the latest version of Windows NT, has plug-and-play support, better administration tools, and other improvements. Microsoft offers certification for Windows NT administrators, and training courses and materials are widely available (11).

The Macintosh

The Apple Macintosh set the standard for user-friendly personal computing with a revolutionary graphical user interface and plug-and-play capabilities long before Microsoft offered these features in their Windows operating systems. Since its release in the 1980s, the Macintosh has enjoyed a very loyal following and continues to be the preferred computer amongst visual artists and desktop publishers.

The Macintosh OS (MacOS) (12), like Microsoft Windows, has gone through many versions and has become more feature rich over time. Originally designed for the Motorola 68000 line of CPUs, the MacOS has never been confined to 640 KB of addressable memory like DOS. Until 1999, however, MacOS did not support advanced operating system features such as preemptive multitasking, memory protection, multiple users, or symmetric multiprocessing. It has also been inferior to Windows 95/98 in memory protection and multitasking capabilities. Apple has addressed these deficiencies by combining the core of a UNIX operating system with traditional MacOS technologies to create the MacOS X operating system.

MacOS X combines the advanced OS features of UNIX, including preemptive multitasking, server, and multiuser capabilities, with the advanced, easy to use MacOS GUI and other traditional MacOS programs. Additionally, MacOS X is the first multi-platform Macintosh operating system capable of running on its native PowerPC platform as well as those based on newer Intel microprocessors. Combined with powerful Macintosh computers, MacOS X is a very capable operating system. With MacOS X, the iMac, a commitment to high-powered desktop computing, and a focus not seen at Apple since the 1980s, the future of the Macintosh appears promising.

OS/2

OS/2 is a single-user, multithreaded, preemptive multitasking operating system developed by IBM that features protected-mode operation, virtual memory, a high-degree of stability, and the ability to run Windows 3.1, DOS, and native OS/2 programs (13). The latest version of OS/2, called OS/2 Warp, comes in client and server versions, much like Windows NT, and offers dual-boot capability, a sophisticated GUI, a DOS command line, and a full complement of networking capabilities.

The main difference between Windows 95/98 and OS/2 is that OS/2 can preemptively multitask DOS, Windows 3.1, and OS/2 programs all at once, whereas Windows 95/98 can preemptively multitask 32-bit Windows programs but must cooperatively multitask 16-bit programs such as Windows 3.1 and DOS programs. Windows NT can preemptively multitask 16-bit applications but does not support DOS applications as well as OS/2 or Windows 95/98. Unfortunately, OS/2 does not support 32-bit Windows 95/98 and Windows NT programs.

A hallmark of OS/2 is its stability and reliability. This has led to its prominence in banking and manufacturing where PCs are used for mission-critical operations.

Novell NetWare

Novell NetWare (14) is an operating system for LAN servers that, before Windows NT, controlled a large share of the PC-based server marketplace. NetWare still has a large, skilled following facilitated by its certification training programs that predated those offered by Microsoft and now Linux vendors.

NetWare 5, released in 1998, has full support of TCP/IP in addition to the standard proprietary Novell communication protocols. It also has native Java support, a 64-bit file system, SMP support, and a 5-user license of the Oracle 8 database. Windows 95/98, Windows NT, MacOS, and UNIX can all act as NetWare clients.

Programming Languages

Programming languages, like operating systems, are a cornerstone of modern computing. Thousands of programming languages have been created, and entire texts are devoted to the subject. In this section, some programming language basics are presented and several popular modern programming languages are surveyed.

Many programming languages were created with specific applications in mind. For example, FORTRAN was designed for science and engineering, Lisp and Prolog for artificial intelligence, C for operating system development, COBOL for business, BASIC to teach programming, and Java for Internet and network computing. Other languages were developed not for a particular application domain but to express new programming paradigms. Prominent among these are the object-oriented languages C++ and Smalltalk. Java is also an object-oriented programming language.

Machine and Assembly Languages

A computer program is a set of instructions executed by hardware to perform a specific task. To hardware, a program is simply a sequence of bits that, when interpreted in small pieces, directs the hardware to perform simple operations such as add two numbers (two sets of bits), store some bits in memory, or illuminate a certain pixel on the display screen. These programs are in *machine language* and are therefore *executable*, which means they run directly on the CPU. They are, however, except for very simple programs, prohibitively difficult to write.

Machine language is machine-specific and depends entirely on the *instruction set* of the CPU. A machine language program that runs on a Dec Alpha will not run on an Intel x86, a PowerPC, or any other type of CPU. Machine language programs, as a rule, are not *portable*. Exceptions to the rule occur within families of microprocessors. For example, the Intel x86 microprocessors are backward compatible (i.e., each CPU supports the instruction set of its predecessors). Therefore, a machine language program that runs on the 80286 will run on the 80386, 80486, Pentium, Pentium II, Pentium III, and Pentium IV. The reverse, however, is not true. Machine language programs that take advantage of features (and instructions) of newer microprocessors cannot run on older ones.

Assembly language is a low-level programming language, one step removed from machine language. Unlike machine language, which uses only numbers for instructions and data, assembly language uses text to represent machine instructions and allows the programmer to assign names to variables. Still, each instruction, or line, in an assembly language program is translated by a program called the *assembler* into a single machine language instruction. Therefore, assembly language programs, like machine language programs, are not portable.

Assembly language allows for very precise control of hardware, and is useful when such control is necessary or can be used to optimize a program's speed or size. Before UNIX, which was written in C, many operating systems were written in assembly language. Today, pieces of operating systems and other types of embedded systems are written in assembly language, although C is usually the language of choice.

Even though relatively few programs are now written in assembly language, assembly language is nonetheless vitally important because it acts as the gateway to machine language, which is the only language understood by hardware.

Compilers and Interpreters

In general, programmers do not write in assembly language. Instead, high-level programming languages like C, C++, or Java are used.

There are three general schemes by which a program in a high-level programming language can be run. It can be translated into machine language; it can be interpreted by another program without any translation; or it can be translated into an intermediate language that gets interpreted. Each approach has advantages and disadvantages, and each programming language supports one or more of these approaches.

Programs that are translated to machine language can be executed directly on the CPU. Translation occurs by running a program called a *compiler* to translate a source code program into assembly language, which is then assembled into machine language. Since most programs depend on calls to the operating system for I/O as well as other services, the machine language program is then *linked* by a program called the *linker* to the operating system code to form an *executable image*, which can be run directly on the CPU.

Compiled programs run on the CPU and are fast compared with interpreted programs. Before they can be run, however, they must be compiled, which can be time consuming depending on the size of the program. Also, compiled programs are CPU specific (i.e., an executable for one machine will generally not run on another). Therefore, when porting a program in a compiled language from one machine type to another, the program must be recompiled and reassembled. C, C++, FORTRAN, and COBOL are compiled programming languages.

Compiler principles and construction are interesting subjects and are necessary for the construction of new compiled programming languages.

An excellent treatment of compiler principles can be found in Aho et al (15).

At the opposite extreme of compiled languages are the interpreted languages. A program in an interpreted language is not run directly on the CPU like a compiled program but instead is read by an *interpreter*, an executable program that acts as a go-between for the source program and the CPU. The source program that gets interpreted, however, is not executable. Therefore, interpreted programs do not need to be compiled before they are run. As a result, the source code of an interpreted program is portable without the need to recompile, which makes testing and debugging more efficient than with compiled programs.

Because interpreted programs are not directly executed but depend on an interpreter to run, they are significantly slower than their compiled counterparts. This makes interpreted programs inappropriate for some computationally intensive tasks and tasks that depend on very fast execution speeds. For most applications, however, especially with modern computers, interpreted programs are fast enough. BASIC is the best-known interpreted programming language.

Between compiled and interpreted schemes for running programs are hybrid implementations that use both compilers and interpreters. The most popular programming language that uses this approach is Java. A Java program is compiled by the Java compiler into Java *byte code*. Java byte code is then interpreted by the Java interpreter, called the Java Virtual Machine. Both the compiler and the interpreter are machine-specific executables. Java byte code, however, is portable and can be run on any hardware/operating system platform that supports the Java interpreter.

The hybrid approach to programming language implementation is a compromise between a purely compiled and a purely interpreted implementation. The intermediate representation of the source program produced by the compiler (e.g., Java byte code) is easier and faster to interpret than the original source language program. This makes for faster program execution speed and simpler interpreters. Programs in languages with hybrid implementations, however, are still significantly slower than their purely compiled counterparts. Again, for most programs, however, this is not significant.

Object-Oriented Programming

Object-oriented programming is a powerful paradigm facilitated by object-oriented programming languages of which C++ and Java are the most popular. Object-oriented programming languages facilitate efficient program construction, maintenance, and reusability by supporting the five fundamental concepts of object-oriented programming: objects, classes, inheritance, polymorphism, and dynamic binding. Although a detailed discussion of each is beyond the scope of this text, all except dynamic binding will be briefly explained. Extensive treatments of these concepts can be found in other texts (16-18).

An *object* is like a variable that has, in addition to data, associated semantics and functionality. Each object has a state, described by its *member data*, and each can be selectively manipulated by its interface, which is composed of its *member functions*. For example, an object is like a telephone. It is not necessary to know how it functions in order to use it. In this way the internal workings of the phone are hidden from the user but the user can use the phone by simply operating its interface.

A *class* is like a blueprint for an object that specifies how each object is to be constructed, or *instantiated*. It specifies the types of member data, which can be objects themselves, and the member functions. For each type of object, there exists a class.

Classes can be related to each other by *inheritance*. This is useful when objects of one class are "kinds-of" objects of another class. For example, in a graphics program that draws geometric figures on the screen, a class *Shape* with a member function draw() may exist. *Circle*, *Rectangle*, and *Triangle* can then be created through inheritance as *child classes* of *Shape*.

Each child class must support every function of the class from which it was derived, the *parent class*. This is accomplished in one of two ways. If the function implementation of the child class is no different from the parent's, then the parent's implementation can be used by default. If, however, special requirements exist for the child class implementation, or if the parent class does not provide an implementation for the function, then the child class can specify the function implementation itself. For example, since the method for drawing a circle differs from the method for drawing a triangle, both the *Circle* and *Triangle* classes provide their own implementations for the parent-class function draw().

Polymorphism allows objects of a child class to be used as objects its parent class. Continuing the previous example, a function that moves a shape on the screen can be specified broadly to use a *Shape* object. Since shape has child classes *Circle*, *Rectangle*, and *Triangle*, polymorphism allows the same function to move a circle, rectangle, or triangle. This eliminates the need for different move functions for each type of shape. If another shape class is added in the future (e.g., *Ellipse*), then it too can use the same function. This is an extremely powerful feature that allows for an old code to use objects of future classes.

Developer's Toolkits

Software developer's toolkits (SDKs) and integrated development environments (IDEs) are software packages that contain everything needed to build application programs. SDKs and IDEs contain a compiler or interpreter, a debugging tool, an editor, libraries of reusable source code, and a GUI builder that allows the programmer to easily add graphical elements such as buttons, display boxes, and drop-down lists to user interfaces. Although SDKs and IDEs are not necessary to build software, they usually make the process much easier.

A Survey of Popular Programming Languages

C

C is a compiled programming language developed at Bell Labs for the construction of the UNIX operating system. Many of C's features were borrowed from ALGOL 68, including block structure, recursion, dynamic memory allocation, machine independence, conditional expressions, and *for* loops.

C is a very popular programming language, and much of its success can be attributed to its free distribution with UNIX. C is not, however, a beginner's programming language, because it requires familiarity with pointers and dynamic memory management. Still, C is very flexible, powerful, and popular. It also forms part of the basis of C++. Additionally, C compilers are widely available, including the free GNU C/C++ compiler *gcc* distributed with UNIX and Linux.

C++

C++ is a compiled, object-oriented programming language developed at Bell Labs. C++ was not designed as an object-oriented programming language from the ground up. Instead, C was used as the foundation, and object-oriented programming features were added. As a result, C is a subset of C++, and C++ compilers and SDKs can be used to develop C programs.

To program in C++, it is helpful to have knowledge of C but not necessary. For those that do, the temptation to write C programs instead of object-oriented C++ programs must be avoided. For long-time C
programmers, this is sometimes difficult.

Like C, C++ requires knowledge of pointers and memory management,
which is often difficult for beginning programmers, and the cause of errors
even for experienced ones. If learning object-oriented programming is a
goal, Java is probably a better initial choice. Since C++ is compiled and
not interpreted, however, its programs are faster than equivalent ones in
Java, which are interpreted.

Many good resources are available for the C++ programmer. Excellent
books for both the motivated beginner and more experienced programmer
include *Thinking in C++* by Bruce Eckel (19, 20). Advanced authoritative
texts include *The C++ Programming Language* by Bjarne Stroustrup, the cre-
ator of C++ (17).

C++ compilers, SDKs, and IDEs are available for nearly all computing
platforms including UNIX, Linux, Windows, Mac OS, DOS, and OS/2.
Microsoft Visual C++ (21) and Borland C++ Builder (22) are IDEs available for Windows and Mac platforms. UNIX and Linux users have the
GNU C++ compiler, *gcc*, in addition to freely distributed reusable code libraries. They also have access to traditional UNIX development tools including *make*, *vi*, *emacs*, and *gdb*.

Java

Java is an object-oriented programming language for creating platform-independent, Internet, and Intranet applications. Developed by Sun Microsystems in the early 1990s, Java is an interpreted language that
resembles C++ but removes pointers and manual memory management
while at the same time adding such features as operating-system–independent multithreading, a singly-rooted class hierarchy, and platform-independent GUI classes.

The success of Java has been remarkable, and this can be attributed to
several factors. First, Java is a full-featured, object-oriented programming
language. Second, it resembles C++, only simpler. Finally, it was designed
from beginning with platform-independent network computing in mind.

While Java is ultimately an interpreted language, Java source code is
initially compiled into an intermediate language called *byte code*. Byte
code, in turn, is run by the Java interpreter, known as the *Java Virtual Ma-*

chine, which is included in popular Web browsers such as Netscape Navigator, Microsoft Internet Explorer, and the Sun HotJava browser. The Java Virtual Machine is also available as a *plug-in* for browsers that do not have one built-in and as a stand-alone executable for UNIX, Linux, Windows, OS/2, and MacOS.

A Java program that runs in a Web page is called an *applet*. When a Java-capable browser requests a Web page that has an associated applet, the server sends the applet to the browser as byte code. The browser then starts the Java Virtual Machine and runs the applet, which appears on the Web page. Therefore, a Java applet can run on any hardware/operating system platform so long as a Java-capable Web browser is available for that platform. This browser-facilitated portability makes Java programs accessible across the Internet and allows program maintenance and distribution to occur at a single location. When a new version of a Java program is released, it can be stored on one server and all users have access to it across the network. This paradigm of software development and distribution is very attractive for organizations that have many users of an application program. Instead of installing a copy of the software on each user machine, the program can be made available as a Java applet stored on one Intranet server.

Java also supports platform-independent database access through JDBC (Java Database Connectivity), a programming interface that allows Java programs to access data in relational databases such as Oracle, SQL Server, and Sybase. JDBC functionality is provided through the JDBC class library.

Java is an interpreted language. Therefore, programs in Java are slower than their C++ counterparts. For most programs running on modern computers, however, this slowdown is not significant. If faster execution speed is needed, however, Java compilers that generate fast machine language executables are available. Unfortunately, the resultant executable programs, like C and C++ executables, are machine-specific and are not portable.

Java compilers, browser plug-ins, stand-alone interpreters, class libraries, online books, and documentation are all available free of charge from Sun Microsystems at www.java.sun.com. The Java Developer Kit (JDK), available at the same site, contains the latest compiler, interpreter, debugger, and class libraries all in one package. It is available for Windows 95/98/NT and Sun Solaris operating systems. In addition to the free developer tools from Sun, popular Java IDEs are available from Borland (22), Symantec (23), Microsoft (24), and Metrowerks (25). Excellent books including *Thinking in Java* (18, 20) and an ongoing series published by Sun Microsystems Press (26) are readily available.

Visual Basic

Visual Basic (VB) is a popular programming language from Microsoft used exclusively to develop Windows-based applications. It is not object-oriented. A descendent of BASIC (Beginner's All-purpose Symbolic Instruction Code), Visual Basic is relatively easy to learn and contains few of the complexities of C-like languages that confuse some beginning programmers. Like Java, VB is both compiled and interpreted with intermediate byte code that is run by a VB interpreter. Unlike Java, the VB interpreter is not used with Web browsers. The Visual Basic IDE from Microsoft supports sophisticated application development including database access through the use of ODBC. Microsoft also offers Visual Basic training and certification (27).

MUMPS

MUMPS (also known as M) is an interpreted, general-purpose programming language developed at the Massachusetts General Hospital Laboratory of Computer Science in the 1960s. MUMPS was designed to facilitate medical records processing and supports some unique and sophisticated data handling features such as persistent variables, multi-dimensional associative arrays, and excellent string-handling capabilities. MUMPS maintains a loyal following in the medical community and is now used in other fields such as banking.

Although MUMPS maintains its own database and is used for database development, it is not a relational database management system (RDBMS) like Oracle, Sybase, or Microsoft SQL Server. MUMPS does, however, support RDBMS access through embedded SQL and ODBC, like other popular programming languages. MUMPS databases, which are really persistent associative arrays, are highly-portable because they are composed of and indexed by a single data type: character strings. Therefore, a MUMPS database can be shared between MUMPS programs on radically different hardware/operating system platforms.

Versions of MUMPS are available for many popular operating systems including Windows, UNIX, and MacOS. Free versions are also available. Most versions of MUMPS are now compiled and interpreted, much like Java and Visual Basic. A guide many MUMPS resources can be found at www.mcenter.com/mtrc/.

Web Scripting Languages

Web scripting languages such as JavaScript, VBScript, and Tcl/Tk are supported by Web browsers and browser plug-ins. Although they are not programming languages *per se*, they are convenient and useful for creating interactive user interfaces on Web pages. Although the same could be accomplished with Java, scripting languages are simpler, easier to learn, and easier to implement for certain routine Web programming problems. Many books and online references are available for JavaScript, VBScript, and Tcl/Tk.

Summary

Operating systems and programming languages have a rich history in computer science and form a significant part of the foundation of modern computing. The reader should now have a basic understanding of each so that new technology can be put in perspective and additional independent study can be pursued.

REFERENCES

1. **Silberschatz A, Galvin P.** Operating System Concepts, 4th ed. Reading, MA: Addison-Wesley, 1994.
2. **Deitel HM.** Operating Systems, 2nd ed. Reading, MA: Addison-Wesley, 1990.
3. http://www.standards.ieee.org
4. http://metalab.unc.edu/mdw/linux.html/
5. http://www.opensorce.org
6. http://www.caldera.com
7. http://www.redhat.com
8. http://www.dell.com/linux/
9. http://www.lineo.com/products/drdos.html/
10. http://www.microsoft.com
11. http://www.microsoft.com/train_cert/
12. http://www.apple.com
13. http://www.software.ibm.com/os/warp/
14. http://www.novell.com/netware/
15. **Aho AV, Sethi R, Ullman JD.** Compilers: Principles, Techniques, and Tools. Reading, MA: Addison-Wesley, 1986.
16. **Cline MP, Lomow GA.** C++ FAQs. Reading, MA: Addison-Wesley, 1995.
17. **Stroustrup B.** The C++ Programming Language, 3rd ed. Reading, MA: Addison-Wesley, 1997.
18. **Eckel B.** Thinking in Java. Upper Saddle River, NJ: Prentice-Hall PTR, 1998.
19. **Eckel B.** Thinking in C++. Upper Saddle River, NJ: Prentice-Hall PTR, 1995.

20. www.bruceeckel.com
21. www.msdn.microsoft.com/visualc/
22. www.borland.com
23. www.symantec.com
24. www.msdn.microsoft.com/visualj/
25. www.metrowerks.com
26. www.sun.com/books/javaseries.html
27. www.microsoft.com/traincert/

4 / Data Repositories, Data Marts, and Data Warehouses

Bryan Bergeron

C ompetition, cost, market pressures, and the permeation of afford-able computer technology throughout the health care industry are fueling the outcomes management movement (1). Paradoxically, the process of collecting, storing, analyzing, and reporting clinical and financial data to determine what practices yield the best results and the lowest cost is most commonly based on data collected from paper surveys and reports (2). Why, after a decade of massive spending on the IT infrastructure of health care enterprises nationwide, isn't computer-based data universally used as the basis for outcomes analysis?

One answer is that health care data exist in disparate pockets throughout a health care enterprise, often residing in autonomous, minimally connected departmental applications. Furthermore, each application may be supported by a different operating system, use a different underlying database, and execute on a completely different hardware platform. For example, the Pharmacy system might run under UNIX on a Sun Server, using a Sybase database, whereas the ADT system might run under VMS on a VAX server with an Oracle database. Within each department or clinic, these differences are usually irrelevant and, except when data from other systems are needed, rarely even noticed.

The traditional way of gaining some insight into efficacy and cost of treatment is to archive transactional data from departmental applications on a routine basis. For each application, a variety of custom reports can be generated, often with considerable effort, that provide some indication of how resources and costs are being managed. However, from the perspective of outcomes management for the entire health care enterprise, the unsynchronized system of individual, transaction-oriented, departmental applications represents a major speed bump on the road to computer-enabled outcomes management.

The best solution to date for this outcomes data conundrum is to create one or more central databases, derived from, and yet completely independent of, each of the transaction-oriented application databases, and to optimize these databases for analysis. Clinical Data Repositories, Data Marts, and Data Warehouses are technologies that represent the current state of development for these analysis-oriented databases. These three terms can be somewhat misleading. From a technical perspective, there is considerable overlap in each technology; significant differences tend to be operational and content dependent. Regardless of the terminology or technology involved, the ultimate goal is to keep the right information flowing to the right people in the most intelligent form as timely and efficiently as possible.

Definitions

Clinical Data Repository

A Clinical Data Repository (CDR) is generally considered to be a structured, systematically collected storehouse of patient-specific clinical data (3). CDR data are most commonly distilled or mirrored from a single clinical application, such as a radiology reporting system or clinic EMR, sometimes supplemented with data from other clinical systems. For example, laboratory values, radiology reports, and clinical orders specific to a particular patient could be combined in a CDR.

Because virtually all patient information in the host application is mirrored and stored in the CDR, longitudinal studies are possible. For example, although it might be virtually impossible to perform even limited longitudinal queries for multiple patients in the original database, such operations may be commonplace on the CDR. In addition, because the data tend to originate from one source and there is little-to-no minimal data manipulation required, near-real-time retrieval of clinical data by clinicians is a reality.

In its simplest form, the CDR is a replication of a single transaction-oriented database, minimally adjusted for errors (4). The advantage of using a CDR instead of the original database is that it offloads query functions, and the associated performance degradation, from the application to the CDR database engine.

Data Mart

A Data Mart is a storehouse or database that contains data extracted or mirrored from one or more clinical and nonclinical applications. That is, a Data Mart containing only clinical data could be considered a CDR. Although some authors consider Data Marts to contain only summary data (4), this distinction tends to be one of degree in that CDRs, Data Marts, and Data Warehouses each typically contain summary data (5).

Data Warehouse

The term Data Warehouse (DW) is usually reserved for an enterprise-wide, central repository of information that reflects activity within most, and ideally all, applications running in a health care enterprise. A DW is usually considered to be a managed database that is subject oriented, integrated, time-variant, and nonvolatile. The ideal DW system captures the processes, not simply the data elements, involved in the application in a way that will aid in decision making. A Data Warehouse is integrated in that it combines data from a variety of application-oriented databases into a single system. This requires cleaning, encoding, and translation of data so that analysis can be performed. Furthermore, unlike most transactional databases, a DW is time-variant in that the data stored is associated with a point in time. In contrast, transactional data are typically valid only at the moment of capture and access. The data in a DW are nonvolatile in that new data are appended to the database and never replace existing data.

Data Warehouses are also distinguished from application-specific transactional databases in how the data destined for storage in the DW are selected, prepared, and loaded into the DW, and how the underlying database is optimized for use. Once data to be included in a DW have been identified, the data are cleaned, merged, and the original database structures are redesigned to provide a historical perspective (4). Unlike a typical application database, a DW is designed to contain historical, nonvolatile data that has been adjusted for transaction errors. In addition, data redundancy may be intentionally built-in to maximize the efficiency of the underlying database engine (e.g., by minimizing the number of relational tables to be joined in a typical DW query).

Figures 4-1 to 4-3 (pages 98 and 99) illustrate the conceptual differences between CDRs, Data Marts, and Data Warehouses. These figures illustrate that, when the marketing hype and the specialized vocabulary are peeled away, CDRs, Data Marts, and Data Warehouses are simply databases. Like any other database applications, there are the usual issues of database design, provision for maintenance, security, and periodic modification. The distinguishing features of these database technologies are not the database management systems, the size of the databases, or the hardware platform requirements. For example, all three technologies could conceivably be implemented on a single floppy disc, running on an ordinary PC, using the simplest of database engines. In practice, however, Data Warehouses require huge amounts of storage, Data Marts often reside on a desktop PC, and CDRs require even less storage and computational power.

For the sake of simplicity, the following discussion will refer to Data Warehouses, but the information applies to Data Marts and, to some degree, CDRs as well.

Database Management Systems

Database Technology

A Database Management System (DBMS) is at the core of a DW and virtually every clinical and nonclinical application in the enterprise. There are separate databases containing QA/UR, Case Mix, product costing, patient demographics, laboratory results, medication listings, radiology reports, Diagnostic Related Group (DRG) statistics, diagnostic lists, clinical reports, operative reports, discharge summaries, nursing plans, and billing information. Only a subset of these data reside in the DW.

The DBMS is the software that provides for simultaneous use of a DW by multiple users and provides tools for accessing, manipulating, and sharing what can amount to a huge store of data. In addition to file management, the DBMS provides for security, data integrity, synchronization, failure recovery, and data management.

Security—The DBMS allows only users with the right and need to know to have different types of access to particular files. Multi-level user password protection schemes can be used to allow, for example, only clinicians to view sensitive medical content and only administrators to view financial information.

Data Integrity—The DBMS imposes data consistency constraints such as requiring numerical data in certain fields and allowing free text in others.

Synchronization—The DBMS can guard against database corruption that might result from two simultaneous operations on a given data item (e.g., one user attempting to change a value being read or used by another user).

Failure Recovery—The DBMS can support quick recovery from hardware or software failures by recording all transactions in a journal file.

Data Management—A properly configured DBMS provides efficient storage that maximizes performance on a given hardware platform.

Perhaps the most important role of the DBMS component of the DW is that it allows researchers conducting outcomes research to interact with raw data elements in abstract, meaningful terms. That is, the DBMS shields the user from the details of the underlying algorithms and data representation schemes employed by the DW. Although it is only the physical database that actually exists, it is often useful to deal with the database system in various levels of abstraction. A DBMS is often described in three levels of abstraction: the physical, the conceptual, and the view.

The *Physical Database* comprises the data and framework that reside on secondary storage devices such as disks and tapes. The physical database abstraction is a useful representation tool for DBMS designers (i.e., those designing a DBMS *de novo* with conventional programming languages). This low-level abstraction is most useful when dealing directly with records and files, logical records within the operating system, and physical addresses on storage devices.

The *Conceptual Database* is often described in terms of a data model. The conceptual database, at a somewhat higher level of abstraction than the physical database, is more closely tuned to the needs of database designers dealing with DBMS data representation and efficiency issues (e.g., the Data Dictionary design). At the conceptual database level, relevant issues include

1. The most appropriate data structures to use in implementing the specific physical database.
2. The properties of the data to be manipulated.
3. The physical structures used to represent the data.

Two decision-support tools commonly used when working with the conceptual database are the entity-relationship model and the data model. These models will be discussed in more detail later.

The *View* is in effect a context-specific window into the database environment. At the highest level of abstraction, views are abstract models of portions of the conceptual database. Each view describes some of the database entities, attributes, and relationships between entities in a format convenient for a specific class of user or application. For example, users of a laboratory results reporting application do not need to know about personnel files or patient scheduling. Users in the personnel department, using a personnel application, do not need to know patient laboratory results but do of course require access to personnel files. Thus, there may be one view of the database for the laboratory department and one for the personnel department. The view abstraction is most useful in the user- and application-interface design process.

Entity-Relationship Models

An entity-relationship model is an idealized standard that can be used to compare the capabilities of the DBMS to represent and manipulate realistic data. The entity-relationship model defines the database in terms of entities and relationships, where an entity is a person, place, thing, or event about which data are recorded. Every entity has some basic attributes that characterize it, such as name, address, diagnosis, height, or age. A group of entities with similar attributes may form an entity set (e.g., the entities in the entity set "patients" may have NAME as an attribute).

Relationships within the entity-relationship model may be classified according to how many entities from one entity set can be associated with entities from another entity set. These relationships, or conceptual links, can be described as one-to-one, many-to-one, or many-to-many. In a one-to-one relationship between two entity sets, for each entity in either set, there is at most one associated member in the other set. When one entity in set 'B' is associated with zero or more entities in set "A", but each entity in set "A" is associated with at most one entity in set "B", the relationship is said to be many-to-one from set "A" to set "B". A many-many relationship describes the case in which there are no restrictions on the sets of pairs of entities that may appear in the relationship set.

For instance, one would normally expect PATIENT ID - SOCIAL SECURITY NUMBER to be a one-to-one relationship. In contrast, PATIENT NAME - HEMOGLOBIN VALUE would likely be a one-to-many relationship, because a given patient might have dozens of hemoglobin values, from multiple admissions, within the DW. The entity-relationship model, in effect a conceptual scheme, can be used to justify the kinds of data structures and data models utilized in the actual DW implementation.

Data Models

Data models, like entity-relationship models, are abstractions of the real world against which to measure the capabilities of the DBMS. Data models have features that make them better tuned to the physical structures that are used to actually implement a DW than are entity-relationship models.

In general, data models consist of two components: 1) a mathematical notation for expressing data and relationships, and 2) operations on the data that serve to express manipulations of the data (6). In some cases, data models may also contain a collection of integrity rules that constrain the valid sets of database states (7). Together, these various components provide a formal means of representing information and a formal means of manipulating such a representation.

Within a database, a small group of related items is commonly referred to as a *record* and each item within the record is referred to as a *field*. The record is retrieved from the database by means of a key, or label, that may consist of a field, part of a field, or a combination of several fields. The ultimate goal of the DBMS employed to manage the information is to make it easy to search for the record that contains the particular value of the key.

Data management has undergone an evolution from early file and record management techniques to hierarchical, then network, relational, and, more recently, to object-oriented systems. These data models are somewhat arbitrary in their definition in that many DBMS packages do not fit cleanly into any one model classification. In addition, the procedural languages included with some database programs allow for mixed model types (i.e., by defining a network structure within a relational database). In this way, the structure of any database can be supplemented with secondary indexes that make it possible to efficiently answer queries that do not follow the underlying organization.

It is the data model that specifies the varying relations among records, fields, and keys. Different database management systems organize the data in the database in different ways, including those patterned after the network, hierarchical, relational, and object-oriented data models.

Hierarchical Model

Within the hierarchical database model, the smallest data entity is the record. That is, records within a hierarchical database are not necessarily broken up into fields. Unlike the relational model, in which connections or links between files depend on the data, connections within the hierarchical model do not depend on the data. Connections are defined when the database is created and remain fixed for the life of the database. As the name implies, the nature of these permanent connections is hierarchical. The hierarchical links, sometimes called the *structure of the data*, can best be thought of as forming an inverted tree, with the parent file at the top and the child files below. Child files have only one parent (i.e., a one-to-many connection exists between the parent and child files).

The basic operation on the hierarchical database is the tree walk, preceding from parent to child. Data can be retrieved only by traversing the levels of the hierarchy according to the path defined by the succession of parent fields. This unidirectional convention causes certain relationships to be difficult to extract from the database, even though they may be explicit in the data.

Network Model

The network model is comparable to the entity-relationship model, with relationships restricted to binary, many-one relationships. In addition, logical record types are roughly equivalent to the entity-relationship model concept of entity sets. The network model is more flexible than the hierarchical one because multiple connections can be established between files. These multiple connections enable the user to more effectively gain access to a particular file without traversing the entire hierarchy above that file.

Relational Model

The relational model is the most popular technology used in DW implementation. In the relational model, relations are used to represent both entities and relationships. Facts are represented in a relational database management system as instances, or tuples, of a relation (8). Flexibility is achieved by abolishing the hierarchy of fields. In addition, all fields can be used as keys to retrieve information.

A relational model is based on the concept of a data table in which every row is unique. The records or rows in the table are called *tuples*; the fields or columns are variably referred to *attributes, predicates,* or *classes* (9). Database queries are performed with the selection operation, which asks for all tuples in a certain relation that meet a certain criterion. To connect the data of two or more relations, an operation called a *join* is performed.

A very useful feature of the relational model is that records from different files can be combined as long as the different files have one field in common. Theoretically, records with a common field can be combined or joined with an unlimited number of files (9). The price paid for this ability to design a relational database without much regard for how it will be used is extended access time. That is, in a database design that does not take likely use patterns into account, performance suffers. A large amount of time will be spent getting the information out of the system as the database program searches through the files, makes proper combinations, and records the results. This performance penalty is a reason for not simply polling a series of application databases for outcomes data. It is far better, from a performance perspective, to move the data into a new database that is optimized for the desired analysis.

The attraction of the ubiquitous relational model is that it is mature, stable, reliable, well understood, and well suited to a number of different application environments. The basic concepts involved with the relational model are easily grasped; data are populated into rows and columns in a table, and tables are associated with one another by joining fields that match in the two tables. Because the software industry has a great deal of experience with relational models, database engines built on this model tend to be very fast.

Because the relational model is based on rows and columns, it is most efficient working with scalar data such as names, addresses, and laboratory values – and therein lies the rub. The most significant drawback of the relational model is that all relationships between objects must be based on data values. This limitation often requires the database designer to create additional relations to describe logical associations between data elements (10).

Object-Oriented Model

The modern practice of medicine involves much more than text and numerical values. The need to store medical images, sounds, and other multimedia, as well as interest in the Web, has rekindled interest in database systems based on the object-oriented model (11). In contrast to DBMSs based on the relational model, Object Database Management Systems (ODBMS) are best suited for non-record-oriented data such as free text, images, voice, and video data (12).

In the object-oriented model, complex structures are represented by composite objects, which are objects that contain other objects. These objects may contain other objects in turn, allowing structures to be nested to any degree. Furthermore, objects communicate with each other through methods, which are procedures contained within objects for the purpose of requesting services of that object.

The object-oriented model can support any number of alternative structures for the same set of data. As such, the major advantage of the object-oriented model is that it can be used to represent complex medical information in a way that does not compromise flexibility. Many medical relationships do not fit nicely into tables but are instead hierarchical and complex. With an ODBMS, it is possible to use arbitrary data types, and complex relationships can be queried without having to create resource-intensive joins between tables.

Outcomes measures requires data be complete, unambiguous, and relevant. For example, structured data and free-form text coexist, but the analysis of free-form text requires specific tools. Object-oriented technology may soon make it possible to analyze physicians' free-text natural language notes (13). Although the object-oriented approach holds great promise in future DW designs, it still lags far behind relational technology for practical DW implementations.

The Data Dictionary

With the possible exception of user passwords and other sensitive materials, individual data elements deemed of sufficient value to be included in the DW, such as PATIENT NAME, must be readily and unambiguously accessible. To that end, standard data element names and formats must be defined and used consistently within the DW, regardless of variations within individual applications. A Data Dictionary, typically in the form of multiple relational tables, provides for this standardization.

Moving data into a DW from a variety of applications – or into a Data Mart from a single application – usually involves a considerable amount of translation of data into standard values. The Data Dictionary is, in simplest terms, a collection of information about naming, classification, structure, usage, and administration of the data within a Data Warehouse. This information is usually referred to as *metadata*, or "data about data".

Conceptually separate, yet intimately related to the Data Dictionary, is the Data Directory. The Data Directory specifies the location of data within a Data Warehouse as well as the most appropriate and/or efficient path to be followed during data access or retrieval. The Data Directory, in effect metadata about the Data Dictionary, contains descriptions of translation tables, record or file definitions, and transactions (14). As such, the Data Directory can be developed only after the implementation of the Data Dictionary. The resulting complex, composed of both the Data Dictionary and its metadata, is referred to as the *common Data Dictionary/directory*. However, for the purposes of this discussion, the complex is referred to as simply the Data Dictionary.

A Data Dictionary can be either active or passive. Passive Data Dictionaries, which simply hold descriptions of data, are most appropriate when there is no way of avoiding the use of multiple files that contain the same data. Passive Data Dictionaries have application in Data Warehouse development and maintenance, where they support the massive integration effort. In contrast, Active Data Dictionaries provide a mechanism by which programs can actually extract data definitions as a program source code for use in semi-automatic application generation. An Active Data Dictionary is most appropriate in the setting in which heavy in-house development of a Data Warehouse is planned.

Structure of a Data Dictionary

Within the Data Dictionary, data items may represent elements or groups of elements. An individual element is normally considered to be at the atomic level of data; that is, it cannot normally be decomposed into smaller pieces. For example, the data item NAME may represent the patient's first, middle, and last names. In this case, NAME is said to represent a group composed of three elements: the first, middle, and last names. The first name would not normally be decomposed into its constituents (i.e., ASCII characters).

A group definition provides a detailed description of the component data elements that compose the group and the relationships among them. For example, a group definition for patient name might include the elements first, middle and last name. In addition, the relationship between these elements is specified; that is, the element first name appears before the element middle name which appears before the element last name. A standard set of relational operators is commonly used to formally define the compositions of such group data elements.

The information that is maintained for each data element defined within the Data Dictionary is largely a function of enterprise-specific Data Warehouse requirements. The minimal information recorded for each element commonly includes naming, classification, representation, usage, and administrative identifiers.

Naming the information element is essentially listing all aliases for the given element throughout the HIS. For example, possible aliases for PATIENT NAME might be PAT_NAME, PAT_ID, PATIENT_NAME, PAT_NAM, NAME, etc. Each alias may be used by different applications to identify the same data element.

Classification information includes a text description of the item, its ownership, item type (e.g., element or group), as well as privacy and security considerations. The text description, analogous to a comment in conventional programming language parlance, is simply a sentence or two describing the item. The ownership information includes a description of which applications within the IHIS make use of the data element. Privacy and security considerations include information relevant to allowing only certain users or applications access to a given item; that is, user passwords can be viewed/manipulated by only the actual user or the system administrator.

The representation information for each item within the Data Dictionary includes item length and, for a group of items, its composition. PATIENT NAME, for example, might be represented by a text string with a maximum length of 24 characters. The item PATIENT ADDRESS might be composed of a group of five text strings, each with a maximum length of 24 characters.

Usage information includes a quantitative description of range of values, frequency of use, and conditional values for each element. For example, the item DOSAGE might represent a group of two elements: drug amount and administration modality. Drug amount may have a defined range from 1.00 to 999.99 mL. Administration modality might have a limited number of valid conditional values, including "IM", "IV", and "PO".

Administrative information can include the resources used by the element and the processing mode(s) available. For example, a given element might be accessible through a specific server, through the use of batch, time sharing, or transaction processing.

Data Dictionary Implementation

A central task in Data Dictionary development is that of establishing the assertions and correspondences among data elements manipulated by individual applications within the enterprise. The first step in this process is to identify naming correspondences for groups and elements. A common problem associated with this initial step is that synonyms occur when elements or groups with different names represent the same concept. For example, the element PATIENT-ID in one application might correspond to the NAME element in another. Similarly, homonyms that occur when the names are the same but different concepts are represented must be dealt with (e.g., within one application NAME might refer to patient first, middle, and last name, whereas in a second application NAME may refer to last name only).

The second step in establishing assertions and correspondences among data elements is to specify the precise relationships between the domains of pairs of elements, or groups of elements, from different applications. Data relationships can be specified as identical, contained, overlapping, or disjoint (15).

An identical relationship is one in which a particular element or group is the same in all applications. Ideally, all relationships within a Data Dictionary are identical. In practice, however, identical relationships are relatively rare within a Data Dictionary, given the nature of the typical health care enterprise.

A contained relationship is one in which an element (or group of elements) defined in one application is a subset of an element (or group of elements) within another application. For example, in one application, application A, the element NAME might have as an attribute the patient's first, middle, and last name. Within a second application, application B, the element PT - NAME might refer only to the patient's first name. In this scenario, the attributes for PT - NAME in application B are said to be contained in the attributes for NAME in application A.

In an overlapping relationship, groups defined within one application share attributes with groups defined within other applications. That is, not only does a group within an application have attributes common to groups defined within other applications, but there are unique attributes within each group as well; that is, the disparate groups are subsets of each other. For example, within a radiology reporting system, patient age might be an attribute in a group also containing attributes for patient height and weight. In the ADP system, the patient age attribute might coexist within a group with attributes for security clearance.

A disjoint relationship describes the case in which elements or groups within an application have no attributes in common with other elements or groups utilized by other applications. For example, a billing application within the health care enterprise may have a data element INSURER with an attribute of insurance company. The laboratory application, however, may make no reference to the patient's insurance company in any element or group.

The final step in Data Dictionary development involves specifying the mappings between equivalent attributes of corresponding element or group classes. That is, if two corresponding elements contain similar attributes, but the attributes are expressed in different units, then a mapping must be specified between the two attributes. For example, if the age attribute of element AGE in the pharmacy system is expressed in months, and the age attribute of element PATIENT - AGE within the radiology system is expressed in years, then a mapping function converting months to years (and vice versa) must be specified.

The Data Warehouse

The Driving Forces: Location and Time

A DW makes sense whenever data that have more value when compared together than when examined separately are stored in different databases. For example, demographic data in an ADT application database, when combined with test results from a laboratory application, are much more valuable to outcomes researchers than either database alone. It does not matter if the disparate databases are running on the same computer, on different computers in the same room, or in different countries. Unless the data are compiled into a single database, there will be extra work involved in using relationships within the data for outcomes analysis.

Even if a health care enterprise is built around a single, central, common database, a DW is not ruled out. The enterprise may merge with another enterprise or may become part of a massive health care network that links providers, insurers, and patients.

Taken one step further, even if an entire health care enterprise were to standardize on a database scheme that allowed sharing of data between departments and applications, the state and federal government might want to get into the act of outcomes analysis. For example, it is conceivable that the federal government could one day require that insurer, procedure, and outcomes data be made available to any number of government agencies. The governmental DW could require feeds from every enterprise-wide DW. Similarly, researchers in the World Health Organization might one day want to compare outcomes and medication used on a nation-by-nation basis. That is, even if the United States were standardized on a medical database scheme, an international DW could conceivably be beneficial.

A major motivation behind creating a DW is usually lack of time. If time were not a scarce resource, a tenable solution to working with data from disparate sources would be to manually transfer the data from application databases to compatible media and then import the data into a DW. Depending on the amount of data and the amount of massaging required to get the data to a DW, the effort could take minutes or months. The result is that queries to the database probably would not be very helpful in making day-to-day decisions, and even long-term forecasts could be in error because of the time lag.

In contrast, when properly implemented, data warehousing automates the transfer and translation of data so that the DW contains data from other databases almost instantly. In the ideal scenario, data are moved from disparate databases to the DW in near-real-time. Decisions based on current data have a better chance of reflecting reality than do decisions based on data several months old.

Development

Data Warehouse development usually entails six stages: planning, data consolidation, data transformation, selective archiving, data distribution, and ongoing maintenance (16).

Planning
In the planning stage, arguably the most important phase of DW development, administrative, clinical, research, and IT representatives decide exactly what to include in the DW. DW content should reflect the questions likely to be asked. For example, clinicians might want to correlate laboratory values with specific diagnoses, administration might want to compile summaries of length of stay for each diagnosis, and researchers might want to compare medication dosages with diagnosis. Because of practical cost, resource, and performance limitations, it is not normally possible to store every data element from every application in a DW. The planning phase directly impacts the eventual cost and functionality of the DW.

Consolidation
In the consolidation stage, the selected data from each application database are restructured. This typically involves de-normalizing tables and adding fields and relations to reflect how the data will be used in the DW. The goal in the consolidation stage is to provide an efficient framework that supports outcomes research and any other queries likely to be asked, as determined in the planning stage.

Transformation
The data transformation stage of DW development involves transforming the consolidated data into a more useful form through summarization and packaging. In summarization, the data are selected, aggregated, and

grouped into views more convenient and useful to users. Packaging involves using the summarized data as the basis of graphical presentations, animations, charts, and spreadsheets.

Archiving
Selective archiving involves moving older or infrequently accessed data to tape, optical, or other long-term storage media. Archiving saves money by sparing expensive magnetic, high-speed storage, and minimizes the performance hit imposed by locally storing data that are no longer necessary for outcomes analysis.

Distribution
Distribution is making data contained in the DW available to administrative, clinical, and research users. Providing for distribution encompasses front-end development so that users can easily and intuitively request and receive data, whether real-time or in the form of routine reports. Push technologies, including email alerts, can be used to distribute data to specific users. The Web is also a major portal for the data.

Maintenance
Maintenance is the final, ongoing stage of DW development. Creating a DW involves much more than simply designing and implementing a database. Even if there is a process in place for extracting, cleaning, transporting, and loading data from transactional systems, and distribution tools are both powerful and intuitive, the DW may not be sustainable. First, there is the economic issue. Extracting, cleaning, and reloading data can be prohibitively expensive and time consuming. A DW that provides a real benefit to users is an ongoing proposition that requires continual redesigning and evaluation. It must also be able to continually change and expand to make allowances for application vendor changes and rising expectations from internal staff. The DW must also be robust enough to scale to meet demands.

Role of the Data Dictionary in Data Warehouse Design

Reduced Data Inconsistency
Descriptions of data are usually included in the applications that process the data. A billing program, for example, typically contains definitions for all data used within the program. By creating a single, gold-standard data element description in a Data Dictionary, the problems associated with multiple files that contain potentially conflicting data definitions can be

avoided. A Data Dictionary ultimately makes data descriptions independent of program logic used in individual applications.

Access Control

The possible inconsistency resulting from unrestricted use of similar or partially overlapping record definitions can be reduced with a Data Dictionary. This central repository for data definitions can

1. Provide a method of controlling access to each data definition (i.e., access to a directory or to a particular data element can be controlled through an access control mechanism).
2. Record information about the location of each data definition (i.e., through the use of hierarchical subdirectories).
3. Provide a means of tracking what happens to each definition (i.e., through the generation of an audit trail for each data element).

Reduced Data Element Ambiguity

The Data Dictionary is perhaps most useful in addressing the problem of data element ambiguity. That is, within a health care enterprise composed of a variety of commercial and in-house applications, a given data element may be defined differently within different applications. For example, patient age might be defined in months within the pharmacy system, whereas patient age within the radiology reporting system and the Data Dictionary might be represented in years. The Data Dictionary can be used to reconcile the two systems, providing an appropriate data transform between the two representations; for example, appropriate transforms to move between the representations used by the pharmacy and radiology systems for patient age might be

$$PatientAge\ (Rad) = PatientAge\ (Pharm)/12$$

$$PatientAge\ (Data\ Dictionary) = PatientAge\ (Pharm) = \\ PatientAge\ (Rad) \times 12$$

Summary

When properly implemented, the Data Dictionary can be an invaluable tool throughout the DW development life cycle. In the analysis phase of the DW, the use of a Data Dictionary minimized data element ambiguity by improving communications among system analysts, application vendors, users, and hospital management. In addition, a Data Dictionary can clarify the flow and content of data items through the system during the design phase of the Data Warehouse. The Data Dictionary also supports maintenance efforts in mature systems by providing detailed documentation of the information complex.

The Challenge of Multiple Environments

A DW can simplify the tangled web of application data to the point that a user interested in outcomes analysis only has to remember and work with one database system. The ideal DW system automatically downloads a subset of individual application databases and combines them into a central database, having performed any necessary conversions and other translations needed. As noted earlier, a properly constructed warehouse takes care of timing issues, automatically performs any conversion in data representation, and populates a central database in such a way as to support the most likely queries to be asked.

Getting a DW to this stage of functionality is no easy task, however, especially when multiple software and hardware environments are involved. One of the greatest hurdles in creating a DW is that the data often reside on multiple machines and in different programs. The underlying database systems used by different vendors and in different niches have been designed independently to meet specific application needs. Data may be entered separately in, for example, the medical record systems, case management system, risk management system, financial system, or some form of decision support system.

Moving health care data from a variety of disparate applications into a single, centrally managed database is usually complicated by variations in data representations between applications. For example, one application might store the admission data as "day/month/year", while another might store it as "month/day/year". For the DW central database to be searched by date, data from one or more application databases would have to be translated into the standard representation used in the DW. Only then can the data be sorted, massaged, translated, and reformatted to support data mining to discover patterns in the data, compile outcome statistics, or perform *ad hoc* queries.

Even if all clinical, administrative, and research applications were built around a single database system, there would be a need for a DW. Much more common is the situation in which administrative, clinical, and research computing are separate in funding, organization, design, hardware, physical location, and database system. Even in the clinical realm, the most likely scenario is to have disparate computer hardware and software systems, integrated at some incomplete level through an HL7 or similar interface. In these circumstances, querying data across multiple departmental systems is expensive and time consuming.

After translating data onto physically compatible media, loading the data into a single database that can be queried typically presents additional challenges. For example, there is the issue of timing and synchronization. Ideally, all data entering the DW represents a snapshot – an instant in time – when all transactions are frozen and data edits and modifications are halted. However, even if the data are downloaded from each transactional database at the same instant, they may be out of sync because of how the applications are written. For example, a radiology reporting system might write data out to disc only periodically, whereas a dermatology reporting system might write the data to disc immediately after each transaction.

The Process of Data Warehousing

An important distinction in data warehousing is the process of managing the flow of information versus collecting data. The process of data warehousing can be time consuming, expensive, and, without proper planning, of little or no value to the health care enterprise. Data warehousing encompasses a variety of processes, most of which can be supported by specific software tools. The most prominent exception is the planning stage, where the data to be warehoused are identified. Other processes, such as incorporating legacy data, are heavily dependent on technology tools. For example, legacy data are often inconsistent, incoherent, redundant, and therefore of questionable value for outcomes analysis. To move these data into a DW to compensate for this lack of organization, a variety of tools must be employed to efficiently process the data.

Other software-dependent components of the data warehousing process include the creation of data models, implementing a database management system, formulating a Data Dictionary, building interfaces, creating data access tools, and DW management (17). For example, a variety of software tools are required to clean the legacy data, map the data to the DW database, and load the databases. There are also database management systems for storing and manipulating data, and data access tools for query, reporting, and analysis. A Data Dictionary tool, described in more detail below, is required for tracking and reporting data definitions and for data translation.

Interface software provides for connectivity between systems and the databases. Data access software tools are required for query, reporting, and analysis functions. Finally, there are a variety of warehouse management tools that can support data collection, archiving, backup, security, and authorization.

Selectivity

In many respects, the processes involved in the design of a DW are not significantly different from those used in any significant database project. There are the usual issues of database vendor selection, establishing overall design criteria, determining hardware requirements, normalizing the database design, providing for adequate security, designing a realistic maintenance plan, and determining how to best handle software updates. A unique factor, however, is the need to determine which data from disparate databases really need to be moved into the DW, becaise moving and storing data costs time, money, and computer resources.

It is important during the planning phase of DW design to exercise constraint in moving data from disparate clinical, administrative, and research computer databases into the DW. For example, in looking at data stored in a laboratory system, individual creatinine values for every patient probably have less value, from an outcomes perspective, than positive HIV results.

The goal in creating a DW is to have a maintainable database, not simply a collection of data that could potentially answer any question that has a possibility of being asked. It is far more efficient to formulate a plan, projecting questions that will have to be answered, than it is to blindly include every data element possible.

One reason for being selective in identifying which data to transfer into the DW is simply the time involved in the transfer process. Ten thousand creatinine values take up finite space on a hard drive and take time to transfer. In addition, if the laboratory system stores the values in milligrams per decalitre and the DW is designed to accept values in micromol per litre, then an extra step and associated computer resources surrounding the translation exist as well.

Planning a successful DW project requires input from clinical, research, and administrative experts. Each group that will eventually be querying the DW should have a good idea of the questions they are going to be asking and a relative ranking of their importance. From a practical perspective, the IT group may simply set an upper limit on the number of elements that can be moved from each application, based on a cumulative ranking of data from the DW design committee.

Data Transfer

Once data to be moved to the DW have been identified, the next step is to move the data from the application databases. At one extreme, this process may consist of manually keying the data into a DW. For example, in a private practice with a clinical and administrative computer system, it is conceivable that the office manager could manually transfer diagnosis information from the clinical system, combine it with insurance data from the administrative system, and store the data in a third database. More likely, especially in a hospital setting, is that interfaces between application databases and the DW are constructed to automatically move selected data into the DW.

An important issue in the data transfer process is that of determining which standard(s) to use in mapping application data into the DW. For example, the American Medical Informatics Association (AMIA) recommends using a patient's Social Security number for a personal identifier. There are problems, however: infants and some noncitizens are not issued Social Security numbers, some patients have two or more numbers, and some numbers are used by multiple patients (18).

In transferring data into a DW, there is the issue of which coding system to use. Unfortunately, there are literally dozens of standards, each addressing a particular aspect of the patient data. For example, SNOMED III has a rich catalog of signs and symptoms, whereas ACR/NEMA is supported by most radiologic imaging systems.

Which vocabulary to use in the DW is another long-standing key issue. The UMLS (Unified Medical Language System) project (19) holds promise, but it is not yet at the point where it can be of practical benefit as a combined clinical, administrative, and research vocabulary (20).

Data Warehouse Issues

Myopia

One of the major obstacles in creating a Data Warehouse system is near-sightedness. It is easy to get so wrapped up in creating a Data Warehouse, in terms of time and budget, that the value of the Data Warehouse – a tool that helps data analysis flow smoothly and easily – often gets obfuscated. The challenges of extraction, transformation, and loading of data can become so resource consuming that data analysis takes a back seat to these tasks. One solution is to use the right tools to provide all of the necessary transformations on the data before loading it into the Data Warehouse, thereby shortening development time.

The Numbers

Every legacy and operational system destined to feed data into the Data Warehouse represents a unique set of challenges, usually requiring special tools for extraction and transformation routines for each combination of source system and target application. For example, if there are four different application databases that feed the DW, there are four sets of data extraction and translation challenges. Just as the rate-limiting step in the implementation of the electronic medical record is typically interconnect development, deployment, and testing (21), interfaces also limit the development of Data Warehouses.

People, Not Technology

In the end, the success of any Data Warehouse project – or IT project in general – is a function of the people and the processes in place to work with the system. The organizational dynamics are as much a key to a successful implementation as are the technical capabilities of the technology used.

Too Much, Too Soon

Another potential pitfall is attempting to build the perfect system and then to release it in one glorious presentation. It is far better to salami-slice the Data Warehouse issue, addressing selected application databases initially, and constantly and consistently adding new data to the stores.

Confidentiality

The goal of Data Warehouse is to have the data you need to make decisions at your fingertips. Unfortunately, the fingertip owners could be unwelcome guests. As such, security procedures, such as multi-level password controls, may be needed.

Scalability

A key issue in tool selection is how the tool will perform a year or two after initial implementation, when the data swell to hundreds of thousands of megabytes. An object-oriented database might work well on a single application and with limited data, but when the system is extended to cover an entire health care enterprise, the poor performance of such a database may render the system useless.

Transformation

Clinical, administrative, and research data must be converted into a common representation in order to be useful. At the database level, this involves a common representation scheme such as normalized data structures. At the content level, this involves special transformations of complex data, from patient names and addresses to diagnostic study results. It is often the case that unstructured data must be parsed into a structured form, validated against known standards, matched and consolidated as necessary, and then formatted into a standard representation. Matching and consolidation often involves fuzzy matching because of missing data, misspellings, and other errors.

As an example of the potential complexity of the transformation issue, consider a hospital in which most departments use an EMR that accepts free-form text entries from clinicians. Consider also that the hospital ER recently installed a voice-recognition-based dictation system that creates structured text entries. Or, conversely, consider a hospital in which most of the EMR activity is through structured text entries, and a rouge department has yet to evolve past free-text entry. How are free-text and structured data combined in the Data Warehouse in such a way that supports outcomes analysis? Most relational database systems do not handle free text very well, and parsing text into key words and phrases is fraught with errors. An object-oriented approach may eventually solve this problem.

Challenges

Standard Vocabulary

By far, the greatest challenge remaining in the arena of DW development is that of establishing a standard vocabulary. Currently, mapping data from individual applications to the central DW database is accomplished best through a Data Dictionary facility. Although data mapping and transformation can be accomplished effectively through a Data Dictionary, the vocabulary used in the DW has yet to be standardized. It is more likely to be an *ad hoc* vocabulary, modified as necessary to minimize translation from the individual application databases. However, as DWs become larger and are combined to form even larger searchable systems, it makes sense to have one, universal standard for vocabulary.

There have been numerous attempts at creating standard vocabularies for a number of niche areas in medicine. For example, the Digital Imaging and COMmunications (DICOM) in Medicine Standard specifies a nonproprietary data interchange protocol, image format, and file structure for biomedical images and image-related information (22). As discussed earlier, the UMLS project (23), sponsored by the National Library of Medicine, may eventually prove to be at least part of the universal standard vocabulary in medical computing.

Part of the fundamental challenge of designing or selecting a standard vocabulary or medical representation language is determining the appropriate level of granularity needed in a CPR, and the level of granularity required by an administrative, intraclinic, third-party payer, or government reporting agency (24). This challenge is intensified with the current shift in the medical record from conclusions and diagnoses to the overall process of care, including the processes of decision making related to care (25). The ideal vocabulary must therefore not only link the patient's experience of care but be capable of adequately describing a wide range of outcomes, functional status, and patient satisfaction issues.

Object-Oriented Technologies

The functionality, flexibility, efficiency, and speed of the database engine underlying a DW defines the usability of the DW system for outcomes analysis purposes. Although the relational model currently dominates the DW arena, the complexity of medical data is driving many vendors and health care enterprises to seriously consider other DBMS technologies, such as Object-Oriented database management systems. Although there is a great deal of interest in object-oriented approaches to supporting the DW, there is more than a modicum of caution in the IT community toward the technology. This is partly because early OODMSs were incomplete in that they lacked backup and recovery functions, object-oriented data models were conflicting, the languages supported by vendors were proprietary, scalability to something on the order of a DW was unproven and therefore of major concern, and the early systems required huge amounts of memory (26). In the past few years, vendors have done a good job at fully addressing these and other limitations of ODBMs (11), but performance and scalability are still major concerns.

The three approaches to using an object-oriented model as the basis for a database system that could be applied to DW development are object/relational databases, semantic databases, and C++ persistent databases (12). C++ persistent databases are closely integrated with C++. Semantic databases provide a pure object-oriented approach and the ability to store and execute methods inside a database.

An object/relational database combines object and relational technologies and therefore supports many of the best features of object and relational database products. It provides a good mix of performance and flexibility with unstructured data, with the speed and SQL support found in relational systems. One way to create an object/relational database is to put an object model on top of a traditional RDBMS.

External Involvement

The Data Warehouse market is maturing. In 1998, it accounted for 23% of IT dollars world-wide (27). However, even in this maturing market, change is commonplace. For example, although the approach seems inherently foreign to medicine, more companies are leveraging their DW to get the most value from their information from those outside of their organization. The latest trend is sharing the data with outside vendors so that suppliers can forecast internal demand for their products and services and be more responsive. For example, in some industries, such as the overnight package delivery system, customers can track orders or the status of their shipments. Inevitably, pharmaceutical and hospital supply companies will have access to the health care enterprise DW in order to create a symbiotic relationship that minimizes paperwork and unnecessary delays associated with replenishing hospital supplies. It is even conceivable that patients will eventually be able to track their laboratory results directly from home, using a Web browser.

In the current medical-legal milieu, it would be difficult to give individuals access to their laboratory results and other clinical and nonclinical data as they are made available to the hospital staff. There are confidentiality and security concerns related to opening the DW to outsiders. One solution is to limit access to batch reports that can be viewed by verified patients and to block *ad hoc* access. Firewalls, passwords, user IDs, IP address verification, and timeout features that cut a session off after a certain amount of time passes without any activity can be used to minimize security risks.

Summary

Clinical Data Repositories, Data Marts, and Data Warehouses are direct responses to the cry for more data, more timely data, and more accurate data. The current approaches to creating these historical archives that are optimized for outcomes research involve a variety of database technologies, including Data Dictionaries, as well as an arsenal of tools that can clean, transform, and import data into a DW as needed. To make technical progress in this arena, designers and decision makers must be aware of current and pending database technologies and more formidable challenges such as the lack of a standard vocabulary. With the Web and other technologies bringing the patient closer to technology and information sources, it is only a matter of time before patients will be tracking the results of their clinical studies as closely as they track the stock market.

A Glossary of frequently used terms appears on pages 100 and 101.

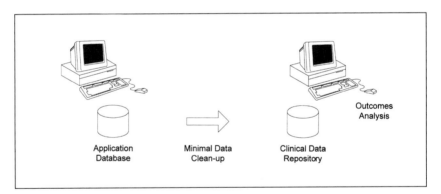

Figure 4-1 Clinical Data Repository Architecture. The transactional data from a single application is imported, with minimal error checking, into a separate database. There tends to be little, if any, summarization, and most of the data are moved to the second database, which is optimized for historical data analysis. By maintaining a separate database, configured specifically to support decision analysis, the application database engine is spared computational loading, and the response time to a particular query should be substantially improved. Error checking or cleaning, for example, entails checking for duplicate entries on the same day. Note that there are usually only two different databases involved: one for the CDR and one for the application. If the database engines are from the same vendor, then mirroring and importing data are usually greatly facilitated.

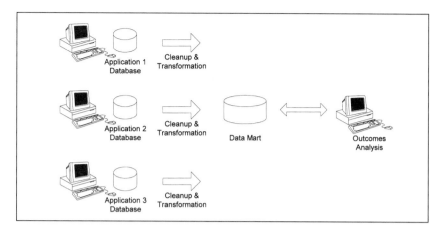

Figure 4-2 Data Mart Architecture. In a Data Mart, data from multiple transactional applications are checked for errors, summarized, and imported into a central database. Because multiple applications are involved, not all data elements from every application can be moved to the Data Mart. Data Marts tend to be developed and run on the departmental level and isolated from the rest of the health care enterprise. The distinctions between a Data Mart and a Data Warehouse are often size, and, more importantly, the scope of operations for the owner of a Data Mart.

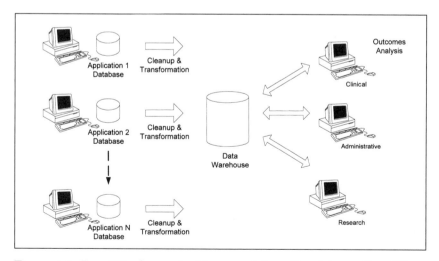

Figure 4-3 Data Warehouse Architecture. Like a Data Mart, a Data Warehouse holds the records of several applications. Unlike a Data Mart, however, these applications extend beyond the boundaries of a department and encompass the entire organization. As data are moved from applications into the DW, they are cleaned, translated, and made available to users.

Glossary

Ad Hoc Query—A query that cannot be determined before the moment the query is issued.

Atomic Data—Data elements that represent the lowest level of detail.

Central Warehouse—A database created from operational extracts that adheres to a single, consistent, enterprise data model to ensure consistency of decision-support data across the health care enterprise.

Client—A single-user computer that is connected via a network to, and works in conjunction with, one or more shared computers, with data storage and processing distributed between them.

Data Dictionary—A database about data and database structures. A catalog of all data elements that contains names, structures, and information about usage.

Data Element—The most elementary unit of data that can be identified and described in a dictionary or repository which cannot be subdivided.

Data Extraction Software—Software that reads one or more sources of data and creates a new image of that data.

Data Flow Diagram—A diagram that shows the normal flow of data between services as well as the flow of data between data stores and services.

Data Loading—The process of populating the Data Warehouse.

Data Management—Controlling, protecting, and facilitating access to data in order to provide information consumers with timely access to the data they need.

Data Management Software—Software that converts data into a unified format by taking derived data to create new fields, merge files, and summarize and filter data.

Data Mapping—The process of assigning a source data element to a target data element.

Data Mining—The process of using statistical techniques to discover subtle relationships between data items, and the construction of predictive models based on them.

Data Model—A logical map that represents the inherent properties of the data independent of software, hardware, or machine performance considerations. The model shows data elements grouped into records as well as the association around those records.

Data Transformation—Creating information from data, such as decoding data and merging of records from multiple DBMS formats. Also known as *data scrubbing* or *data cleansing*.

Data Warehouse Management Tools—Software that extracts and transforms data from operational systems and loads it into the Data Warehouse.

DBMS—DataBase Management System. Used to store, process, and manage data in a systematic way.

Drill Down—A method of exploring detailed data that is used in creating a summary level of data.

DSS—Decision Support System. An application for analyzing large quantities of data and performing a wide variety of calculations and projections.

Dynamic Dictionary—A Data Dictionary that an application program accesses at run time.

Entity Relationship Diagramming—A process that visually identifies the relationships between data elements.

ETL—Extraction, Transformation, and Loading. Activities required to populate Data Warehouses and OLAP applications with clean, consistent, integrated, and probably summarized data.

Gateway—A software product that allows SQL-based applications to access relational and nonrelational data sources.

GUI—Graphical User Interface. The buttons, windows, and icons that the user interacts with, usually by pointing a cursor with a mouse. The Apple Macintosh is credited with popularizing the GUI, which is now used by the dominant desktop operating system, the various flavors of Microsoft Windows.

HOLAP—Hybrid OLAP. A product that can provide simultaneous multidimensional analysis of data stored in a multidimensional database and in an RDBMS.

MDB—Multidimensional DataBase. A product that can store and process multidimensional data.

Metadata—Data about data. How the structures and calculation rules are stored; provides information on data sources, definitions, quality, transformations, date of last update, and user access privileges.

Normalization—The process of reducing a complex data structure into its simplest, most stable structure.

Object—A person, place, thing, or concept that has characteristics of interest to an environment. In terms of an object-oriented system, an object is an entity that combines descriptions of data and behavior.

OLAP—On-Line Analytical Processing. A category of applications and technologies for collecting, managing, processing, and presenting multidimensional data for analysis and management purposes.

OLTP—On-Line Transaction Processing. Operational systems for collecting and managing the base data in an organization.

OO—Object-Oriented. A method of application development that allows the re-use of program components in other contexts.

Query Response Times—The time it takes for the warehouse engine to process a complex query across a large volume of data and return the results to the requester.

Query Tools—Software that allows a user to create and direct specific questions to a database.

RDBMS—Relational DataBase Management System. Used to store, process, and manage data arranged in relational tables.

Scalability—The ability to scale to support larger or smaller volumes of data and more or less users.

Semantic Mapping—The mapping of the meaning of a piece of data.

SQL—Structured Query Language. The standard data structuring and access language used by relational databases.

Summary Tables—Often used in RDBMSs to store pre-aggregated information, rather than holding it in the same table as the base data. Used to improve responsiveness.

VLDB—Very Large Databases.

REFERENCES

1. **Aron L.** Approaching outcomes: the debate. Imaging Economics. 1997;Dec:49-54.

2. **Gilbert J.** Outcomes. Health Data Management. 1998;April:66-75.

3. **Johnson R.**(1997). Today's CDRs: an elusive complete solution. Healthcare Informatics. 1997;14:57-60.

4. **Gagnon G.** Data Warehousing: an overview. PC Magazine. 1999;March:245-6.

5. **Humphries M, Hawkins M, Dy M.** Data Warehousing Architecture and Implementation. Upper Saddle River, NJ: Prentice Hall PTR, 1999.

6. **Ullman J.** Principles of Database Systems. 2nd ed. Rockville, MD: Computer Science Press, 1982.

7. **Date CJ.** An Introduction to Database Systems. Reading, MA: Addison-Wesley, 1983.

8. **Kellog C.** From data management to knowledge management. Computer. 1986;Jan:75-84.

9. **Krajewski R.** Database types. Byte. 1984;Oct:137-42.

10. **Hartzband HJ, Maryanzki FJ.** Enhancing knowledge representation in engineering databases. Computer. 1985;Sept:39-45.

11. **Celko J, Celko J.** Debunking object-database myths. Byte. 1997;22:101-6.

12. **Blake J.** ObjectStore delivers. Advanced Systems. 1995;8:30-6.

13. **Myers D.** When all you have is a hammer: the use of free-form text in the electronic medical record takes another approach. Advance for Health Information Executives. 1997;July/Aug:33-4.

14. **Aktas A.** Structured Analysis and Design of Information Systems. Englewood Cliffs, NJ: Prentice-Hall, 1987.

15. **Navathe S, Elmasri R, Larson J.** Integrating user views in database design. Computer. 1986;Jan:50-62.

16. **Simon A.** Data Warehousing for Dummies. Foster City, CA: IDG Books Worldwide, 1997.

17. **Lewis B.** Leveraging legacy data in health care. Advance of Health Information Executives. 1999;3:55-60.

18. **American Medical Informatics Association.** Standards for medical identifiers, codes, and messages needed to create an efficient computer-stored medical record. JAMIA. 1994;1:1-7.

19. **Humphreys B, Hole W, McCray A, Fitzmaurice J.** Planned NLM/AHCPR large-scale vocabulary test: using UMLS technology to determine the extent to which controlled vocabularies cover terminology needed for health care and public health. JAMIA. 1996;3:281-7.

20. **Campbell J, Carpenter P, Sneideman C.** Phase II evaluation of clinical coding schemes: completeness, taxonomy, mapping, definitions, and clarity. JAMIA. 1997;4:238-51.

21. **McDonald C.** The barriers to electronic medical record systems and how to overcome them. JAMIA. 1997;4:213-21.

22. **Bidgood W, Horii S, Prior F, VanSyckle D.** Understanding and using DICOM, the data interchange standard for biomedical imaging. JAMIA. 1997;4:199-212.

23. **Lindberg D, Humphreys B, McCray A.** The Unified Medical Language System. Methods of Information in Medicine. 1993;32:281-91.

24. **Hammond E.** Call for a standard clinical vocabulary. JAMIA. 1997;4:254-5.

25. **Bruegel R, Rothwell D.** Clinical vocabularies: the missing link in CPR systems. Advance for Healthcare Information Executives. 1998;Feb:67-9.

26. **Taylor D.** Object-Oriented Technology. New York: Addison-Wesley, 1990.

27. **Davis B.** Data Warehouses open up. Information Week. 1999;June 28:42-8.

5 / Internet/Intranet Technologies

Daniel R. Masys

O f all the information technologies that affect modern life, none is more emblematic of the times in which we live than the Internet. As a communications medium, the Internet holds both promise and peril for electronic medical records. This chapter provides the reader with an overview of how the Internet works, its technical vocabulary, and the strengths and weaknesses it brings to medical applications. Special variations on Internet technology, called Intranets and Virtual Private Networks, are described, along with current and evolving standards for communicating both data and computer programs over the Internet.

History

As outlined in Chapter 2, much of the power and usefulness of computers derives from the ability to share and retrieve information as needed via computer networks. The term "Internet" is a short form of "internetwork," and was originally used to describe any network that connected two or more computer networks to each other. Internetworks and today's Internet have their historical roots in the 1960s when computers were expensive and few and far between. The problem of creating communications to and among computers that did not suffer from single points of potential failure was the subject of a series of seminal theoretical papers by researchers at the Massachusetts Institute of Technology and the RAND Corporation in 1961 and 1962 (1). These treatises proposed the idea of "packet-switching" networks, built on the idea of an electronic envelope or packet containing a destination address, a return address, and up to a few hundred bytes of data. These packets would be passed via what might be thought of as a "bucket brigade" of specialized computers called *routers*, whose job would be to read the address information on the packet and send it to the next router on the route to its final destination. Multiple routes would be available to each router, so that if a single line failed, the router would simply re-route the packet via a different route.

In 1968, the Advanced Research Projects Agency (ARPA) of the U.S. Defense Department initiated a project to build a network using these design principles. This new network (the ARPANET) became a reality with the connection of computers at four research sites: UCLA, the Stanford Research Institute, UC Santa Barbara, and the University of Utah. In 1971 there were fifteen "nodes" (i.e., participating computers) on the ARPANET; by 1972, thirty-seven. By the second year of operation, however, an interesting phenomenon emerged. ARPANET's users developed tools to turn the computer-sharing network into a dedicated, high-speed, federally subsidized electronic post-office. The main traffic on ARPANET was not long-distance computing. Instead, it was news and personal messages. Researchers were using ARPANET to collaborate on projects, to trade notes on work, and to engage in informal "conversations". This unexpected and personal focus of network usage was a harbinger of events that would occur on a much larger scale two decades later.

The technical building blocks of the Internet as we know it today evolved quickly. In 1974, a set of rules for movement of packets throughout the network, the Transmission Control Program/Internet Protocol (TCP/IP), was developed and published as an open standard that replaced the original ARPANET technology in 1983; it flourishes today as the basis for communications among hundreds of millions of computers worldwide.

The technologies supported and used by the Defense Department in the original ARPANET became the essential data communications infrastructure of research universities in the United States and throughout the world during the 1980s. In recognition of the importance of these technologies to colleges and universities, the National Science Foundation in 1986 established the NSFnet, which linked five university-based supercomputer centers and provided support to regional networks that connected over 10,000 computers at university and industrial research sites by 1988.

The specifications for network functions essential to today's Internet were also developed during this time. These included the Domain Name Service (DNS), a form of "white pages" directory service that translates human-readable computer names (e.g., yahoo.com) into the computer-readable string of numbers representing the unique address, called the *IP address*, of each computer reachable by the network. A set of rules, called *protocols* in engineering terms, was also created for newsgroups (named *nntp* for Network News Transport Protocol) posting messages on electronic community bulletin boards. The standard for error-free transfer of computer files, called *ftp* for File Transfer Protocol, was developed and formed the basis of the "click to download" functionality now ubiquitously available.

The turning point that propelled the Internet beyond universities and into homes and businesses occurred in 1991 with the development of the HyperText Transport Protocol (*http*) that underpins the functionality of the World-Wide Web. The idea of Hypertext is based on linkages between related information sources, where those related sources may be additional "pages" (downloadable files, each representing a "page" of information) located anywhere on the network, whether on the same computer or on another network-connected computer tens of thousands of miles away. The World-Wide Web is based on the notion of "server" computers, which make information available on request, and "client" computers, which make requests, receive information, and display it.

A simple set or rules for describing the content of pages, the HyperText Markup Language (HTML), was developed with the concept of a "hyperlink", which is a word, phrase, or picture that is associated with the address on the Internet of another, related page. The user of a World-Wide Web browser program generally sees the hyperlinked text or image highlighted in a way that, when he or she clicks on the link, the browser program makes a request of the server whose name is "hidden" behind the link.

This remarkably powerful set of ideas was embodied first in a World-Wide Web viewing program called Mosaic developed at the University of Illinois and now available on virtually every Internet-connected computer in the form of browsing programs such as Netscape and Microsoft Internet Explorer. The ease and low cost of both publication and viewing via the World-Wide Web have made it the foundation of electronic commerce (i.e., online shopping) and fueled an explosive growth in both server and client computers. As of this writing, the Internet is used by over 150 million people in the United States and Canada, and more than 300 million worldwide; industry analysts predict one billion users worldwide within the next five years.

Beginning in 1991, the federal government began to withdraw its subsidies of the Internet to transition it to a set of commercial data communications providers. Currently, federal support is directed solely to universities and research organizations developing the "Next Generation Internet" which provides faster communications speeds and additional functions not currently available on today's Internet. The decade of the 90s saw the emergence of thousands of local Internet Service Providers (ISPs) offering a variety of ways for individuals and organizations to connect their computers to the global Internet. Connections based on dial-up phone lines were supplemented by a growing array of technologies capable of communications speeds in the millions-of-bits-per-second range. The pace of change and innovation continues to accelerate, and the near-term future promises a veritable alphabet soup of communications alternatives from phone, cable, and wireless communications companies, all holding the promise of higher communications speeds and lower costs.

How the Internet Works

Since the Internet may be thought of as a telephone system for computers, one enabling them to "talk" to one another in the way that we use the telephone system for voice communications, it is useful to compare the Internet to the phone system to highlight its strengths and weaknesses.

The design of the phone network has its roots in the original model developed by Alexander Graham Bell. Two or more phone devices that convert audible sound into electrical signals are connected by a set of wires (a circuit). In early phone systems, these connections were physical wires connected via physical switches that could make an electrical pathway between any two phones for the duration of a single phone call. Now, switching is done electronically but the notion of a dedicated circuit—a channel used solely by the communicating parties for the duration of the call—persists as a design feature of the phone network. This "circuit switched" model guarantees a certain amount of *bandwidth*, which is the term used for the transmission capacity and speed of a particular connection between two devices (in this case, telephones) connected to the network. In the circuit-switched phone network, one either gets a full allotment of bandwidth, or none, resulting, for example, in the familiar "I'm sorry, all circuits are busy" message on Mother's Day, the heaviest calling day of the year. If a circuit is lost, all communication ceases. A complex, centralized control scheme is required to maintain the proper operation of local and long distance phone circuits.

In contrast, the Internet was designed to have no central authority and to be tolerant of disruptions of parts of the network. The principles of this "fault-tolerant" network are simple. The network is assumed to be unreliable at all times. All of the specialized router computers that serve as the hands in the bucket brigade that pass packets are equal in status to all other routers, and each has its own authority to originate, receive, and forward messages. The messages themselves are divided into packets; each packet is separately addressed. Each packet begins at some specified source computer and ends at some other specified destination computer, but each packet can potentially wind its way through the network on an individual basis.

The particular route that a packet takes is unimportant; only final results count. Each packet is tossed like a hot potato from router to router, more or less in the direction of its destination, until it ends up in the proper place. In the Internet, the TCP (which started as the Transmission Control Program and is now the Transmission Control Protocol) converts messages into streams of packets at the source, then reassembles them back into messages at the destination. The IP (Internet Protocol) handles the addressing, seeing to it that packets are routed across multiple router computers and even across multiple networks with multiple standards for exchange of information worldwide.

By design, Internet networks can be loosely characterized as either *access networks* or *backbone networks*. Access networks are those to which users connect directly and often serve a limited geographic region. These include dial-up networks that serve consumers who access the Internet using the public telephone network and a variety of emerging network technologies described below. Backbone networks typically have wide geographic scope and are used to interconnect the access networks as well as large corporate customers. One important consequence of this architecture is that a packet moving through the Internet will normally traverse networks owned and operated by many different providers en route to its eventual destination. This has implications for two aspects of the network especially important for health care: Quality of Service and security, both of which are discussed later.

The Internet Backbone

Within the United States, the Internet backbone is currently operated by a small number of independent companies. The major backbone providers interconnect with each other at numerous points, some of which are "private" (typically a connection between only two providers), others of which are public. The public interconnection points are used not only by backbone providers but also by local providers to gain access to the backbone.

Backbone networks carry highly aggregated traffic, which represents the combined traffic flows of millions of customers connected to access networks. Backbone networks connect to access networks and to each other at Points of Presence (POPs). PoPs are locations where service providers house switching hardware and transmission equipment. PoPs are interconnected by long-distance transmission lines. They are also the places where providers make connections to each other and to their customers.

A useful metric of backbone bandwidth is the capacity of a single *inter-PoP trunk*, a link from one Point of Presence to another. Providers typically have PoPs in major urban areas; a large provider might have 30 or more PoPs in the United States. Within the backbone networks, today's trunk speeds are typically on the order of 600 million bits per second (Mbps) to 2.5 billion bits per second (Gbps). Providers upgrade link capacity constantly, either replacing slower links with faster ones or installing new links. The key driver for backbone providers is to enlarge capacity to keep up with demand in order to avoid congestion in their networks. Current traffic measurements on the Internet indicate that such efforts are not always successful (i.e., some of the backbone links are at or near capacity).

The Last Mile

"Last Mile" is the term used to describe the access link to end-users, especially residential users. The overwhelming majority of residential users connect to the Internet using a dial-up connection; that is, they use a modem connected to a conventional telephone line to connect to an ISP. These consumer-oriented ISPs then aggregate traffic from large numbers of residential customers and provide connectivity to the rest of the Internet by interconnecting with other ISPs.

The fastest modem connections are capable of providing 56,000 bits per second, or about 5600 characters per second (56 kbps) connections. Many residential users connect at 28.8 kbps or less. Options for connecting at higher speeds are the exception today but will become more prevalent in the future. Limitations on bandwidth have important implications for some types of health care applications. While having a bottleneck in the access link will always prevent one from achieving high end-to-end throughput, the converse is not necessarily true. Even with a high-speed access link, congestion at other points in the network may limit the throughput to a small fraction of the access speed. The issue of obtaining assured end-to-end bandwidth is one of the essential components of Quality of Service.

Businesses have a range of options for connecting to the Internet, depending on their ability to pay. At the low end, they have the same options as residential users. At the high end, many businesses connect over *dedicated lines* (i.e., not dial-up) at speeds ranging between 1.5 million bits per second, called "T-1" in communications parlance, and 155 million bits per second, called "Optical Communications Standard 3", or "OC-3", because it uses and requires fiber optic lines. The number of businesses at the higher end is small as of this writing, but a few high-profile Web sites connect at these high speeds. Prices charged for these services vary by geographic region and depend to some extent on market forces within local regions. Prices for dedicated lines are generally high enough to preclude use by residential customers (hundreds to thousands of dollars per month).

In between these two extremes, the Frame Relay and the Integrated Services Digital Network (ISDN) are popular methods of connection for businesses. Frame Relay connections are typically sold at speeds from 56 kbps to 1.5 Mbps. Unlike a dedicated line, the bandwidth on a Frame Relay connection may be shared with other customers. Thus, for example, a business with a T-1 (1.5 Mbps) Frame Relay circuit might only be able to send 100 kbps at a certain time. ISDN is sold in units of 64 kb channels, which can be combined ("bonded") to create channels of higher capacity.

Internet Limitations

As noted above, the Internet is a "best effort" network that provides no guarantees with respect to several key communications parameters. The most important of these from a health care perspective are assured Quality of Service and security.

Quality of Service (QoS) refers to the ability of a network to provide a range of levels of assurance of performance. Performance is characterized by metrics that include:

- *Bandwidth*–The throughput that is actually obtained between two points in the network (which may be dramatically less than the link speeds in the path between those points due to resource sharing and contention).
- *Packet Loss Rate*—The percentage of packets transmitted that are dropped inside the network.
- *Latency or Delay*—The time taken to get a packet from one point in the network to another.
- *Jitter*—The variation in delay over time.

Note that these metrics are not independent of each other. For example, a high packet loss rate is likely to lead to low throughput. Note also that QoS is distinct from reliability. Reliability refers to the likelihood that a service remains available at all times. A network may be highly reliable in the sense that it is always possible to obtain connectivity to a given destination, but the same network may lack any assurance of performance and thus QoS as defined above.

A few numbers will help to illustrate the nature of best-effort service. For example, while round trip times (or latency) from East to West Coast across the Internet are frequently in the range of 100 milliseconds (ms), latencies in the range of a second are not unheard of. Although this amount of delay is not significant for asynchronous applications such as e-mail, it makes interactive applications such as videoconferencing unusable. There is nothing that a customer of an ISP can do today to ensure that this type of latency will not be encountered. This variation in latency might even be observed in the lifetime of a single connection, making it hard for a user or application to adapt to the prevailing latency. Similarly, packet loss rates range from fractions of a percent to tens of percent, which results in degradation of quality or the need to re-transmit packets. Re-transmission, in turn, results in increased latency. In addition, many applications reduce their sending rates in response to lost packets as they attempt to reduce congestion. As a result, packet loss directly affects the time taken to complete a transaction such as an image transfer over the network. While some links are chronically congested (e.g., between the United States and Europe), some links display high loss rates only sporadically. There are no mechanisms deployed in the Internet today to address this issue, but it is high on the list of issues to be addressed soon, as discussed below.

Quality of Service is important for any application that involves interactive audio or video motion. Audio is the more sensitive of the two to delays and disruptions. For example, in transmitting normal speech, a pause of 50 ms is noticeable to the speaker and listener but does not disrupt communications. Difficulty understanding speech increases as pauses or periods of silence lengthen, until at 300 ms of pause, speech becomes largely unintelligible to the listener. Thus the necessary quality of signal provided by the circuit-switched phone network is simply unavailable in the current packet-switched Internet. Although voice-over-IP "Internet telephone" programs exist and may be useable over certain Internet paths at certain times of the day, they are currently unreliable as an alternative to standard telephone voice service.

Because the Internet lacks QoS guarantees, a variety of adaptations have been developed for time-sensitive information such as audio and video. So-called "streaming media" players are based on the sending of a continuous series of packets containing audio and/or video data by a server computer. The client computer program receives and stores ("buffers") several seconds worth of data before beginning to play or show it, and continues to play the audio or video at a precise and regular pace while accumulating additional data, often irregularly, in the background due to the unpredictability of packet delivery from the Internet.

Security

Security is a fundamentally important aspect of health care data communications, and the Internet presents special challenges and vulnerabilities in this regard. First, it is important to understand the basic functions that are needed to make an information system of any type secure. These include:

1. *Identification* of the persons and computers that will be involved in the acquisition, storage, and communication of information within the system is the first stage. Identification is a process that computer security professionals refer to as "out of band". An example of such a process would be a human being that compares an identifying document such as a passport with your person to establish for the system that you are authorized to have access in some way. As a general rule the network itself cannot be used to identify parts of the network.

2. *Authentication* is the function that assures that the user or system, at the time of each use of the system, is who they represent themselves to be. In contrast to identification, that occurs once or at relatively long intervals (e.g., renewal of a driver's license), authentication in a secure system occurs every time a person or machine makes their presence known to the system, such as during a system log-on.

3. *Access Control* is the set of functions that assure that people, computer systems, and processes, once authenticated, can use only those resources (e.g., files, directories, database records, computers, networks) that they are authorized to use and only for the purposes for which they are authorized.

4. *Confidentiality* is provided by functions that assure that sensitive and/or private information is protected from unauthorized disclosure. While access control mechanisms define what one is autho-

rized to see, and thus what the system *should do*, confidentiality mechanisms provide assurance that the system is not doing what it *shouldn't do*.

5. *Integrity* is maintained by functions that assure that data, computer programs, and system resources are as they are supposed to be and that they cannot be modified by unauthorized people, software, or computer equipment.

6. *Attribution* (also called *nonrepudiation*) comprises functions that assure that information and actions that occur in the system are reliably traceable to the users and/or computers involved.

These six functions are required of any information or communications system that is designed to be secure, ranging from tin cans on a string to computer networks. In contrast, the Internet was designed to support open communications and collaboration between mutually trusting entities. Thus, authenticating the identity of computers and users and protecting the contents of IP packets simply were not issues that the IP protocol needed to address.

The Internet as it exists today has a number of vulnerabilities:

- The Internet provides no positive means of identifying systems. No reliable means exists to positively bind IP addresses to specific computers. Indeed, there is an Internet standard for a Dynamic Host Configuration Protocol (DHCP) that has capitalized on this "vulnerability" by enabling IP addresses to be assigned in real-time. Using this approach, ISPs generally maintain a pool of assignable IP addresses. As users dial in to initiate a session, an IP address is temporarily assigned to that user's account; after the session is complete, the IP address is made available to the next caller as needed.

- The Internet provides no positive means of identifying users. In fact, the Internet does not recognize the concept of the individual "user".

- The Internet provides no protection for confidential information. Information is loaded into the IP packets and passed from router to router ("node to node" in computer network parlance) in the clear. A "sniffer" program on any node through which the data passes can see the contents as it passes through, even packets containing sensitive information such as user passwords or medical test results.

- Vulnerabilities in attached systems can be exploited to further reduce the presumed security of the Internet. "Trojan horse" programs, for example, provide some useful and visible services while performing actions in the background that are neither desired nor known to the user, such as transmitting information to malicious host computers on the Internet (2).

Encryption

The technology that makes it possible to authenticate users, protect the confidentiality and integrity of information, and assure attribution or non-repudiation over a network is *encryption*, the age-old practice of re-arranging a message to make its contents difficult to interpret. Two forms of encryption are in common use in the Internet: *symmetric*, or *conventional* or *private-key*, and *asymmetric*, or *public-key*.

Symmetric encryption is based on the principle that the code or "key" used to scramble a message (formally called a *ciphertext*) is the same key used to unscramble it; in one form or another private-key encryption has been used since the time of the Romans. Popular symmetric encryption algorithms include the Data Encryption Standard (DES) (3), which uses a 56-bit encryption key and its proposed successor, the International Data Encryption Algorithm (IDEA), which uses a 128-bit key (4). Private-key encryption has the problem that the parties must agree upon the key to be used before the encrypted communication is exchanged. If the key can be intercepted in the same way that an encrypted message can be intercepted, then little or no advantage of secrecy is gained by using encryption.

Asymmetric encryption is based on a two-part key. What one part of the key pair encodes, only the other part of the key pair can decode; even the original key will not decode the message. This asymmetry has very useful properties. If one key of the key pair is kept private and the other, "public" key is made available to others, then a message successfully decoded by the public key must have been encoded by the private key. This effect makes public-key cryptography well suited to creating digital signatures, establishing user authentication, and exchanging private (symmetrical) session keys in a way that does not permit eavesdropping. The RSA algorithm (5) was one of the first public-key encryption algorithms to be widely adopted. Named for its developers, Ron Rivest, Adi Shamir, and Leonard Adleman, RSA relies on the difficulty of factoring large numbers for its security.

In general, conventional private-key encryption is used for protecting the confidentiality and integrity of large amounts of data, whereas public-key encryption, which imposes a greater processing burden and, depending upon key length, may be a thousand or more times slower to decrypt, is often used for user authentication purposes and for exchanging private keys. The difficulty of attempting to decipher an encrypted message without use of the key, as might be attempted by an attacker, is proportional to the length of the key relative to the message; the longer the encryption key, the more possible combinations exist that must be tried to unscramble the message simply by guessing at all possible solutions. A 128-bit encryption key, which is currently considered "strong encryption" and limited by U.S. State Department export controls, generates a ciphertext that has 300,000,000,000,000,000,000,000,000,000 (a three followed by 26 zeroes) times as many possible key combinations as there are for 40-bit encryption, which is the current international export standard.

Secure HTTP

The Hypertext Transport Protocol (HTTP) that underpins the functioning of the World-Wide Web lacks protections for confidential data. The Secure HTTP Protocol (SHTTP), developed for secure and private exchange of information such as credit-card numbers, has become an essential tool for Web-based communication of health care data. SHTTP is an application-level protocol (meaning that it is a set of procedures executed by the server program and the client browser program, not by the network) that provides encryption of messages transmitted in both directions between client and server and for encapsulation of the message in a "wrapper" specifying the encryption method used, thus ensuring confidentiality. Any of a number of encryption mechanisms can be used; the particular mechanism is negotiated between client and server at the time the connection is made. An encrypted message may also incorporate a message digest, which guarantees the integrity of the data in the message, and a digital signature, which guarantees the authenticity of the sender. SHTTP is designed to be backward compatible with HTTP, so browsers that do not implement SHTTP can still access data on SHTTP servers.

Secure Sockets Layer

SSL is a secure communication protocol implemented as a layer between the transport layer (usually TCP) and applications that send and receive messages. It provides for message encryption and certification of public-key authenticity, data integrity, and server authentication; client authentication is optional. It can provide these services to any application protocol, such as HTTP, telnet, or even SHTTP. When SHTTP and SSL are used together, SHTTP encrypts data at the application layer and passes it to SSL, which encrypts it a second time. As with SHTTP, SSL performs security services independently from the operating system and the network.

Public Key Infrastructure

As described above, an essential component of Internet security is based on public key cryptography, the two-part encryption scheme where one part of the key is held privately and one is made public. This technology has given rise to a small but growing industry that provides Certificate Authority (CA) services. These companies verify that a server computer's public key is valid and combine it with their own public key to create a unique *digital certificate*. A digital certificate is simply an electronic "statement", signed by an independent and trusted third party, in a format that is standardized so that its contents can be decoded by client programs such as Web browsers. Certificate Authority services are built on a combination of out-of-band identification (e.g., calling individuals associated with the organization to verify the authenticity of the request for a public key certificate) and technology that "wraps" the public key of a given server with the Certificate Authority's own cryptographic key. The most common digital certificates on the Internet follow a standard named X.509 (6). In health care, State Medical Boards are responsible for certifying and licensing practitioners within their jurisdiction; thus it can reasonably be expected that in the future such regulatory agencies will perform the functions of a medical Certificate Authority for practitioners and institutions. The technical and documentary relationships for certifying the authenticity of the public keys of server (and potentially also client) computers on the Internet is referred to collectively as a *public key infrastructure*.

Encryption of Health Data on the Internet

In 1999, the Health Care Financing Administration (HCFA) issued an Internet Security Policy that requires encryption of all person-identifiable health data communicated to HCFA (7). The policy specified a minimum level of encryption as "triple DES", which means encrypting a message with the DES 56-bit key, and then encrypting the resulting message twice more. A single 128-bit encryption is equally acceptable; this is important for Web-based clinical systems because commonly used domestic Web server programs (such as Microsoft Internet Information Server, which is available as a no-added cost option for Windows NT servers) are capable of being made compliant with the HCFA 128-bit standard.

In contrast to Web-based communication of health data, the use of Internet electronic mail is currently problematic. Recent surveys of Internet usage indicate that approximately half of the U.S. adult population now uses e-mail. In a 1999 study of 10,000 physicians conducted by Healtheon, 63% of physicians reported using e-mail daily, and 33% used it to communicate with patients; this represented a 200% increase in one year. Electronic communications between patients and doctors did not even register as a significant behavior when physicians were surveyed in 1997. In this same survey, more than 34% of respondents cited security as a concern in the use of e-mail or other interactive Internet services (8).

The growth in the use of electronic messaging for clinical care highlights an important set of risks. Standard (smtp – simple mail transport protocol) e-mail is passed in cleartext format over the Internet, which makes the "snooping" of message contents trivially easy to do using a variety of network management and hacker tools. Although encryption utilities such as PGP and standards for privacy-enhanced e-mail exist, they are as of this writing not widely installed or used. The American Medical Informatics Association's Internet Working Group published in 1998 a set of guidelines for e-mail communications between patients and providers that emphasize the establishment of orderly procedures for the handling of provider-patient e-mail (9). A partial list of the recommendations of that White Paper are summarized here for they provide a reference point for some of the challenges and difficulties associated with electronic health care communications:

- Establish a turnaround time for e-mail responses to patient inquiries; do not use e-mail for urgent matters.
- Inform patients about privacy issues (e.g., who sees e-mail in the practitioner's office, how that e-mail becomes part of the medical record).
- Establish types of transaction (e.g., prescription refills, appointment scheduling) that are appropriate for e-mail and set limits on message content in terms of sensitivity (e.g., HIV test results).
- Instruct patients to put category of transaction in e-mail subject line (e.g., "Med refill").
- Acknowledge receipt of all messages and request that patients do the same.

- Print all messages, replies, and confirmation of receipt and place in paper chart.
- Request patients to put name and MRN in body of message.
- Use encryption as soon as it is feasible and practicable.
- Do not use unencrypted wireless communications for patient-identifiable information

While representing a pragmatic approach to the management of clinical messages that are now flowing in increasing numbers between patients and providers, the guidelines advise practices that heighten the risk of breeches of confidentiality (e.g., putting patient name and MRN in the body of the message). They also serve to highlight the lack of currently available security mechanisms and the lack of tools to integrate electronic messages easily into the increasingly electronic medical record.

Intranets

The networking technologies developed for the open Internet can also be applied to a private network. The term *Intranet* is given for a local area network that is configured to use the networking protocols (TCP/IP) and services (World-Wide Web, smtp e-mail, ftp file transfer protocol, etc.) of the larger Internet. An Intranet can either be isolated unto itself or connected so that information can also be transmitted to and received from the Internet (Fig. 5-1). In the case where an Intranet is connected to the Internet, it inherits the security challenges and difficulties (such as the risk of unauthorized access by malicious users) of the larger network. As a result, most Intranets are designed to have only a single point of contact with the Internet, through which all incoming and outgoing communications streams must pass. At this point, a specialized communications filtering computer called a *firewall* is installed. As the name implies, firewalls are designed to protect an internal network from external threats. A variety of rules regarding the types of incoming and outgoing messages allowed, and how the machine identities (IP addresses) authorized internal and external computers, can be implemented via software programs. Rules can relate both to types of services (e.g., no incoming file transfers except from specific 'trusted' sources) and to the contents of the IP packets (e.g., no e-mail attachments that are executable programs). Firewalls can also inspect the communications stream for patterns that indicate malicious programs such

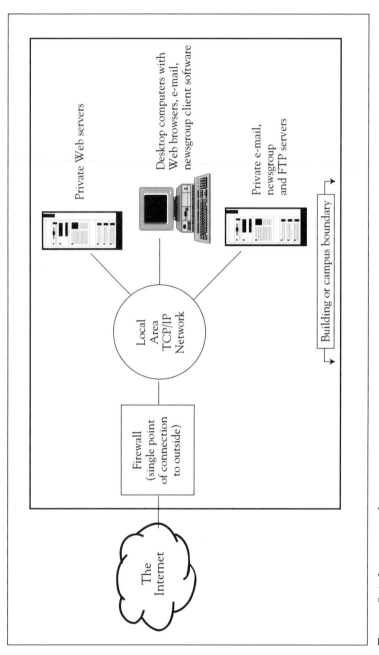

Figure 5-1 Intranet architecture.

as computer viruses. Most large corporations and a growing number of health care enterprises have some form of corporate Intranet.

Extranets and Virtual Private Networks

The popularity of Intranets gave rise to the idea of extending the same forms of private communications found within an Intranet to selected sites (e.g., branch offices, affiliated clinics, or business partners) using the open Internet to pass data communications traffic between two or more geographically distant Intranets. The general idea of this has been called an *Extranet*, but this term does not imply a specific set of technologies (Fig. 5-2). In some cases what is called an Extranet is simply the use of open Internet protocols, such as secure HTTP and Secure Sockets Layer (SSL), between organizations known to one another.

In contrast, a Virtual Private Network (VPN) has a specific technical definition. Like an Extranet, it involves passing communications between Intranets using the open Internet. However, a VPN is based on specially configured routers that are programmed with a private encryption key and the IP addresses of the other routers comprising the VPN. The router computers perform "link level encryption" of packets and may adopt a private and nonstandard messaging protocol known as a "tunneling protocol", so-called because it effectively creates a tunnel for communications that can only be interpreted correctly by the routers of the VPN. VPNs provide strong security and predictable paths (unlike the open Internet where packets are passed in a generally unpredictable series of hops) but have the disadvantage that the specialized routers must be preconfigured with the security keys and destination information of the other members of the network.

Extending the Web via Markup Languages

The World-Wide Web began as a publication metaphor, one based on servers providing electronic data representing individual pages with content encoded in the Hypertext Markup Language (HTML). HTML is a formatting language based on the Standard Generalized Markup Language (SGML) developed by the publishing industry to specify page layout and text appearance. SGML and HTML use simple text tags of the form:

<TAG>This is text affected by the instruction in the tag</TAG>

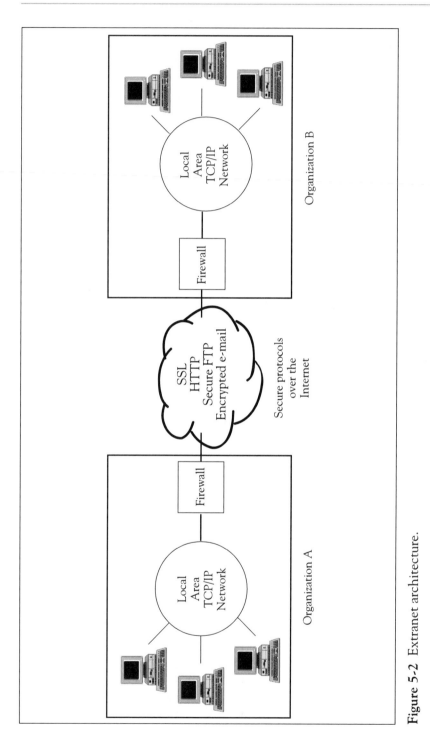

Figure 5-2 Extranet architecture.

The tags themselves are not displayed but provide instructions to a Web browser on how to treat the information contained between the tags, so that an HTML construction such as

This is <B>Bold</B> text and this is <I>italic</I>.

will be displayed as

This is **Bold** text and this is *italic*.

HTML is a limited and "improper" subset of SGML. This means that an SGML document can be translated to HTML, but information is lost in the translation so that an HTML document cannot be translated back to SGML, which has additional requirements for specifying a formal document type description (DTD) and structure.

The power and utility of specifying document structure and content via embedded tags has given rise to an evolving set of standards called Extensible Markup Language (XML). XML is a flexible way to create common information formats and share both the format and the data on the World-Wide Web, Intranets, and elsewhere. There is intense activity underway to develop XML specifications for elements of health care records (12, 13). Using XML as a standard for representing documentation of clinical encounters, laboratory results, dictated operative reports, and so on facilitates both the consistent formatting of this information by Web browsers and the ability to analyze content via computer programs that look for and extract specific tagged elements.

XML is "extensible" because, unlike HTML, the markup symbols are unlimited and self-defining. Thus, XML tagging of an initial history and physical could include health care relevant tags such as <CHIEF COMPLAINT>....</CHIEF COMPLAINT> as well as the formatting information carried by standard HTML tags.

Extending the Web with Downloadable Computer Programs

In addition to these evolving standards for describing viewable "document" or "page" content on the Web, there is no barrier to a servers sending executable computer programs to a client upon request. The idea of transmitting on-demand programs to a client computer has given rise to a variety of programming languages developed specifically for use via computer networks, the most widely deployed of which are Java and Javascript.

Java

Java is a programming language developed by Sun Microsystems specifically to expand the interactive possibilities of the Web. Java is similar in syntax to C++ but has special adaptations for a networked environment, including security limitations that can limit its ability to cause inadvertent or intentional damage to files on the client computer. Java is intended to be "platform independent" (as is HTML) so that a program written in Java will run correctly regardless of the type of client computer receiving it. Java programs are converted to a compact common format called *bytecode*, which is interpreted by a piece of software known as a Java Virtual Machine (JVM). Most of the major Web browsers include JVM functionality, and almost all major operating system developers (IBM, Microsoft, and others) have added Java compilers as part of their product offerings. As is often the case with computer languages, the full potential of "platform independence" has not yet been realized due to the emergence of variant "dialects" of Java developed and promoted by competing companies (in this case, primarily Sun and Microsoft).

Java can be used to create complete applications that may run on a single computer or be distributed among servers and clients in a network. It can also be used to build small application modules called *applets* that are downloaded to a client computer as part of a Web page (for example, an interactive Body Surface Area calculator displayed within a page providing guidance on drug dosage) .

JavaScript

Although it has a similar sounding name, JavaScript is a more limited "scripting language" than Java, with a much different syntax. JavaScript can be embedded within an HTML page. Originally called "LiveScript", JavaScript was developed by Netscape and soon modified and renamed in order to tap into the Java craze sweeping the Internet. As with Java, most major browsers provide support for interpreting its scripts. It is used primarily for animating and enhancing navigation on Web pages; the now-familiar Web motif of buttons which "glow" when the mouse cursor is passed over them is most commonly implemented by JavaScript scripting within the Web page.

CORBA

Providing access to and control over network-accessible programs is the goal of another set of emerging standards called CORBA (Common Object Request Broker Architecture). It is an architecture and specification for creating, distributing, and managing distributed program objects in a network. It allows programs at different locations and developed by different vendors to communicate in a network through an "interface broker", a set of software functions that examines requests coming from programs running on client computers and determines how and where to route those requests to the appropriate server. CORBA was developed by a consortium of vendors through the Object Management Group (OMG), which currently includes over 500 member companies. Industry-specific committees and working groups are developing standards for CORBA, including a CORBA MED group focussed on the functionality unique to health care computing (11).

A notable hold-out from CORBA is Microsoft, which has its own distributed object architecture, the Distributed Component Object Model (DCOM). However, CORBA and Microsoft have agreed on a gateway approach so that a client object developed with DCOM will be able to communicate with a CORBA server (and vice versa).

Internet-Accessible Medical Records

The description of the various Internet-related technologies described above serves as a preamble to a discussion of the use of the Internet for communicating person-specific clinical data. Vendors of electronic medical record (EMR) systems have been under increasing pressure from purchasers to create Web-based information access methods to complement their existing products. The Health Care Financing Administration's implementation in 1999 of a set of security standards for transmission of person-identifiable health data established an acceptable set of technical measures for satisfactory information security, opening the floodgates for a vast array of new commercial products. Today, it would be exceptional if a vendor did *not* have a Web interface to its EMR product either available or in development. As with most new technologies that eventually achieve widespread acceptance, the first applications tend to be evolutionary and incremental modifications to existing systems. Later, revolutionary applications appear that support a redefinition of roles, responsibilities, and workflow. The Internet is currently being used to support the former but will almost certainly change the very nature of EMR as the latter emerge. Examples of both are provided below.

Web Interfaces to EMR Systems

The most common approach to making EMR data from existing systems available via the Internet is to create an accessory "wrapper" system that accepts queries from client computers via HTML forms and translates those queries into a syntax compatible with the existing (often mainframe-based) Clinical Data Repository (CDR). The CDR responds as it would to a request originating from any workstation in the existing system architecture and sends back data to the Web-server machine. The server then re-encodes that data as a dynamic-generated HTML page and sends it to the requesting Web client. If the client is located outside of the organization's local area network, the Web client-server communications are encrypted and travel though the firewall computer to the open Internet (Fig. 5-3).

The strength of such a model is that it does not require a fundamental redesign of the CDR, because the incoming transactions appear to the existing system to be "just another workstation" sending and receiving data. The weakness is that, because designs of this type have several additional layers of information processing and reformatting, they are as a result relatively inefficient and difficult to scale up.

New Internet-Based EMR Designs

Though most Web interfaces to EMR systems are "grafted on" to the existing architecture using the design described above or a variant of it, the emerging technologies and growing ubiquity of the Internet will enable a new genre of EMR designs that include

- Java-encoded EMR client programs that connect directly via the Internet to an organization's CDR database without the need for an intermediary Web server, thereby improving data access efficiency while giving an organization control over the user interface and the security aspects of the data communication. Because the Java code is downloaded each time a user session is initiated, this design has the additional benefit that all client workstations are guaranteed to be running the most up-to-date version of the client program. An example of a Java applet-based EMR access program

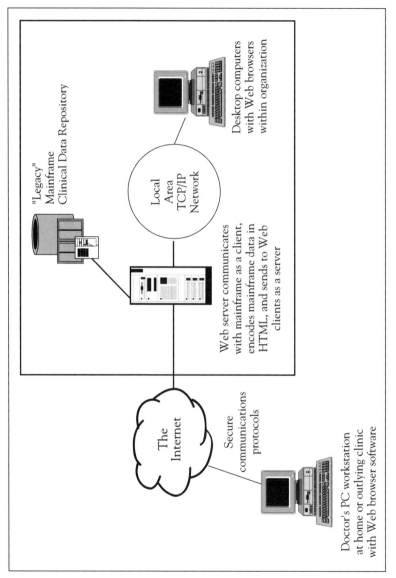

Figure 5-3 Web "wrapper" architecture.

is the PCASSO (Patient-Centered Access to Secure Systems On-line) research project of Science Applications International Corporation and the University of California, San Diego. This experimental system uses a Java client to create a high assurance encrypted communications protocol over the Internet that enables both providers and their patients to view the contents of their records contained in a clinical data repository (2).

Clinical data repositories that are in reality just a logical view of data that are physically located on many different servers located at geographically distant sites. The Internet will provide, via "middleware" services such as CORBA, an environment where requesting client computers do not need to know or be concerned about the location of servers. Though health care organizations have historically viewed their computer systems as a necessary local resource, computer networks loosen the requirement for physical facilities and enable strategies such as outsourcing to medical "data warehouses" located hundreds or thousands of miles from the hospital or clinic. The most provocative (and perhaps inevitable) model would locate the electronic records of care delivered in a network-accessible "neutral repository" database, encrypted with a private key unique to each patient, and with access controlled by the patient. On entry into a health care plan or system, the patient would grant access privileges to their providers via a public key infrastructure as described in the Encryption section above.

The Future of Health Care Data Networks

The importance of the Internet and Internet-associated technologies for EMR systems will continue to grow for the foreseeable future, driven by the dual forces of innovation and societal change. It can be reasonably predicted that four key areas of data networking that affect health care will see substantial change and improvement over the next several years. They are bandwidth, quality of service, security, and ubiquity.

Bandwidth

The first and most obvious difference between the current Internet and the networks that will evolve from it in the future is a dramatic increase in transport speeds. Speeds of OC-3 (155 Mbits/s) to OC-48 (2.5 Gbits/s) are being deployed in research settings and are expected to become commercially available in some metropolitan areas within the next several years. From a health care perspective, requirements for bandwidth of this magnitude tend to derive from the aggregate traffic of dozens to thousands of data streams, rather than from individual applications that have stringent requirements for extremely high bandwidth. One might assume that many data-intensive clinical transactions require very high bandwidth communications. However, empirical telemedicine studies conducted over the past decade have concluded that by and large a relative minority of clinical applications, such as cardiac cineangiography, require application bandwidth in the range of 768 kb/s (e.g., 6 bonded ISDN channels). Most interactive video telemedicine, such as telepsychiatry and routine general medical follow-up, can be effectively delivered with bandwidth as low as 128 kb/s (14-17). More importantly, very high bandwidth alone will not be sufficient for interactive telemedicine unless it is accompanied by guarantees of Quality of Service.

Quality of Service

As noted previously, best-effort service is the only option available via the Internet today; a range of different services will be available within the next several years. The two main approaches to offering Internet QoS are typically referred to as "integrated services" (int-serv) and "differentiated services" (diff-serv). Both int-serv and diff-serv improve upon the current best-effort service model.

As the name implies, in diff-serv the intention is to deliver a differentiated set of qualities of service beyond best-effort. As a simple example, a clinic might purchase "Premium Service" from an Internet Service Provider at a certain transmission rate, say, 128 kbps. Such an agreement would mean that the organization could send up to 128 kbps of packets into the network and expect them to receive "better" service than a best-effort packet would receive. Exactly how much better would be determined by the provider. An important limitation of differentiated service is that it goes only as far as the boundary of a single ISP network.

The term "integrated services" is used to refer to an overall architecture for providing QoS in IP networks such as the Internet. An important component of the architecture is the signaling protocol, the Resource ReSerVation Protocol (RSVP); the int-serv model is sometimes referred to as the RSVP model. Unlike diff-serv, int-serv attempts to provide quantifiable end-to-end guarantees to applications of the form "This video conference from host A to host B will receive 128 kbps throughput and 100 ms end-to-end latency." It also includes a signaling mechanism (RSVP) to provide "on-demand" guarantees, which appears to be ideal for many health care applications.

The major concern that has prevented widespread deployment of int-serv and RSVP is scalability. As currently defined, every connection (e.g., a single video call) needs its own reservation, and each reservation requires information about the connection to be stored at every router along the path that will carry the application data. The prospect of having per-application state in backbone routers is not attractive to ISPs, for whom scaling is a major concern. In addition, an ISP would need to have mechanisms to control which users were able to make reservations and to bill for such reservations. In spite of these problems, an int-serv model remains attractive. It provides a service model that more closely resembles that of the telephone network than diff-serv does. Service is requested as needed: If resources are available to provide the requested service, then the service will be provided; if not, a negative acknowledgement (equivalent to a busy signal) is returned. For this reason, int-serv is already being used in "Voice over IP" networks that are small enough to avoid the scaling issues mentioned above.

Security

"IPSec" refers to a security architecture and set of standards currently undergoing standardization within the Internet Engineering Task Force. The standards provide for a variety of services such as encryption and authentication of IP packets. One of the main areas of deployment of these technologies has been to support Virtual Private Networks (VPNs) across the Internet. A number of products are now available to enable the establishment of an "encrypted tunnel" across the Internet. Such a tunnel is created between a pair of IPSec gateways, which might be located at two geographically separated locations of a single health care organization. Each gateway encrypts the data sent from one site to the other and sends the encrypted data as the payload of a standard IP datagram to the other gateway. The receiving gateway then decrypts the data before passing it on to the final recipient at the second site. Because the data are encrypted using a key that is known only to the two gateways, it cannot be "snooped" as it crosses the Internet. Furthermore, the receiving gateway can authenticate the data as having come from the sending site and not some other source in the Internet. Thus an IPSec tunnel provides a viable way to build a VPN. Like other approaches to VPNs, it requires *a priori* knowledge of where connectivity will be required, because the gateways must be configured with appropriate keys and routing information to create the tunnel.

Ubiquity

The importance of understanding and taking advantage of Internet technologies comes more from their projected future growth than it does their current functionality. Global computer data networks will become ubiquitous to a degree that equals or surpasses voice telephone service (and in fact will likely become carriers of both voice and data as networking technologies converge). Surveys of Internet users in the United States show that the demographics are "regressing to the mean" so that access to the Internet, once the province solely of the affluent and well educated, will be the norm in most or all segments of society.

A major trend that will help propel the Internet into homes and offices is the appearance of "smart" appliances and machines that communicate over IP data networks. Recently devices such as "Internet refrigerators" have been announced that record food items as they are removed from the refrigerator in a shopping list database that is automatically transmitted to an online grocery as needed. The tongue-in-cheek vision of "toaster net" that is a current joke among Internet aficionados will have an analogous impact in the medical office, where a vision of "sphygmomanometer net" will become a reality in an increasingly paperless health care environment.

One prominent computer company has had for over a decade a slogan that states "The Network *is* the Computer" (18). The impact of the Internet, though already substantial in health care, is at an early stage along a path that may lead eventually to a similar assertion: The Network *is* the Health Care Organization. Internet-based EMR systems will be an important component of that future.

REFERENCES

1. For a complete technical history of the Internet, the Internet itself is not surprisingly a rich source of information. Readers interested in pursuing this may wish to navigate the Internet subject area of catalog sites such as http://www.yahoo.com or the Electronic Commerce Resource Center site at http://www.becrc.org/nethistory.htm.
2. **Masys DR, Baker DB.** Patient-Centered Access to Secure Systems Online (PCASSO): a secure approach to clinical data access via the World-Wide Web. J Am Med Inform Assoc. 1997;4: Fall Symp Supplement:340-3.

3. Federal Information Processing Standard Publication No. 46-2, Data Encryption Standard (DES), available from the National Institute of Standards and Technology at http://www.itl.nist.gov/fipspubs/fip46-2.htm.

4. http://csrc.nist.gov/encryption/aes/aes_home.htm.

5. http://www.rsa.com.

6. For more information on Public Key Infrastructure and digital certificates, see the National Institutes of Standards and Technology PKI site at http://csrc.nist.gov/pki/

7. HCFA Internet Security Policy, available online at http://www.hcfa.gov/security/isecplcy.htm

8. http://www.healtheon.com

9. **Kane B, Sands DZ.** Guidelines for the clinical use of electronic mail with patients. The AMIA Internet Working Group, Task Force on Guidelines for the Use of Clinic-Patient Electronic Mail. J Am Med Inform Assoc. 1998;5:104-11.

10. For a comprehensive overview of Java, consult the Sun Microsystems Java page at http://java.sun.com

11. The Object Management Group provides introductory tutorials and additional technical information on CORBA, including activities of the CORBA MED group, at http://www.omg.org/

12. **Kahn CE Jr, de la Cruz NB.** Extensible Markup Language (XML) in health care: integration of structured reporting and decision support. In Chute C, editor. Proceedings of the AMIA Symposium. 1998;725-9.

13. **Dolin RH, Rishe W, Biron PV, et al.** SGML and XML as Interchange Formats for HL7 messages. In Chute C, editor. Proceedings of the AMIA Fall Symposium. 1998;720-4.

14. **Anogianakis G, Maglavera S, Pomportsis A, et al.** Medical emergency aid through telematics: design, implementation guidelines and analysis of user requirements for the MERMAID project. Int J Med Inf. 1998;52:93-103.

15. **Stewart BK, Carter SJ, Cook JN, et al.** Application of the advanced communications technology satellite to teleradiology and real-time compressed ultrasound video telemedicine. J Digit Imaging. 1999;12:68-76.

16. **Stoloff PH, Garcia FE, Thomason JE, Shia DS.** A cost-effectiveness analysis of shipboard telemedicine. Telemed J. 1998;4:293-304.

17. **Phillips CM, Murphy R, Burke WA, et al.** Dermatology teleconsultations to Central Prison: experience at East Carolina University. Telemed J. 1996;2:139-43.

18. Sun Microsystems, Inc., at http://www.sun.com

SECTION II

Understanding Processes and Outcomes

6 / Identifying and Understanding Business Processes

Blackford Middleton and John J. Janas III

I n this chapter, we discuss the essential business processes that underlying the clinical practice of medicine. We review the "business" of clinical practice and identify opportunities for business, and clinical, process re-engineering using clinical information management technology. The core clinical workflows and business processes in a typical ambulatory clinical environment are presented, and opportunities for using clinical information systems to support these business processes are reviewed. Essential features of clinical information systems to support the management of a clinical enterprise are also discussed. This chapter focuses on clinical information management technology, as opposed to financial or accounting systems, which may also exist in clinical departments. While we recognize that these systems are also important for effective business management within a clinic, we focus on the clinical information management technology, or electronic patient records, which fundamentally drive the clinical business, and related information systems. We next discuss essential features of an electronic patient record required to support advanced business and clinical process management. The chapter closes with an example of how to integrate clinical and business processes for advanced process management and re-engineering.

The "Business" of Clinical Practice

In this section we review the "business" of clinical practice. Business pressures facing the average practitioner in clinical practice at the turn of the millennium are highlighted. Critical office workflows that drive the clinical enterprise, and the business processes that support them, are reviewed with the aim of understanding how these processes might be supported by clinical information management technology. Next, the basic principles of process re-engineering are presented, and the role of the computer in business process re-engineering is highlighted.

Business Pressures on Clinical Practice

The contemporary practice of medicine has changed greatly from the practice of medicine in years gone by. After World War II, the biomedical industry emerged as one of the fastest growing sectors of the health economy, fueled by an extraordinary amount of research funding from the federal government, fee-for-service reimbursements in private practice settings, and cost-plus accounting in hospital environments. With the advent of prospective payment in the mid-1980s, the emergence of managed-care and health maintenance organizations, and the increasing number of federal regulations, today's physician often feels beleaguered by administrative pressures. Many physicians have opted to leave independent practice settings and join staff model HMOs or other medical organizations to relieve themselves of administrative responsibilities. Nevertheless, the vast majority of physicians remain in small-to-midsize medical group practices in a variety of organizational models. Whether affiliation is with an independent practice association (IPA), preferred provider organization (PPO), or other organizational structure, the pressure remains on the physician to run an efficient practice.

Critical Office Workflows

There are four critical office workflows in the clinical practice environment: communication, documentation, scheduling and time management, and knowledge management workflows. Each is central to the practice of medicine and integrating these successfully leads to an efficient practice.

Communication
The practice of medicine is largely dependent upon effective communication between physician and patient and between physician and the rest of the clinical and administrative staff. In the average clinical office, the shear volume of communications between members of the staff and patients through telephone calls, mail, and office visits is staggering. In fact, many clinics have difficulty keeping up with patient demand for telephone or mail information and office visits. A typical physician may receive more

than a hundred telephone calls at the office in a single day for everything from a prescription refill, an insurance information request, and billing issues, to referrals and consultation requests. Similarly, there may be dozens of pieces of mail each day. In a typical clinic of three to five physicians in a small group, the number of calls and pieces of mail can quickly swamp all the ancillary staff and the physicians themselves. In addition, clinical practices have state and federal reporting requirements for such things as communicable diseases and, if they are participating in a managed care contract, they have other reporting requirements to fulfill as well. Clearly, all of this may affect the efficiency of the clinic in seeing the patients on the schedule that day.

In response, many clinics have added ancillary administrative staff dedicated to giving and taking telephone messages. Many clinics now have "practice management systems" that can help support the administrative component of the practice, such as payroll, accounts payable, scheduling, managed care coordination, and other administrative functions. Some clinics have established complicated phone triage systems to handle high call volume. Many physicians use dictation systems to communicate effectively with their colleagues whether they are physicians referring from primary care settings or consultants providing specialty opinions or performing procedures.

Documentation

A second critical workflow that occurs continuously throughout the day in the clinical environment is the documentation workflow. The contemporary practice of medicine calls not only for comprehensive and accurate documentation of clinical encounters to support the practice of medicine but also, regretfully, for appropriate documentation to ward off malpractice claims and assure appropriate reimbursement for services rendered. The central documentation workflow for the physician is to record a progress note for each clinical counter. At the same time, however, physicians typically are communicating routinely with other office clinical and administrative staff to get things done for the patient. Physicians may call upon their nursing support staff to assist with the clinical assessment of the patient and in performing clinical procedures. Physicians may call upon the administrative staff less directly, but the clinical encounter documentation serves as a communication vehicle to the administrative staff for purposes of generating a bill, coordinating insurance, and scheduling.

Recently, very detailed requirements for clinical documentation requirements have emerged from the Health Care Financing Administration

(HCFA) due to recurring fraud and abuse in claims for reimbursements from Medicare and Medicaid. These evaluation and management (E&M) documentation requirements place an extraordinary burden on clinicians to properly document multiple components of the clinical note to support the claim for a level of service. The E&M rules are arcane and difficult to remember for every possible visit type. Generally, physicians "undercode" defensively as routine practice. That is, a physician may indicate a level of service less than that actually rendered due to the difficulties in documenting the visit properly for the appropriate service level.

Schedule

A third critical workflow in the clinical practice environment is that of time management or, more simply, scheduling. A busy practitioner may see anywhere from 25 to 40 or more patients per day—some will be new patients, others may be scheduled for office procedures. This clinical volume generates an extraordinary amount of primary and secondary scheduling requirements. Primary scheduling requirements refers to the need to schedule patients appropriately for new or follow-up visits within a single clinic or functional group of doctors. Secondary scheduling refers to scheduling needs for patients who will have tests or procedures in other settings or patients being referred to a colleague. Effective management of these scheduling tasks includes the ability to match the availability of clinicians and other resources with the clinical needs for acute or follow-up visits. A common difficulty in scheduling arises when the clinical groups do not have access to the office schedules of their colleagues or to the schedules of an x-ray or other department where tests and procedures are to be performed. The scheduling processes in effect at most offices today, therefore, are inefficient because the patient ofttimes must be the "go-between" who must actually schedule the visit or procedure.

Knowledge Management

The fourth critical workflow in the clinical practice environment is that of knowledge management. Physicians are obligated to provide the highest quality of care possible to their patients. This means that not only must physicians pay critical attention to appropriately documenting the clinical care delivered for outcomes, or practice, analysis, but also that physicians must stay abreast of the latest medical developments that may apply to their patients. To keep their medical licenses, physicians must comply with continuing medical education (CME) requirements for states in which they are licensed to practice. Fulfilling annual CME requirements, however, does not always translate into applying the most recent insights from the medical literature to each and every clinical decision.

Certain aspects of medical practice require knowledge that is never obtained in medical school or CME settings. Knowing the various formularies for different insurance plans, or the appropriate specialists or primary care practitioners in various referral networks, is critical to the daily practice of medicine but difficult to learn and use appropriately. Other aspects of medical knowledge, like medication interaction assessment, are so complex that they are best suited for a computer that can monitor potentially adverse medication interactions, or allergies, and alert the clinician when a problem exists.

Basic Business Process and Information Management

In this section we describe basic business process management in the clinical environment. We focus on the outpatient, or office-based practice, setting because it is beyond the scope of this chapter to address business process management in the inpatient setting . Nevertheless, the core issues discussed below operate in both settings.

Given the four critical workflows described above, it is clear that effectively running a clinical practice requires attention to managing processes and managing information. The practice of medicine is one of the most information intensive occupations of the modern era. The amount of information that may apply to an individual patient is enormous when one considers all of the administrative and clinical information gathered and used in the course of the clinical encounter. Effectively managing basic business processes requires that the relevant information for each process be available. Below, we describe the six essential business processes that operate within the clinical setting to support the critical workflows described above and give examples of how electronic patient records may be used to support these processes. Table 6-1 shows how these business processes support the critical workflows.

Registration
The process of registration in the clinical environment typically means acquiring from the patient all the relevant demographic information to reliably identify that patient to the clinic and to indicate the nature of the complaint for the current visit. Critical information to be gathered in the

Table 6.1   Relationship Between Critical Workflows and Business Processes in the Clinical Environment

	Communication	Documentation	Time	Knowledge
Registration/ Check-in	X	X		X
Schedule			X	
Clinical encouter	X	X	X	X
Patient education	X	X		X
Billing	X	X		X
Patient checkout	X		X	

registration process includes information pertaining to the patient's insurance program, or guarantor, in the fee-for-service reimbursement model, or information identifying the patient as a member of a particular managed care plan in the capitated reimbursement model. In either case, good business process management includes the ability, at some level, of correlating real costs of providing care with the amount reimbursed so, ideally, the clinic managers can determine whether they are providing cost-effective care, or providing a service in a managed care contract that is profitable. Also, if the patient has any co-payment obligation on his insurance plan, these fees are received during the registration and check-in process.

It is beyond the scope of this chapter to describe in detail the information gathered by clinics during the registration process. It goes without saying, however, that there most be sufficient information regarding patient identify, demographics, primary and secondary insurance coverage, employer, important personal contacts such as next-of-kin, family members, and contact information.

Today, many clinics have both a *practice management system* that serves principally to support the administrative management of the office and a *clinical system* (or electronic medical record [EMR]) that serves to support its clinical management. Whether from a single vendor or from two vendors, these applications typically require a systems interface to allow sharing of the registration information gathered in one system with the other system. In this situation, one system is typically designated as the "master" system, the second as the "slave" system, to allow information to be gathered once and shared as appropriate.

Scheduling

The clinical schedule, whether managed with a practice management system, a clinical system, or a paper system, determines the volume of patients seen in a day, and thus is the most important determinant of the amount of work to be done. Scheduling can be accomplished using practice management software or through the clinical system. In most settings, only one system serves as the "master" scheduler; the other system (whether a practice management system or EMR) is "slaved" to the master scheduler, as is done with the registration information.

Critical scheduling issues include matching the appropriate resources and people with the clinical need, scheduling the appropriate amount of time for the clinical need, leveling scheduling requirements across resources or people, and monitoring the schedule to report on clinical productivity, appointment no-shows, on-call schedule, etc. One advantage of scheduling through a clinical system is the ability to link clinical encounter types to specific documentation forms or templates. Some EMR systems will automatically launch encounter-specific information when the patient has arrived, which can save time and improve patient care.

Clinical Encounter

The clinical encounter is at the heart of the process of delivering health care and thus the key process that drives all the business processes of medicine. During the clinical encounter, information is exchanged between patient and practitioner, decisions are made regarding a therapeutic plan and possible clinical interventions and diagnostic testing, and, hopefully, a therapeutic result is achieved for the patient. It is often reported that decisions made by the physician during the clinical encounter are responsible for >80% of the costs attributed to the health care economy.

The practice of medicine requires documentation, at a summary level at least, of the information gathered by the clinical team and the decisions made regarding the assessment and treatment of the patient. Historically, documenting the clinical encounter was primarily intended to serve as a memory jog for the physician who maintained a medical record to chronicle the events, observations, decisions, and outcomes on the patient's behalf. Additionally, the medical record served as a repository of information, which, with the patient's permission, could be reviewed for the purposes of medical research. Often, the medical record consisted of very abridged notes, abbreviations, and code words, which had meaning to the author but often not to anyone else.

Today, the medical record must serve all the foregoing functions as well as be the source document to support claims for reimbursement, legal inquiry, disability assessment, outcomes analysis, and more. Often, a patient may have many different medical records, all maintained by different clinicians, each with a partial view of the patient's comprehensive health status and history. The E&M requirements from HCFA, described above, place a considerable burden on the physician to document all components of the clinical encounter appropriately to garner proper reimbursement for the level of service.

EMR systems support the clinical documentation process through a variety of techniques and, often in the process of supporting clinical documentation, create a rich clinical database to support practice management. Most EMR systems now allow data entry through dictation and unstructured document import, free-text data entry, facilitated data entry with templates, or structured data entry using electronic forms to guide the user. These methods are described in detail in the section on Critical Clinical Information System Features That Support Business Process Re-Engineering.

Patient Education

Another essential business process in clinical practice is patient education. Physicians are obligated, along with their professional nursing colleagues, to inform patients about their health status, tests and procedures, methods for primary prevention of disease, and medical therapy. Regretfully, this process is often an afterthought and poorly addressed during the clinical encounter. Most clinics have a variety of handouts that may be given to the patient, but often they are not comprehensive or do not address the more unusual conditions. Information technology is well suited to managing such handouts, and patients themselves are searching the Internet in vast numbers to find information about their medical conditions and well-being.

EMR systems can generate most of the handouts, letters, reminders, and reports to patients and health plans that had to be manually created in the past. A few examples include camp and school physical forms, workers' compensation reports, laboratory result letters, preventive care reminders, disability forms, and HEDIS (Health Plan Employer Data and Information Set; from the National Commission of Quality Assurance) compliance reports.

Billing

After the clinical encounter, the business process of billing is central to the financial health of a clinic. As described above, practice management systems are available to support all of the financial aspects of managing a clinical office. A clinical system can assist in billing issues on several levels. Utilizing E&M software available with some systems can increase revenue and decrease risks associated with audits through proper documentation and coding. Time spent on coding is reduced when the EMR is configured to require that a coded diagnosis be entered at each visit, thus minimizing time spent looking up ICD-9 codes by providers or coders. The ultimate integration between EMR and a practice management system is an interface that allows coding and diagnosis to be entered in the exam room by the provider and then to cross directly into the billing software, thereby eliminating the need for manual entry. This can decrease labor costs and shorten claim turnaround time when properly implemented.

Patient Checkout

The last business process, which closes the clinical and administrative cycles in the clinic, is patient checkout. At checkout, a patient may be required to pay any fees beyond a co-pay that were not gathered during registration and check-in. Many other activities typically must be coordinated at patient check-out: prescriptions, scheduling and coordination of diagnostic tests and procedures, additional therapy, consultations and referral, among others. Using a clinical information system, one can improve the process of checking out by saving time and improving compliance with appropriate coding and documentation. As a physician completes a visit in the exam room, several processes can be automated or included in the provider's encounter. Instead of writing on encounter sheets or going to various staff and giving oral instructions to schedule labs, diagnostics, referrals, or follow-up, the physician can accomplish these steps while in the exam room or at a sign-out area by automatically documenting the encounter.

Using a clinical system, which includes order management, one can order lab tests, diagnostics, referrals, and follow-up appointments through point-and-click technology. The orders are automatically entered into the physician's files, then can be printed, faxed, or, using an interface, electronically communicated for completion. Time is saved and errors reduced because the codes required for billing (CPT [Common Procedural Terminology]) can be generated by the system automatically, and making duplicate forms or documentation by ancillary staff is eliminated. Referrals can be printed and given to the patient before leaving and/or bulk faxed or electronically transferred to the specialist and managed care companies. This process can be centralized and coordinated by one or many referral coordinators, thus reducing time and expense associated with managed care referral compliance.

In many clinics, the most common result of a clinical encounter is for a patient to receive a medication prescription. Another time-saver at patient checkout built into the EMR is prescription completion. The clinical encounter note automatically charts medications and prescriptions; these can be printed and given to the patient or faxed or electronically delivered to the pharmacy. This is especially useful with multiple prescriptions or the frequent vendor changes associated with managed care.

The Role of the Computer

Most of what has been written on information technology has focused on billing, coding, and practice management applications. Claims data derived from such systems are the basis for most HMO and major insurer Utilization Management (UM) and Quality Assurance (QA) programs. Because these systems rely on claims information, the granularity of the information often does not reflect the true clinical scenario, and one is limited to retrospective reviews. One can determine past utilization and track trends, often combining a retrospective review with a concurrent review process to try to manipulate results. The same holds true for quality measurements and assessment. This form of information allows an organization to know how it has done over a period of time and to compare trends, but again one is limited to retrospective, or, at best, concurrent and retrospective review.

Another limitation in utilizing claims information stems from inconsistencies in diagnosis and procedure coding. Some groups try to add another dimension to their UM and QA efforts with costly labor-intensive chart audits or reviews. So what is an organization to do? Those with an eye to being the most competitive while providing the highest quality of care must be willing to invest the time and expense on an EMR information system. This area of information technology continues to evolve but at present is only implemented in a small fraction of ambulatory practice settings. (It is estimated that <6% of all clinics have an EMR system.) EMR is often viewed as a luxury but, as the Institute of Medicine described in its landmark 1991 report and as we will demonstrate below, this technology is quickly becoming essential.

To maximize the tools of an EMR requires process re-engineering, the optimum use of interfaces, and knowledge of the business process. A keen understanding of billing/coding, HCFA regulations, NCQA/HEDIS requirements, national guidelines, managed care contracts, and Quality Improvement Process techniques is also required. Some basic and advanced process improvements are detailed below.

Critical Clinical Information System Features That Support Business Process Re-Engineering

To be competitive and successful in today's changing health care delivery systems, careful evaluation, selection, and implementation of information technology is essential. There are many vendors of software, hardware, and support packages to choose from which sometimes makes it harder to pick the right package for a particular clinic, or medical group. Before making a decision, the clinic should know what information it wants to gather, what it intends to do with the information, and then find the system that can meet the clinic's needs with the most efficiency and lowest cost. It seems easy enough, but many organizations rely on system vendors to tell them what they need instead of making their own informed decisions. What is important or works for one group may not for the next. Certainly, because of the rapidly changing trends in health care, it is difficult to anticipate all the needs of a system.

Unlike traditional paper charts, which limit information collection to free text, the EMR combines free text with data fields that may record clinical findings in a database. Once information is entered in a chart as a data element, it can be retrieved for reporting, tracking, or quality improvement initiatives. Just as there are many billing, coding, and practice management vendors, there are several EMR options to choose from. The sections below list the minimum features one should expect from an EMR system when it comes to information gathering in order to optimize basic and advanced clinical and business processes. More specifics on what can be done or accomplished after choosing and implementing an EMR system and return-of-investment issues are also highlighted.

Clinical Findings and Clinical Data

The heart of effective business, or clinical, process management is data. In any setting, if data cannot be measured, they cannot be assessed. For information to be retrieved, it must be first entered into a computer in data fields, which represent various clinical findings. It is desirable to select not only a system that has a substantial number of structured data elements but a vendor that is willing to create custom data fields for your organizational needs. Taking it one step further, the ideal situation is for the physician to custom-tailor the clinical findings directly at his home site without the vendor.

Efficiency or Ease of Data Entry

Data entry is the first step to an effective EMR system. Any obstacle to data entry will diminish the ability to retrieve the information at a later date. A system should allow multiple ways of entering information, with the least amount of effort, by physicians, nursing and medical assistant staff, or administration staff. This may be accomplished using preloaded, or custom-made, documentation forms, text templates, data flow sheets, problem lists, medication lists, or other methods.

Data Display or Retrieval

Once the information has been entered into the EMR system, it should be displayed in a format that is easy to read, supports quality or utilization efforts, and can be gathered in easy-to-use reports. The system should have built-in protocols and allow customization to prompt for preventive care and quality care based on established guidelines either at the time of service or at a future date. Utilizing these features can proactively improve an organization's HEDIS compliance, ease documenting compliance, and improve reimbursement from HMOs. One can also track internal compliance on a variety of disease management or quality improvement projects such as meeting American Diabetes Association guidelines for quality care of diabetics.

Interfaces

A system interface allows one computer to share or exchange information with another computer. Like language, there are many different ways for messages to be constructed and exchanged between computers. Many computer information interfaces are available, however, and those built on widely accepted informatics standards will be the most reliable. At a minimum, the EMR system should have a demographics interface with the practice management system, and a laboratory interface with the laboratory information system (Fig. 6-1). The time-savings and enhancements in data entry that result from having automatic data flow from the practice management system and laboratory system to the EMR help defray the initial up-front costs of the systems interface. Other interfaces can improve productivity

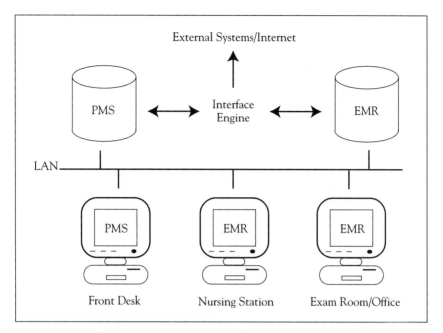

Figure 6-1 Schematic representation of basic clinic computing environment (PMS = Practice Management System; EMR = Electronic Medical Record; LAN = Local Area Network). Other systems may be in place in some settings, such as laboratory systems, dictation systems, and the Internet. If not resident within the clinic, such external systems may exchange information with the PMS or EMR through an interface engine. The schematic does not depict all the work stations in the case study. See text for details.

and decrease overhead: interfaces with the transcription system (if dictation is to remain a data entry option), the hospital information system, and the new Internet-based system interfaces for e-commerce in the health care arena. Health care e-commerce will soon include on-line eligibility determination, prescription fulfillment, referral authorization, and more. Future communication interfaces will allow orders to travel from the patient's EMR during the encounter directly to the laboratory or radiology department, decreasing the errors and time required to complete requisitions. Soon, this technology will be used to send referral requests electronically directly to insurers. Currently, internal tracking of referrals allows organizations to provide internal UM without relying on data provided by the HMOs.

Support and Implementation Issues

An effective EMR system must have strong support. Detailed training at implementation and start-up is essential. Quarterly updates provided by the vendor should be easily loaded with minimal disruption to day-to-day activities. It is important to have physician leadership in the initial and ongoing design of the system and support of the parent health care enterprise (if one exists) to assure buy-in, quality control, and maximization of its potential. The vendor should provide a detailed start-up program that describes all the necessary steps in a system conversion or the implementation of a new system before going "live". This program should be complete in all aspects of staff training, workflow re-engineering, and trouble-shooting and should be geared to all levels of computer competence. Finally, the vendor should have a proven industry track record, one that is a good indicator it will remain in business for years to come.

Integrating Clinical and Business Processes for Advanced Business Process Management and Re-engineering

Once an organization has a handle on the basic process improvements the EMR affords, more advanced opportunities can be addressed. It is important to understand these opportunities early during implementation so that proper data and information can be gathered. One cannot stress enough the importance of specific data collection to providers early in the process, even though a clinic may not use these features until later in the organization's growth. Failure to prepare in advance will delay your ability to maximize these opportunities.

Cost Accounting

Utilizing EMR's reporting features can better account for and manage utilization of services and procedures provided by your group. An example is tracking and evaluating variations in budgetary items and practice patterns. Recently it was determined in the author's clinic (JJJ) that its costs for chargeable drugs were 25% higher than in comparable family practices. Utilizing the reporting capabilities of the EMR system, the clinic was able to account for the variance. Because of recent initiative utilizing protocols, the clinic's compliance rate for pneumovax, flu vaccine, and adult and childhood immunizations was significantly greater, yet the budget was determined utilizing average practice costs. Because the clinic's compliance rate was higher than average, its costs were also higher than average. (There is always a price for improving quality.) Theoretically, these costs should be recaptured by society overall, if not for this clinic, through future prevention of disease.

Clinical Profiling

An EMR can be used for retrospective reporting on referral patterns, formulary compliance, diagnostic test utilization, and preventive care compliance for individuals or groups. The real value of an EMR, however, comes from the ability to be proactive.

Utilizing formulary decision support functions built into an EMR system, the physician's prescribing powers can be enhanced at the point of care. Providers retain ultimate control over prescribing but are able to access quickly information on costs and drug alternatives, which can reduce callbacks from patients, pharmacists, or managed care companies. For those organizations accepting risk on pharmacy costs, the savings can be significant. Recently, the author's (JJJ) clinic, working with a local HMO, implemented an incentive program in an attempt to improve formulary compliance. Taking national statistics showing estimated savings of $0.30 pmpm for each 1% increase in generic or formulary compliance, an incentive program was developed whereby each provider would be credited $0.10 pmpm for every 1% increase in generic usage or formulary compliance. If this percent exceeds 5% in any given year, then $0.15 pmpm would be credited. The HMOs are interested in saving money, but the providers are more concerned about quality and minimal hassle. The formulary decision support system allows for instant identification and notification of formulary compliance when a drug is ordered and also shows acceptable bioequivalent alternatives. The provider does not have to search for alternatives, which often decreases compliance in formulary management. The provider can choose not to substitute if clinically indicated. By maximizing savings on cases where no significant clinical difference exists, nonformulary costs can be offset. Patients, providers, and insurer all win.

Utilizing preventive care protocols built into the EMR, provider compliance with HEDIS and other quality measures can be maximized. At each patient encounter, be it telephone call, prescription refill request, or office visit, preventive care protocol reminders can be displayed and the necessary testing or service ordered. Using these capabilities, our group has been able to achieve and maintain compliance rates consistently above our peer groups. Quarterly reports are also generated for a variety of preventive care services such as adult and childhood immunizations, Pap smears, mammograms, and annual diabetic eye exams. Patients are then notified by phone or mailings generated by the EMR and the services ordered. This again improves quality but at a cost. Our group, following national guidelines established by the American Diabetes Association, has maximized compliance rates with a variety of recommended screenings including number of visits, lab testing, and diabetes eye exams. This in turn has led by word of mouth to more diabetic patients transferring to our practice. Unfortunately, one HMO recently tried to retain our withhold, claiming overutilization. We met with its medical director, armed with data showing a greater number of diabetic patients in our practice, greater compliance with quality measures, and decreased hospitalization and ER utilization rates. Our withhold was returned, and we received the maximum quality incentive bonus offered by this HMO. (One should not be penalized for doing a good job, but if you are not aware of the possible consequences and armed with supporting data to support your claims it can happen.)

Utilizing built-in practice guidelines developed locally or based on national standards, encounter forms or note templates can automatically make available a variety of user-friendly practice parameters to improve quality and reduce variability. Examples include management of chronic disease states such as diabetes, asthma, COPD, and CHF through preventive care or recommended treatment protocols. Implementation of guidelines to assist in clinical decision-making can also be built into the EMR. A few topics developed and implemented in the author's (JJJ) clinic include the management of dyspepsia, utilization guidelines for x-rays in ankle and knee injuries, acute low back pain management, and asthma management including acute and chronic management plans. Many nursing telephone triage protocols improve patient care and access for common problems including UTI, sinusitis, pharyngitis, conjunctivitis, chest pain, and abdominal pain. Taking a proactive approach through teaching and implementation has proven to be more effective than retroactive manipulation of practice patterns based on utilization data.

Contract Management

Through the use of EMR, groups can take steps to improve quality and manage costs through formulary management, diagnostic procedures and referral utilization guided by best clinical practices, reduced variation, and implementation of preventive care and disease state management protocols. Adopting a value-oriented model is fundamental in looking at the quality of care provided by any clinic:

$$Value = Quality/Cost$$

To maximize contract management, a clinic must be able to document its value to insurers (quality and cost measures). The EMR system provides you with the tools to improve and measure quality through outcomes. Opportunities to explore and maximize in managed care contracts include:

1. *Quality incentive bonuses*, based on measurable indicators that a clinic can maximize taking a proactive approach.
2. *Formulary costs*, based on whether to take risk directly on health plan formularies or indirectly through incentives for formulary compliance.
3. *Increased capitation rates or fee schedules*, based on continued documentation of quality, value, or reduced overhead costs for the HMO that manages an organization. The automation that the EMR system lends through interfaces can be used to decrease overhead expenses for the HMO in the areas of referrals, billing, precertification or prior authorization requests, and formulary management.
4. *Self-insuring, direct marketing, or managed care partnerships with HMOs*, an option if the number of providers on the same EMR system (or multiple EMR systems if a central data repository is available and they all have the above features) and the number of covered lives are large enough.

Case Study: Cost and Quality Benefits of EMR

The following case study describes how the clinic of one of the authors (JJJ) used an EMR system to support the business processes of the practice and to begin clinical process re-engineering and workflow redesign.

Clinical Setting

Capital Region Healthcare (CRHC) is an evolving Integrated Delivery Network (IDN) located in central New Hampshire. It includes three acute-care hospitals licensed for 450 beds, two visiting nurse associations performing 160,000 visits annually, an affiliation with a mental health system, and, under construction, a 100-bed assisted-living facility. In the mid-1990s, CRHC embarked upon a strategy for acquiring primary care physicians and their practices. Today, there are 20 primary care practices composed of 75 providers and a family practice residency/clinic composed of 16 residents and 8 faculty. Total revenue for the IDN is $175 million.

Recognizing the need to focus on the productivity of its primary care providers and the qualitative outcomes within those practices, CRHC began an information technology strategy that focused on implementing EMR. The focus of this case study is on the cost reductions and qualitative benefits realized from the reengineered workflows implemented in conjunction with the EMR in CRHC's pilot clinic, Family Care of Concord (FCC).

Family Care of Concord, located in Concord, New Hampshire, is a member of Capital Region Physician Group, a subsidiary of CRHC. It consists of one Board-certified family practitioner, one double Board-certified internist/pediatrician, and two nurse practitioners. Support staff includes three registered nurses, two licensed practical nurses, and three medical assistants. The practice manages 7200 active patients and averages 1200 visits/month. The payer mix is approximately 42% Managed Care, 15% Medicare, 3% Medicaid, 5% Self-Pay, and 35% Commercial Insurance. The practice contracts with seven managed care companies.

FCC opened in April 1996 using ClinicaLogic, a DOS-based EMR from MedicaLogic, Hillsboro, Oregon. In December 1997, the practice converted to Logician, MedicaLogic's Windows-based EMR. The practice uses Medisense from Compusense for its practice management and scheduling needs.

EMR Implementation Overview

Challenges
An information technology project of this magnitude faced social, financial, and technical challenges. Staff resistance to changes in traditional work roles and their readiness to use microcomputers had to be considered. Additionally, the transition team had to be sensitive to the needs and concerns of the patients as the new technology was implemented.

The initial financial investment in 1997 of $87,000 for hardware, software, and implementation was significant. Annual support costs, which include software maintenance fees, upgrades, information technology support staff, and depreciation, are $37,000. Senior management endorsed the pilot system, despite the significant initial investment and the absence of relevant research about EMR benefits.

There were technical challenges with the design and implementation of real-time interfaces. Coordinating efforts between external vendors and information technology staff was time consuming yet critical. Room size, ergonomics, and patient-provider interactions all needed to be taken into consideration when deciding where to place the PCs. Migration from the

DOS-based product (ClinicaLogic) to the 32-bit windows product (Logician) required both an extensive data conversion and a complete re-training effort.

Personnel
To successfully implement the EMR, clinical and technical expertise were required. Technical expertise included network, interface, and project management resources provided by the Information Technology department. The staff of Family Care of Concord provided clinical expertise.

Responsibilities of the technical team included:

- Sizing of server based on number of concurrent providers to accommodate adequate data storage and acceptable response time
- Configurating and installing server, network, software, and microcomputers
- Providing customized training that integrated the newly designed workflows with the application software
- Establishing a project timeline, coordinating project resources, and managing the budget

Responsibilities of the clinical design team included:

- Prioritizing feature implementation
- Creating EMR-based workflows
- Establishing clinical content for go-live and developing templates/encounter forms
- Testing of system to verify functionality and integrity

Workflow Redesign
Productivity enhancements and quality improvements do not occur merely by implementing EMR. A conscientious effort to re-engineer workflow is necessary to optimize benefits. To support the newly created workflows and promote point of care documentation, microcomputers were placed in each exam room (8), each provider's office (4), and at each clinical workstation (7).

Here is a typical patient visit using the newly implemented workflow:

- Support staff schedule patients in Medisense, which uses a one-way demographics interface to upload ADT information to Logician.
- Upon arrival, patient checks in and is acknowledged in Medisense by support staff.

- Fee slip is placed outside exam room door by support staff.
- Nurse checks computer to see if patient has arrived.
- Nurse brings patient into exam room. Customized encounter screens are assigned to the patient's electronic chart based on type of visit; vital signs are entered. Prior clinical results are automatically available.
- Physician enters exam room. By accessing the encounter form the following information is readily available: applicable protocols, medications, current problems, allergies, and directives and vitals entered by nurse. Physician updates any necessary information at the point of care, which eliminates the need for transcription. Prescriptions and patient education handouts are generated and sent to the laser printer.
- Services, tests, and referrals are entered into the system.
- Patient leaves exam room and checks out. Provider delivers prescriptions and patient education handouts. Support staff schedules any follow-up appointments. Fee slip is collected and forwarded to the central billing office.
- All paper-based documents (consult notes, insurance correspondences, etc.) are scanned. For medical/legal reasons, consent forms must be saved; the practice uses a day file system for tracking this information.

Benefits and Results

Elimination of Transcription Costs

The practice has eliminated all transcription costs by utilizing structured flow sheet views, note templates, and point-of-care documentation. The practice generates approximately 14,000 visits per year. The average CRHC practice generates approximately 35 lines of transcription per patient. At a cost of $0.11 per line the practice estimates a yearly savings of $53,900. However, it does take approximately one hour longer per week per provider to generate the documentation. That time at a blended rate of $55 per hour for four providers for 46 weeks equates to about $10,120. The net savings to the practice is thus $43,780.

Chart Pulls

At Family Care of Concord, the traditional paper chart has been eliminated. Assuming one chart pull per visit at 6 minutes each and using the average salary for the practice's support staff of $17 per hour (including benefits) the practice estimates a savings of $24,500 annually.

Prescription Generation

New prescriptions and refills are generated as a by-product of the documentation process. Each prescription takes less than 3 minutes to complete. Electronic steps include creation of prescription from documentation, automatic allergy and interaction checking, flag to physician for review and signature, fax to pharmacy. Prior to the electronic record the average time to complete a prescription was approximately 15 minutes. (A significant difference is that no chart pulls are necessary for prescription refills.) The practice generates approximately 400 prescriptions per week, most of which of are refills. Saving 12 minutes per prescription equates to a total savings of 4200 hours per year. Using the average salary for the practice's support the practice estimates a savings of $71,400 annually. An ancillary benefit of electronic prescription data is the ability to easily regenerate patient prescriptions in the event of managed care formulary changes, which has occurred eight times since the EMR was implemented.

Coding

By using the EMR system, the practice has reduced its coding time. When problems are documented in the EMR, ICD9 diagnosis codes are automatically assigned. At 14,000 visits per year and an average of two codes per visit, the practice generates approximately 28,000 diagnosis codes. Assuming that 15% of the codes needed to be researched, at an average of 5 minutes per code, we estimate that 350 hours of coding time is saved per year. Using the practice's average support staff salary, we estimate that $5950 has been saved. This feature also allows the practice to track and report patient acuity to insurance companies. Insurance companies are beginning to use this information to calculate reimbursements and quality bonuses. In the future, through the use of MedicaLogic's enhanced Evaluation and Management Code module, FCC expects to accurately meet Medicare's coding compliance regulations.

Laboratory Interface

The practice uses a laboratory interface (HBOC Star Lab) to upload results into EMR, thus reducing data entry and filing time. Results are sent every 20 minutes. The practice generates about 6500 laboratory tests annually. It took about one hour to file twenty results; therefore, the practice has saved approximately 325 hours of filing time. Using the practice's average support staff salary, we estimate a savings of $5525 annually. In addition, the system generates letters notifying patients of their results. The average turn-around time has been reduced from two or three weeks to one week, thus improving patient satisfaction.

Referrals

The provider generates referrals during the clinical encounter, eliminating the need to manually fill out paper-based payer forms. The practice generates about 3600 referrals annually. Using the system, an estimated 7 minutes per referral is saved, a total of 420 hours per year. Using the practice's average salary, we estimate a yearly savings of $7140. Overall turnaround time for a referral has been reduced from one day to within an hour. Additionally, using the reporting tools and the documentation database the practice has eliminated payer-based denials and can report provider referral patterns for payer utilization requirements.

Qualitative Reporting

The practice uses the EMR system to report its quality indicators to qualify for managed care incentive bonus programs. Typical areas targeted include Pap smears, mammograms, and diabetic eye exams. For one managed care company, the average compliance is approximately 60% for providing diabetic patients with annual eye exams. By capturing discrete data through the system, FCC was able to document that 199/200 patients received such exams. Compared to the average compliance estimate of 60%, the practice performed approximately 80 more eye exams. Nationally it is expected that about 40% of all diabetic patients tested will have a surgically correctable complication detected. Therefore, the practice estimates that it diagnosed and prevented complications in 32 patients that otherwise may have gone undetected. Based on these results, the practice has qualified for the maximum quality bonuses provided by this payer.

Drug Recalls

The practice can use EMR to generate patient letters in the event of drug recalls. Since opening the practice there have been four recalls affecting 45 patients. All patients received letters within one day of the drug recall alerts.

Hospital Inpatients

FCC generates approximately 760 hospital admissions per year. The EMR system is accessible from the emergency room and inpatient floors. Instead of dictating discharge summaries and having them transcribed by the hospital's medical records department, the physician has his discharge summary produced directly from EMR and a hard copy is forwarded to the medical records department for filing. Having access to the patient's record in the hospital setting allows providers to have up-to-date patient information to support clinical decision-making.

Patient Satisfaction
Throughout the project, concern for patient satisfaction was of paramount importance to the practice. CRHC began performing patient satisfaction surveys in the third quarter of 1997. Results are now available for the past year. The average patient satisfaction for the practices within Capital Region Physicians Group is 88.2%; FCC's average patient satisfaction is 88.9%. FCC concludes that EMR did not negatively affect patient satisfaction and in fact may have contributed to its improvement.

Benefits and Results Summary

Family Care of Concord, a group of four providers, has estimated a net annual cost reduction of approximately $121,300 for the practice, or $30,300 per provider (Table 6-2). Another method for estimating cost reduction is to compare FCC's staff-to-provider ratio to the national average (Table 6-3). FCC has a staff-to-provider ratio of 2.0. The industry average according to National MGMA survey data is 3.4. Based on a difference of 1.4 staff per provider, the practice is saving approximately 5.6 full-time equivalents annually. Using the support staff average salary of $17 per hour, the practice estimates a net annual savings of $161,000, or $40,200 per provider.

The implementation of EMR has also made several quality improvements. FCC has been able to respond faster to prescription refill requests, alert patients to drug recalls, notify patients of laboratory results, and

Table 6.2   Direct Costs Analysis.

	Annual Costs ($)
Total benefits	158,295
Total expenses	37,000
Net benefits	121,295
Net benefits per provider	30,324

Table 6.3   Staff/Provider Ratio Analysis.

	Annual Costs ($)
Total benefits	198,000
Total expenses	37,000
Net benefits	161,000
Net benefits per provider	40,250

quickly initiate referrals. Through its better documentation and reporting, the practice has demonstrated that it has exceeded the quality standards set forth by HEDIS and managed care companies.

In the overall integrated delivery network, CRHC will strive to duplicate the successful use of the EMR in each of its primary care practices. Yearly savings of between 2.25 and 3 million dollars may be achieved if the EMR is successfully implemented in the CRHC practices (75 providers). In addition, and equally as important, CRHC recognizes that numerous qualitative advantages are inherent in using an EMR. It also concludes that a successful implementation of EMR need not negatively affect patient satisfaction ratings and may, in fact, contribute to increased patient satisfaction. However, CRHC recognizes that successful EMR implementation largely depends on multiple factors including provider belief the system will make a difference, provider willingness to promote and accept change, management commitment, technical competence of staff, and leadership and project management abilities. The challenge is to duplicate FCC's success.

Conclusion

We have presented a review of critical clinical office workflow and the business processes that support it. We discussed how computers may be used for business and clinical process re-engineering and workflow redesign. A case study presented the costs of, and economic benefits arising from, implementation of an EMR system. The study demonstrates that a well-implemented EMR system saves money and improves office efficiency and patient care.

REFERENCES

1. **Ziegler R, et al.** Change Drivers: Information Systems for Managed Care. Chicago: American Hospital Publishing, 1998.

2. **Walton M.** The Deming Management Method. New York: Putnam, 1986.

3. **McLaughlin CP, Kaluzny AD.** Continuous Quality Improvement in Health Care: Theory, Implementation, and Applications. Gaithersburg, MD: Aspen Publishers, 1994.

4. **Landholt MD, Thomas F, The Coker Group.** Managing the Outpatient Medical Practice. Chicago: American Hospital Publishing, 1999.

5. **Donaldson MS, Lohr KA, Eds.** Health Data in the Information Age: Use, Disclosure, and Privacy. Washington, DC: National Academy Press, 1994.

6. **Murphy GF, Hanken MA, Waters KA.** Electronic Health Records: Changing the Vision, Philadelphia: WB Saunders, 1999.

7. **The Institute of Medicine.** The Computer-Based Patient Record: An Essential Technology for Health Care. Washington, DC: National Academy of Sciences, 1991.

7 / Identifying and Understanding Clinical Care Processes

Matthew W. Morgan

Successful EMR (electronic medical record) implementation requires a thorough understanding of the everyday activities and work habits of those providing care. This chapter addresses how to identify and analyze clinical care processes for the ultimate purpose of selecting/specifying an EMR system to support them.

Introduction

The need for an electronic medical record (EMR) can be justified on many fronts; however, one of the greatest benefits to both clinicians and patients is its ability to improve clinical care processes. Electronic medical records have the potential to be the clinician's new "black bag". Ever present, reassuring, and useful, EMR systems contain powerful instruments to assist in delivering care with less expense, in less time, and of higher quality. For those who are naysayers, remember the folly of the physician who declared "that it will ever come into general use notwithstanding its value…is extremely doubtful; there is even something ludicrous in the picture… of…physicians using this device." This was reported in *The Times* of London, not recently about the EMR, but in the 1860s about the stethoscope (1). Today the stethoscope remains an important instrument to the clinician. The challenge of the EMR system is to clearly show how it can provide more value than the stethoscope to the clinician, patient, and health care delivery system.

This chapter provides evidence of an EMR's ability to assist in the everyday activities and work habits of clinicians. The chapter offers guidance to the reader in identifying and analyzing clinical care processes for the ultimate purpose of selecting and specifying an EMR system to support them.

Historical Overview

Historically, the paper medical record has been the only medium for supporting clinical care processes. As clinical practice has evolved, however, the paper medical record has not. Paper does not support the shift away from single-physician centered care to multidisciplinary patient centered care. Paper does not allow information to be shared in a timely manner and cannot adapt to the reality that the doctor's office is being replaced by integrated delivery systems. Paper can no longer serve as an effective medium for communication between clinicians, quality control, real-time decision support, outcome analysis, medico-legal protection, and a longitudinal record of care (2). Despite these limitations, there remains a resistance to letting go of the paper medical record. Clinicians find paper to be a fast, comfortable, and user-friendly mechanism for transaction-based clinical care processes such as documentation and test ordering. Although paper provides a great deal of trouble and expense when it comes to storing, retrieving, and reviewing large amounts of data, health records departments staffed with support personnel protect clinicians from many of the mundane information management activities. Simply put, paper is a fast medium for clinicians to use at a single moment in time. It is analogous to the use of a paper day-timer compared with an electronic organizer. Those using a paper day-timer will initially be faster than those using an electronic organizer at simple activities such as finding addresses, penciling in appointments, and entering new contacts and phone numbers. It is not until information management becomes more complex, of greater volume, and required by more than one user that the electronic organizer's advantages become clear. Clinical information management has become complex and is in need of EMR systems that recognize the scarcity of clinician time and are able to replace and improve upon the limitations of the paper medical record.

Electronic medical record systems have been under development for more than 30 years. The classic EMR systems focused on integrating non-clinician-derived data such as diagnoses, laboratory results, and medication lists (2). Character-based user interfaces provided clinicians with the ability to view and trend simple results; however, clinician data entry was difficult and time-consuming. In the 1970s, several organizations developed EMR systems that went beyond this limited functionality and included the ability to document clinician-patient encounters and enable clinical alerting (3). The publication of a 1991 Institute of Medicine (IOM) report, "The Computer-Based Patient Record: An Essential Technology for Health

Care," served as the catalyst that moved the EMR agenda forward (4). The report outlined 180 features divided into 12 key attributes of a computer-based patient record (CPR):

1. Supports problem lists
2. Measures health status and function levels
3. Documents clinical reasoning and rationale
4. Provides longitudinal and timely CPR linkages with other patient records
5. Guarantees confidentiality and audit trails
6. Provides continuous authorized user access
7. Supports simultaneous user views in the CPR
8. Provides timely access to local or remote information resources
9. Facilitates clinical problem-solving
10. Supports direct data entry by physicians
11. Supports practitioners in measuring and managing costs and improving quality
12. Provides flexibility to support existing and evolving clinical needs of each specialty

In 1997, the former director and senior staff officer of the IOM CPR study described five key underpinnings of a CPR (5):

1. Clinical data dictionary
2. Clinical data repository
3. Point-of-care facility
4. Ergonomic presentation facility
5. Anticipation of clinical processes

and nine clinical attributes:

1. Supports images and multimedia data
2. Links with other patient records
3. Supports multiple formulary lists based on each patient's plan of care
4. Checks and documents RBVS (resource-based relative value scale) compliance
5. Supports multiple EDI (electronic data interchange) financial links with concurrent clinical link support
6. Supports automated history and physical examination

7. Supports icon-generated text
8. Supports SNOMED-III (Standardized Nomenclature of Medicine, 3rd ed.) and UMLS (Unified Medical Language System) vocabularies
9. Supports other integrated or interfaced technology

The advances in technology since 1991 have been enormous and rapid. Innovators from the private and public sectors have clearly shown that EMR benefits to clinical care processes are real. And, although their use is not widespread, the number of commercial EMR systems that have the potential to provide the 12 key attributes listed above is expanding and provides hope that EMR use will become the standard of practice for all clinicians. Despite this hope, however, the reader must be aware that EMR development remains in its infancy. No single EMR system can provide comprehensive clinical information management that seamlessly integrates and coordinates clinical care processes across the spectrum of health care delivery (6). A practical and realistic strategy to the selection and implementation of an EMR is required. This strategy should clearly articulate and convince clinicians as well as other stakeholders that it will result in the improvement of care upon implementation and will have the ability to grow, mature, and provide additional value in the years to come. With this caution in mind, successful EMR selection and implementation today *is* possible, and rapid and measurable improvements in clinical care processes can be achieved.

Overview of Clinical Care Processes

Identifying the clinical care processes and understanding how EMR systems can improve patient care are crucial. Without this understanding the selection, purchase, implementation, and utilization of an EMR will at best fall short of expectations and at worst result in clinician rebellion, front-page headlines, and the abandonment of the EMR system (7).

The Institute of Medicine's list of 180 features, 12 categories, 5 key underpinnings, and 9 additional clinical attributes is extensive. However, EMR systems can have over 2000 features and functions that directly or indirectly support clinical care processes (8). To prevent the reader from becoming overwhelmed and to assist in a practical approach to the identification and selection of EMR systems that support clinical care processes, this chapter focuses on those processes or activities that consume the majority of clinician time. The proposed list is not exhaustive and serves merely as an introduction to the clinical benefits of an EMR. Additional sources of information can be found in the References.

As clinicians, we spend most of our time retrieving, reviewing, tracking and trending, documenting, ordering, deciding, communicating, and educating. For the purpose of this chapter the following 10 major clinical care processes will be discussed:

1. Time management and scheduling
2. Reviewing diagnostic test results and clinical documents
3. Diagnostic test ordering
4. Patient encounter documentation
5. Medication prescribing
6. Electronic signatures
7. Clinical decision support
8. Disease guidance
9. Data analysis and report generation
10. Patient education

In evaluating EMR systems, it is helpful to list which of the above clinical processes are of most importance and in most need of change. Table 7-1 can be used to assist in this prioritization exercise when evaluating EMR systems (9).

Time Management and Scheduling

Although time management and scheduling is not by strict definition a clinical care process, without this the delivery of patient care can be slow and painful for clinicians and patients alike. EMR systems should provide time management and patient scheduling capabilities that are truly integrated into clinical care. An example of an EMR integrated scheduling system is depicted in Figure 7-1. As can be seen in this example, patient appointments for the day are accessible from within the EMR system. New appointments, cancellations, and changes, as well as staffing, room availability, and equipment resources, are also viewable. The view can be easily changed from "By Day" to "By Week" or "By Month". Physician notification of patient arrival is automatic. In addition to showing the scheduling function, Figure 7-1 depicts how clinician time management is improved. Flags and alerts inform the clinician of conditions requiring action; urgent

Table 7-1   Checklist for Evaluating EMR Impact on Clinical Care Processes.
(Will the EMR's method of (clinical care process) provide...?; e.g., Will the EMR's
method of reviewing results provide...?)

Factor	Yes	No
Greater chart availability		
Less time-consuming care for clinician		
Less time-consuming care for patient		
Better diagnosis		
Better therapy		
Better patient compliance		
Improved communication between clinicians		
Improved communication between clinician and patient		
Better clinician knowledge		
Better patient knowledge		
Less expensive care		
Higher quality care		

Adapted from Finley SW. The electronic medical record as a tool to improve patient care: hypothetical and practical opportunities. Journal of the Healthcare Information and Management Systems Society. 1997;11:5-11.

documents are flagged in red; and all incoming documents are placed in a clinician "in-box".

This type of solution, offered by many EMR vendors, has been termed the *standard clinical desktop*. The desktop provides the clinician with a complete view of the day's activity and access to the other clinical care processes. From the desktop, the clinician can quickly access the charts of patients scheduled for the day, know the status of the patient encounter (i.e., pending, arrived, cancelled), reserve protected time, and schedule new appointments. In addition, the desktop should serve as the gateway to all other required clinical information management tools such as e-mail and the Internet. Until recently most EMR vendors provided their own scheduling solutions; however, it is now possible to integrate off-the-shelf scheduling systems into some EMR systems. The desktop should also be customizable: A physician's desktop may be different from a nurse's desktop, which in turn may be different from an office assistant's desktop. A

The currently logged-in user is shown in the title bar.

Flags—electronic sticky notes—inform clinicians of conditions requiring action.

Easily add the problems you frequently treat to build disease or specialty custom problem lists on the fly.

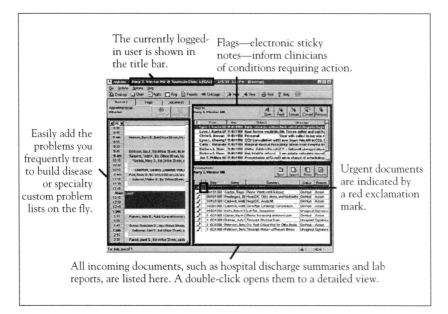

Urgent documents are indicated by a red exclamation mark.

All incoming documents, such as hospital discharge summaries and lab reports, are listed here. A double-click opens them to a detailed view.

Figure 7-1 EMR integrated scheduling system and clinical desktop.

well-designed, easy-to-use clinical desktop will improve patient flow and aid in the delivery of efficient patient care.

Important Point. *When evaluating EMR systems, determine if a standard clinical desktop is offered, whether it can integrate with off-the-shelf scheduling systems and Internet applications, and whether it can be easily customized by the clinician.*

Checklist. The EMR's method of time management and scheduling should provide

✓ Greater chart availability
✓ More time saved by the clinician
✓ More time saved by the patient

Reviewing Diagnostic Test Results and Clinical Documents

Clinicians spend a significant amount of time retrieving and reviewing patient results—up to 25% of a clinician's day (10). Without the dedicated support of health records departments and clerical staff this percentage would increase significantly. EMR systems have been successful at solving many of the problems associated with finding, retrieving, organizing, and reporting patient results that exist with paper medical records (11). EMR systems make it possible to quickly inform not only a single clinician but many clinicians of critical-patient laboratory results, previous ECGs, recent chest radiographs, past hospital discharge summaries, and so on. Important clinical data are available 24 hours a day, 7 days a week when accessed though an EMR. EMR systems can greatly assist in providing the right information, to the right person, at the right place, at the right time.

Leading EMR systems should be able to clearly demonstrate comprehensive result review functionality. Figure 7-2 shows an EMR results reviewing screen. The results are patient centered, well organized, easy to find, and clearly indicated as normal, abnormal, or critical. Results include numerical data, text, and images and may also include audio and video files.

Structured data, such as laboratory results and ECG images, and unstructured data, such as word-processed documents, should be available to the clinician for review. However, comprehensive results reviewing takes careful planning, willingness to change workflow, and a significant amount of work solving the technical and human issues of data entry. Without data input/entry there are no results to review. This can occur through a number of modalities (Table 7-2) (12).

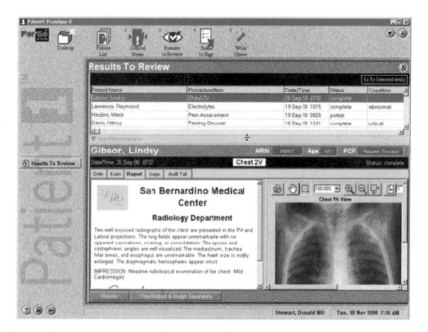

Figure 7-2 EMR results reviewing: clinical notes and images.

Most EMR systems utilize all of the modalities given in Table 7-2 for data input. However, interfaces with departmental systems such as laboratories, pharmacy, diagnostic imaging, and bedside monitors can result in more efficient, less manual data entry. Interfaces allow for the communication of electronic data between systems. For this to work, systems must be able to understand each other or talk the same language; this requires message standards of data exchange. The most common message standards are ASTM, HL7, and DICOM; see Chapter 3 for details. In addition, although point-to-point interfaces are common, a more sophisticated method involves the use of an interface engine that allows HL7 messages to be communicated between numerous systems.

The automatic capture of structured data has many advantages. An alternative approach is to utilize scanning to input documents into an EMR. Although almost any piece of paper can be scanned, this approach has many disadvantages and severely limits its usefulness as a comprehensive approach. Specifically, scanned documents must be indexed to enable efficient retrieval. In addition, an illegible hand-written note will continue to be of little use as a scanned document. More importantly, a scanned document remains a passive document; there is no opportunity for the EMR system to interact and interpret its data, a prerequisite for clinical decision

Table 7-2   Mechanisms for Data Input.

Mechanism (Examples)	Advantages	Disadvantages
Manual (Patient demographics)	Relatively inexpensive	Labor intensive Data entry errors
Automatic (Lab instruments, monitors)	Rapid input No data entry errors	Expensive Interface required
Bar codes (Specimen handling)	Rapid input No data entry errors	Expensive Interface required
Scanning (Hand-written notes)	Rapid input No data entry errors	Expensive Interface required
Word processing uploading (Dictated/transcribed notes)	Rapid input No data entry errors	Expensive Interface required
Voice recognition	Alternative to dictation	Data entry errors Interface required

Adapted from Overhage M, McDonald CJ. Medical records systems for office practice. In: Computers in Clinical Practice. Philadelphia: American College of Physicians; 1995:19-36.

support and data analysis. At best, scanning should be reserved as an adjunct for the entry of clinical data that are either too difficult or too time-consuming/expensive to capture electronically and for data that have little clinical decision support value.

When attempting to determine which modality to utilize for capturing patient data it is helpful to assess the value of the data. Being able to establish by consensus what constitutes core clinical data form noncore clinical data will assist in this valuation. One institution's core clinical data set for inpatients is outlined in Table 7-3.

For this example, a core clinical document was defined as one that was required for "urgent clinical decision-making during a present or future inpatient encounter". The implications of this definition were clinical, to provide rapid access to patient data, and administrative, to allow for the closure of the health records department on weekends and nights. As can be seen from Table 7-3, diagnostic test results were considered core data. This table also illustrates the reality that core clinical data often reside not only on paper but also in more than one electronic data repository. The reliance on hybrid paper-electronic medical records is costly and inefficient. A main objective of EMR implementation should be to provide a reliable infrastructure that does not require such redundancy.

Another useful adjunct approach for the electronic capture and storage of unstructured data is the automatic uploading of word-processed documents into an EMR. Because dictation and transcription of clinician notes contribute significantly to the medical record of most clinical practices, uploading these documents to the EMR is advantageous and replaces the need to store them as part of the paper medical record. Some EMR systems provide automatic upload capabilities that require indexing by the transcriptionist based on a unique patient identifier, the date of dictation, and type of report. However, like scanned documents, uploaded unstructured word-processed documents have minimal clinical decision support capability.

Important Point. *When evaluating EMR systems, determine the best modality for data entry for each data type, realizing that a willingness to change current practices may be needed to take advantage of EMR capabilities. Ensure that vendors are able to provide required interfaces and the needed data entry modalities. Consider all costs for data entry including the development of interfaces, ongoing support of interfaces, scanners, hardware and software, and labor.*

Once the data input issues have been solved, attention can be turned to the data output or viewing functionality of the EMR. Some of the required features are outlined in Table 7-4.

Table 7-3   University Health Network's Core Clinical Data Set.

Document	Exists in EMR	Exists in Other Electronic Databases	Exists on Paper
Admission Summary (Face Sheet)	X		X
Discharge Summary	X		X
Patient Safety Assessment	X		X
Nursing Admission Assessment	X		X
Emergency Services Report			X
Physician Progress Notes			X
Social Worker Notes			X
Home Care Report			X
Radiological Reports (including Nuclear Medicine Report)	X	X	X
Electrocardiogram			X
Echo Laboratory Report		X	X
Current Angiogram Report from Cardiologist		X	X
All Labs Currently on Ulticare	X		
X-ray Images			X
Anesthesia Record			X
Pathology Report (including Bone Marrow Report)	X		X
Operative Note	X		X
Transfusion Record Mount Sheet			X
Medications		X	X
Living Will			X
Letter/Clinic Note	X	X	X
Chemo Flow Sheet			X

Adapted from University Health Network, Toronto, Canada.

Table 7-4   Important Features of EMR Results Reviewing.

Easy to navigate	Patient centered	Summary and details
Searchable	Reference ranges	Normal, abnormal, critical
Trending/graphing	Flagging	Acknowledge/sign
Copy and paste	Print	E-mail

When reviewing results, the key goals are to save clinician time, prioritize results, and ensure that critical information is not missed. To accomplish these goals results must be patient specific and easy to navigate within a patient's chart and from one patient chart to the next. Clinicians should also be provided with a snapshot of the patient (Figure 7-3).

In addition, a summary of the results and further detailed information should be available to the clinician for review. Reference ranges for normal results should be provided, and abnormal results should be indicated. Critical results should be brought to the attention of the clinician immediately. Some EMR systems now use push technology, such as auto-paging and auto-e-mailing of critical lab results, allowing clinicians to be informed of results as soon as they become available (13). Results review functionality should include the ability to quickly trend and graph a series of results, thereby enhancing interpretation and allowing important trends to be identified. Results that require further action should be flagged, and the ability to electronically acknowledge and sign results must be available. Finally, in order to improve communications with others, results in the form of reports should be available for copying and pasting to e-mail and printing to paper. The ability of clinicians to customize results reviewing to meet their own personal workflow is also advantageous.

Important Point. *When evaluating EMR systems, the results reviewing functionality should provide clinicians with flexible and customizable views of patient results. Results should be indexed and stored in a manner that is intuitive to the clinician and provides rapid access. Results should be clearly flagged as normal or abnormal, and mechanisms to immediately alert clinicians of critical results should be available.*

Checklist. The EMR's method of reviewing diagnostic test results and clinical documents should provide
- ✓ Greater chart availability
- ✓ More time saved by the clinician
- ✓ Better diagnosis

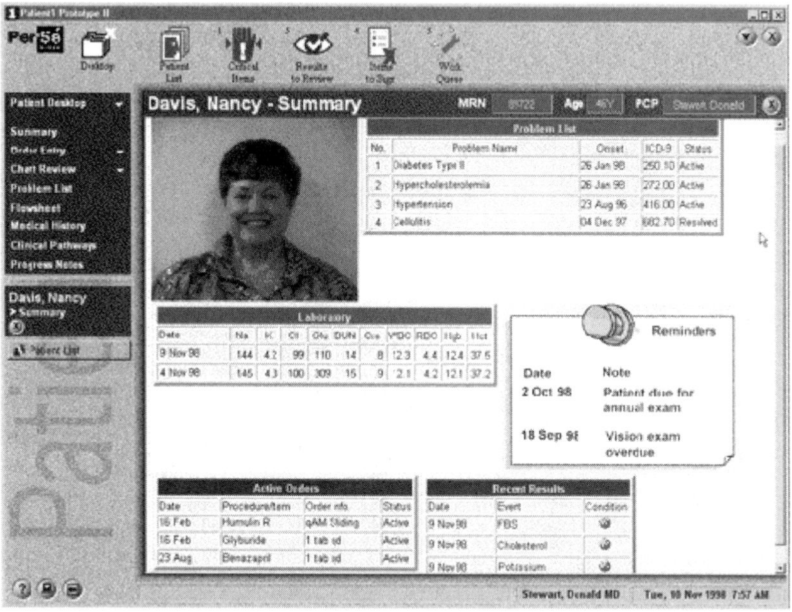

Figure 7-3 EMR results reviewing: lab tests and active orders.

✓ Improved communication between clinicians

Diagnostic Test Ordering

One of the great attributes of EMR systems is the ability to perform direct clinician order entry, which can save time, improve diagnostic test utilization, improve care, and cut costs. Yet one of the main reasons that EMR implementations have failed to live up to expectations has been the unwillingness of clinicians to embrace order entry. The clinicians who historically have been the most unwilling have been those responsible for the vast majority of diagnostic test ordering—that is, the physicians. The main reason for this reluctance has been the negative impact of order entry on physicians' time. Order entry takes time, and it takes longer to order an individual test electronically compared with ordering it on paper, especially if support staff have completed all the necessary patient demographic information and simply hand a paper requisition to a physician for signature. At first glance, from the physicians' perspective, direct EMR order entry appears time consuming, and it has been argued that it is "clerical work".

The arguments in favor of direct order entry by clinicians are numerous. First, if properly designed, electronic order entry of a single test can be easy and quick. Second, if ordering more than one test, the use of EMR order sets and order protocols clearly saves time compared with paper requisitions. Third, there is the ability to suggest or advise the ordering clinician on choice of test at the time of order entry. Fourth, all the benefits of reviewing results, such as at-a-glance trending/graphing, clinical alerting, and flagging are not possible without someone assuming the role of order entry. Fifth, the ability to provide ordering clinicians with regular reports on diagnostic order utilization can be readily accomplished through electronic report writing. Sixth, cost savings can be realized by the elimination of the production, processing, filing, and storage of paper requisitions. Seventh, errors in interpreting hand-written orders are eliminated.

Important Point. *If there is unwillingness to plan for and enforce order entry by physicians as part of the proposed EMR solution, the return on investment from cost, quality-of-care, and patient safety perspectives may be limited.*

Once physician order entry is confirmed as a goal of the EMR implementation, the next step is to evaluate the order entry capabilities of EMR systems. Of paramount importance is the user interface and design of order entry screens. In general, those that are designed by clinicians for clinicians are more likely to succeed. Most EMR vendors utilize clinical specialists to assist in the development of order entry. When evaluating EMR systems the order entry process should be tested with several different types of simple orders (e.g., INR daily × 5 then daily × 3 then weekly and CT head, stat). Counting both the number of screens required to place an entire order and the number of seconds it takes will provide valuable information about the user interface design and the EMR's on-line transaction processing (OLTP) capacity. A simple order like the one above should require the clinician to navigate through only one or two screens and take only several seconds to complete. Moving from one screen to the next should be instantaneous in a production environment for simple transactions. The EMR vendor should guarantee response time of less than a second per screen for simple transactions. Figure 7-4 depicts a well-designed, user-friendly clinician order entry screen.

Besides simple order entry, the ability to order groups of tests, known as *order sets*, is an important feature of the EMR. This provides the opportunity to build disease-specific order protocols (e.g., admission orders for atypical community-acquired pneumonia). Complete protocols require the ability to order not only diagnostic tests but also medications and nursing/allied health orders as well (see Disease Guidance section).

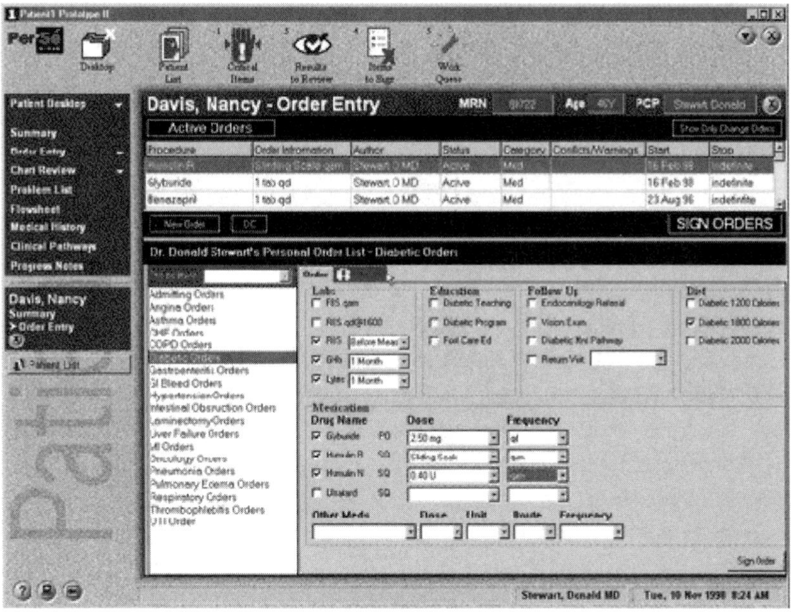

Figure 7-4 Diagnostic test order entry.

Important Point. *When evaluating EMR systems, diagnostic test ordering should be easy and fast. The vendor should guarantee adequate OLTP response times. Simple orders as well as order sets and disease specific protocols should be available. It is strongly recommended that the entire process be thoroughly evaluated in a production environment similar to your own in order to clearly determine the impact on clinician time.*

Checklist. The EMR's method of direct clinician order entry should provide

✓ Better diagnosis

✓ Less expensive care

✓ Higher quality care

Patient Encounter Documentation

As Table 7-2 has shown, there are several data entry modalities for inputting data into the EMR system. Documentation of the patient encounter provides additional challenges for the EMR. Historically, EMR systems have relied heavily on the use of dictation, transcription, and uploading word-processed documents. Scanning of printed patient encounter documents is also possible. As previously mentioned, these two modalities support unstructured reports and do not take full advantage of EMR potential. Table 7-5 summarizes the advantages and disadvantages of structured and unstructured documents.

The ultimate goal is to develop efficient mechanisms to convert unstructured patient encounter documents into structured electronic forms that can be completed before, during, and after the patient encounter by the clinician.

The ease of generating unstructured documents is significantly outweighed by the benefits of structured reports as long as the time required and the effort involved in completing electronic forms are acceptable. EMR vendors that truly understand this have designed electronic forms and tools to achieve this goal. An example of an EMR encounter form is depicted in Figure 7-5.

Electronic forms may contain both structured and free-text entries that can be rapidly completed using input devices such as the keyboard, mouse, pen, scanner, and voice-recognition microphones. The structured data can be coded allowing for real-time clinical alerting and retrospective data

Table 7-5   Advantages and Disadvantages of Structured and Unstructured Documents.

Unstructured Documents (Handwriting and Dictating)	Structured Documents (Electronic Forms)
Free text	Minimizes free text
Uncoded	Coded
Limited searching	Comprehensive searching
Limited clinical decision support opportunities	Maximizes clinical decision support opportunities
Limited data analysis and report generation	Maximizes data analysis and report generation
Supports clinician's historical workflow	Requires changing clinician's workflow
Cannot be uploaded to other databases (i.e., billing and coding)	Can be uploaded to other databases (i.e., billing and coding)
Minimal clinician work	Increased clinician work
Increased clerical work	Minimal clerical work

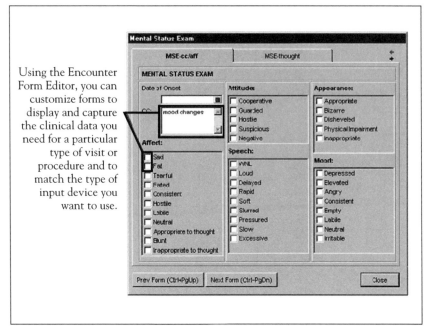

Using the Encounter Form Editor, you can customize forms to display and capture the clinical data you need for a particular type of visit or procedure and to match the type of input device you want to use.

Figure 7-5 Patient encounter documentation.

analysis and report generation. In addition, structured data are searchable and can be automatically sent to other systems that support patient care de-livery such as coding and billing applications.

Electronic forms can be customized to display and capture required data such as those required to meet the Health Care Financing Administration Evaluation and Management guidelines (Fig. 7-6) (14).

Electronic forms work well for encounters that can be easily standard-ized and are relatively brief in duration such as office follow-up visits (e.g., for hypertension), short procedures (e.g., colonoscopy), and progress notes. Electronic forms are also practical for problem list documentation. Problem lists that utilize structured codeable data not only serve to describe impor-tant clinical conditions but can also be proactive in nature, initiating ac-tions such as the launching of disease guidance information, clinical alerts, and health maintenance reminders. An example of an EMR problem list is shown in Figure 7-7. Problem list documentation can also be used for billing and other administrative purposes.

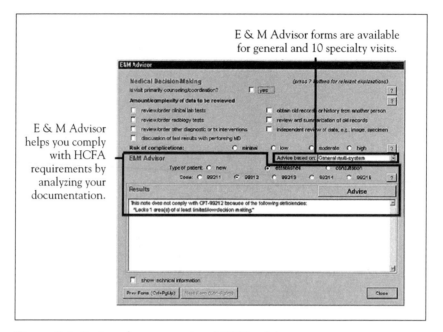

E & M Advisor forms are available for general and 10 specialty visits.

E & M Advisor helps you comply with HCFA requirements by analyzing your documentation.

Figure 7-6 Patient documentation: HCFA advisor.

The complexity of converting unstructured documents to structured reports increases significantly as the length of the document increases. For example, consultant letters, discharge summaries, and surgical reports are often lengthy and complex. It may not be practical to try and convert these to electronic forms. However, the combination of electronic forms with word-processing templates is another option to consider; not only does this decrease the need for transcription services, it provides an opportunity to provide high level coding to otherwise unstructured documents.

Patient encounter documents that are generated outside the organization such as consultants' reports or outside imaging study reports usually arrive on paper. The most practical option for including these reports within EMR is scanning. Another possibility is to request that the reports be sent via e-mail as encrypted word-processing attachments, then index and upload them into the EMR system.

Important Point. *When evaluating EMR systems, the ability to document patient encounters using structured data provides significant added value. These benefits must be balanced by the work required to convert unstructured data to*

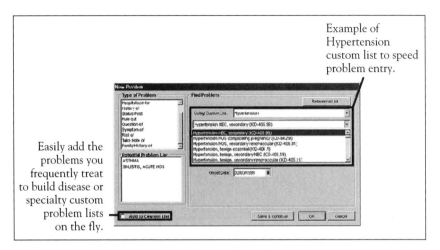

Figure 7-7 Patient documentation: problem list.

structured data and the ability to provide a user-friendly and efficient solution for data capture by clinicians. EMR systems should provide flexible encounter forms and tools to allow for easy customization and come preloaded with an inventory of useful clinical encounter forms.

Checklist. The EMR's method of documenting patient encounters should provide

✓ Greater chart availability

✓ Improved communications between clinicians

Medication Prescribing

Medications account for a significant and growing health care expenditure. The aging population, the approval of an increasing number of new and expensive pharmaceuticals, and the inappropriate and overuse of medications are a just a few of the reasons for this. Adverse drug events are a leading cause of death, and prescribing errors are not uncommon (15). Many organizations have called for direct EMR ordering of medications by physicians (16). Physician order entry using EMRs has been shown to be an effective mechanism for decreasing adverse drug events, decreasing medication errors, decreasing costs, and improving patient care (14, 17).

EMR-enabled prescriptions require the same considerations as diagnostic test order entry and documentation. For physicians to buy in, it must be an easy, fast, user-friendly process that can be successfully integrated into physician workflow in both inpatient and outpatient practice. The additional cost/value must be clearly shown in a form of medication management that includes clinical alerting, medication tracking, automatic renewals, and printing and faxing capabilities. EMR systems should allow for quick and easy viewing of current and previous medications, dosages, and duration of therapy. Writing initial prescriptions and refills should be aided by drop-down menus that contain medications listed on formularies. Suggested dosages, recommended duration of therapy, and additional physician and patient educational information should be easily accessible. Substitutions should be possible, and the ability for prescriptions to be printed, sent electronically to in-house pharmacy systems, or automatically faxed to outside pharmacies should be available. An example of medication order entry is shown in Figure 7-8.

One of the advantages of medication prescribing using the EMR is the opportunity to guide and advise the clinician's therapeutic choices and to alert clinicians about possible adverse interactions. Table 7-6 describes some of the common forms of medication clinical alerting that can be incorporated into EMR medication order entry.

Clinical alerting consists of on-line advice that occurs in real-time as the clinician is prescribing medications. In addition to informing the clinician of potential interactions, it may also suggest alternative medications for consideration. Automatic reference to therapeutic guidelines such as locally developed antimicrobial guidelines for common infections may be in-

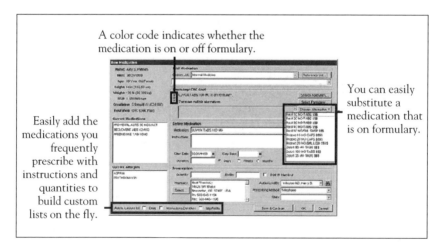

A color code indicates whether the medication is on or off formulary.

You can easily substitute a medication that is on formulary.

Easily add the medications you frequently prescribe with instructions and quantities to build custom lists on the fly.

Figure 7-8 Medication order entry.

corporated. Additional information may also include duration of therapy, route of administration, and cost of therapy where appropriate. Many EMR vendors use medication management programs of other commercial vendors that include clinical alerting. The extent of integration and advantages and disadvantages of such programs should be clearly explained and understood as part of EMR evaluation and selection.

A recent report of one organization's EMR medication management functionality revealed several benefits (18):

1. Reductions in prescription transcription errors
2. Shorter turn-around time from drug order to drug administration
3. Fewer medication errors
4. Shorter time to therapeutic anticoagulation in the treatment of deep-vein thrombosis
5. More appropriate vancomycin use and lower rates of vancomycin-resistant enterococci.

Important Point. *When evaluating EMR systems, medication prescribing can provide many advantages over hand-written prescriptions and can signifi-*

Table 7-6   Medication Clinical Alerting.

Type of Alert	Description	Example
Drug/drug	Identifies drug combinations that may have serious adverse interactions	Warfarin and aspirin
Drug/laboratory	Identifies laboratory values that could affect drug dosages, commonly renal and liver abnormalities	Digoxin-potassium Aminoglycosides-creatinine Liver?
Drug/pregnancy	Identifies drugs contraindicated in pregnancy	Warfarin
Drug/condition	Identifies drugs that may be contraindicated with certain medical conditions	NSAIDS in peptic ulcer disease
Drug/pediatric	Identifies reduced drug dosing in children (BMI)	Antibiotics
Drug duplication	Identifies co-administration of similar classes of drugs	Lorazepam and valium

cantly improve patient safety and reduce costs. Medication clinical alerting soft-
ware should be fully integrated into EMR systems.

Checklist. The EMR's method of direct clinician order entry (pharmacy) and medication management should provide

✓ Better therapy
✓ Less expensive care
✓ Higher quality care

Electronic Signature

EMR systems provide clinicians with the ability to review results, place orders, document encounters, and prescribe medications. Ensuring that these clinical care processes are appropriately authorized and tracked is accomplished with electronic signature. Electronic signature allows the clinician to access information, handle action items, and place orders and requests from any location at which the EMR is available. Electronic signature is achieved by simply clicking on the item's sign button. For viewing numerous results simultaneously (e.g., a trend of INR values), summary electronic signature should be available, allowing all data points to be viewed and acknowledged with a single click. All items for electronic signature may be kept in a queue similar to an e-mail in-box, providing clinicians with an easy-to-use mechanism that ensures important data are not overlooked. Once signed, items become a permanent part of the patient's EMR and are automatically removed from the clinician's in-box. An example of electronic signature is shown in Figure 7-9. Provision of thoroughly integrated/multilevel securities within the EMR system ensures that appropriate authorization occurs.

Important Point. *When evaluating EMR systems, electronic signature from authorized users allows items that require review or action to be easily tracked and signed from wherever the EMR system is available. Items along with signature acknowledgement become a permanent part of the EMR that can be retrieved and audited at later dates.*

Checklist. The EMR's method of electronic signature should provide

✓ Greater chart availability
✓ Less time-consuming care for the clinician

Clinical Decision Support

If the EMR is the clinician's black bag for the 21st century, the most powerful instrument contained within is clinical decision support (CDS). Defined

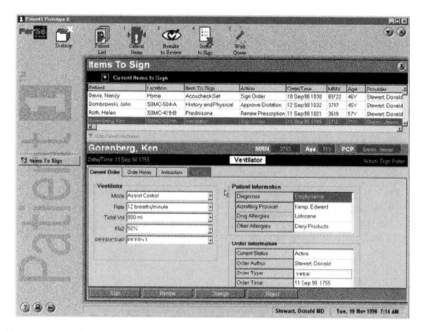

Figure 7-9 Electronic signature.

broadly, CDS systems "can be any automated tool that helps clinicians improve the delivery or management of patient care. In its ideal sense, CDS is a set of knowledge-based tools that are fully integrated with both the clinician workflow components of an EMR and a repository of complete and accurate clinical data" (19). Examples of CDS capabilities designed to improve clinical care processes are highlighted in Table 7-7 (20). Many EMR vendors provide off-the-shelf CDS in the form of simple clinical alerting and reminders. The ability to provide on-line access to guidelines is also available in most EMR systems. More complex CDS such as interpreting, diagnosis, and suggestions requires more sophisticated CDS logic.

The evidence of the benefits of EMR-integrated CDS continues to grow, both in terms of patient care improvement and cost savings. A recent prospective study of an EMR-CDS system designed to disseminate expert knowledge on antimicrobial therapies in an ICU setting reports patient care improvement as well as cost savings (19). Specifically the EMR-CDS cohort had fewer drugs ordered with known patient allergies and experienced less antibiotic susceptibility mismatches and adverse events. In addition, reductions in excessive drug dosages and length of stay contributed to

Table 7-7   Functions of CDS Systems.

Function	Example
Alerting	Highlighting a critical blood potassium level
Reminding	Annual flu vaccine
Critiquing	Rejecting duplicate diagnostic test orders
Interpreting	Diagnosing atrial fibrillation on ECG
Predicting	Predicting mortality risk from a severity-of-illness score
Diagnosing	Listing a differential diagnosis for patient with chest pain
Assisting	Modifying antibiotic choice for patient with renal failure
Suggesting	Generating suggestions for mechanical ventilator weaning

Adapted from Randolph A, Haynes RB, Wyatt JC, et al. Users' guides to the medical literature; XVIII. How to use an article evaluating the clinical impact of a computer-based clinical decision support system. JAMA. 1999;282:67-74

lower overall hospital costs. A time-motion evaluation revealed that it took on average 14 minutes for clinicians to retrieve the same information that the EMR CDS system retrieved in 3.5 seconds. This landmark study clearly showed that CDS systems effectively integrated into the EMR can truly enhance clinical care processes.

A systematic review of prospective controlled studies examined the effects of computer-based clinical decision support systems on physician performance and patient outcomes (21). Although many of the studies used CDS systems that were not integrated into EMR, the results for the most part are encouraging. The review reported that CDS research is becoming more common and the quality of the research is improving. CDS systems were shown to enhance clinical performance for drug dosing (e.g., warfarin dosing), preventive care (e.g., vaccine compliance), and other aspects of medical care (e.g., hypertension management) but were not shown to be effective for diagnostic decision making such as the evaluation of chest pain. The effect of CDS systems on patient outcomes remains mainly unproven due to the lack of published studies in this area.

EMR-integrated CDS systems rely on the ability of the system to gather data, analyze data in relation to predefined rules, draw conclusions, then send this information to the clinician in a predetermined manner. Simply put, it requires computer processing that can perform a series of complex and sophisticated "If this, do that" actions. The most successful EMR-integrated CDS systems have come into existence through decades of work by computer programmers and clinical informatics specialists who have taken advantage of home-grown proprietary systems to build their own CDS systems using rules engines and data dictionaries. An example of this is LDS's Health Evaluation through Logical Processing system (HELP) (22). One of the greatest challenges and disappointments in clinical informatics has been the inability to replicate CDS successes in other institutions. One of the main reasons for this has been the proprietary nature of EMR systems. The languages used and resulting rules and logic operate within a single system and often cannot be applied outside the walls of the institution that developed the CDS system. The need to develop CDS standards that will allow wider applicability is being advanced by numerous organizations and supported by many EMR vendors (23).

Important Point. *Determine what, if any, standards the EMR-CDS functionality supports and how easy it is to build, customize, maintain, and support existing and new CDS interventions. When evaluating EMR systems, a clear understanding of the tools used to build the system is needed to determine if they will meet your needs.*

Historically one of the arguments that has been made in opposition to EMR systems is the notion that CDS systems will dictate to clinicians the only course of action. The resulting disastrous consequences of clinicians being replaced by computers and patients falling prey to technology misadventures makes for good fiction but represents a hollow threat in the real world of clinical practice. CDS systems do not dictate policy; they simply disseminate information and expertise that can be heeded or ignored by clinicians. They represent powerful tools to assist the clinician in the gathering and analysis of clinical data and present information and expertise for consideration in real-time at the point of clinical decision-making. CDS systems should be viewed as on-line advisors available 24 hours a day at the point of clinical decision-making.

There are many obstacles to the implementation of a successful EMR-CDS system. The following critical success factors have been offered to assist in achieving clinician acceptance (24):

1. *Frequent Direct Contact Between the Clinician and Computer*—CDS interventions are most effective when the clinician is the one who is directly exposed to the intervention. Clinicians need to embrace EMR as an essential tool for clinical practice.
2. *Existence of a Rich Clinical Database*—CDS interventions require the analysis of data on many patient factors. EMR systems that

integrate or have ready access to all the necessary data are more likely to succeed.

3. *Leadership Support*—Clinical and administrative leadership must provide strong support for EMR-CDS initiatives. At budget time, these initiatives must not be seen as competing for scarce patient care dollars but rather as initiatives essential for effective care delivery.

4. *Track Record*—Establishing early wins with basic CDS initiatives (e.g., drug allergy alerting) should make clinicians more willing to give more complex initiatives an opportunity to prove their worth.

5. *Software Quality Review*—Ensuring that the CDS software performs in the manner that it is supposed to perform is critical for user acceptance. CDS interventions that result in poor advice or inaccurate advice must be avoided.

6. *Impact Assessment*—Showing clinicians that CDS interventions can improve patient care in their own clinical practice will assist in converting the reluctant volunteer to a committed supporter.

Although these critical success factors are offered for CDS initiatives, they are just as relevant and important for all aspects of EMR implementation.

Important Point. *When evaluating EMR systems, set modest goals for CDS at the outset. Early CDS interactions should be based on clinical priority, opportunities, and EMR functionality. Implementing the entire spectrum of CDS requires expertise, experience, and a significant organizational commitment.*

Checklist. The EMR's method of clinical decision should provide
✓ Less time-consuming care for the clinician
✓ Better diagnosis
✓ Better therapy
✓ Better clinician knowledge
✓ Less expensive care
✓ Higher quality care

Disease Guidance

Clinicians are inundated with clinical guidelines on a daily basis. Thousands of clinical practice guidelines (CPG) have been published in the last decade, yet even the best evidence and resulting guidelines are often ignored. In a survey of physicians' attitudes on CPGs, only 52% reported using them at least once per month, citing difficulty integrating paper-based CPG into clinical practice and the lack of evidence into the impact on outcomes as reasons for infrequent use (25). It appears that in the busy world of clinical practice, guidelines will not be used if they are not believed or readily available when clinical decisions are being made. EMR systems provide an incredible opportunity to disseminate to clinicians CPGs, protocols, pathways, and health maintenance reminders in a manner that can be effectively integrated into clinical care. Figure 7-10 illustrates how high-quality guidelines available on the World-Wide Web (WWW) can be easily viewed while remaining within a patient's EMR chart.

Determining when patients are due for routine health exams can be easily accomplished through built-in protocols. Figure 7-11 depicts an EMR-integrated U.S. Public Health Service protocol.

Reminders for immunizations and screening procedures can also be incorporated into an EMR. Another opportunity for disease guidance is the use of referral guidelines that outline diagnostic workups to be completed before consultation (Figure 7-12).

EMR vendors may provide pre-packaged guidelines, protocols, and pathways; however, it is important that all forms of disease guidance be en-

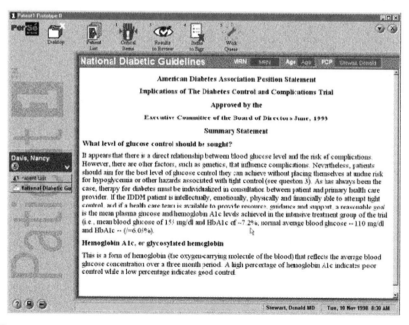

Figure 7-10 Disease guidance: on-line clinical practice guidelines.

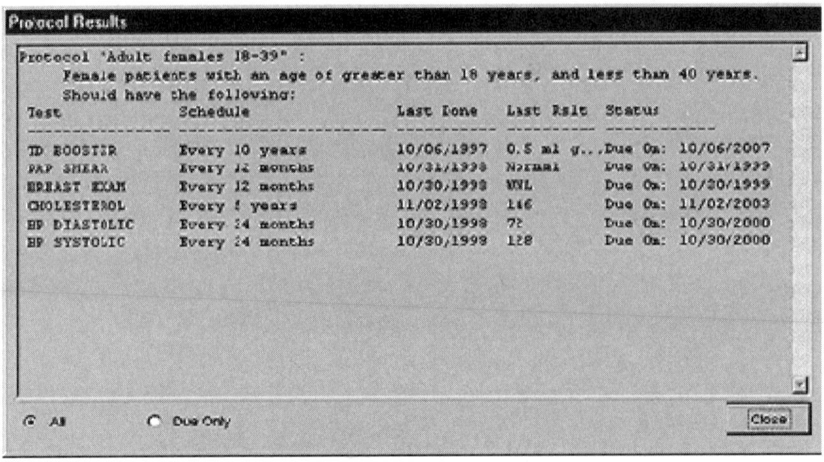

Figure 7-11 Disease guidance: health maintenance protocols.

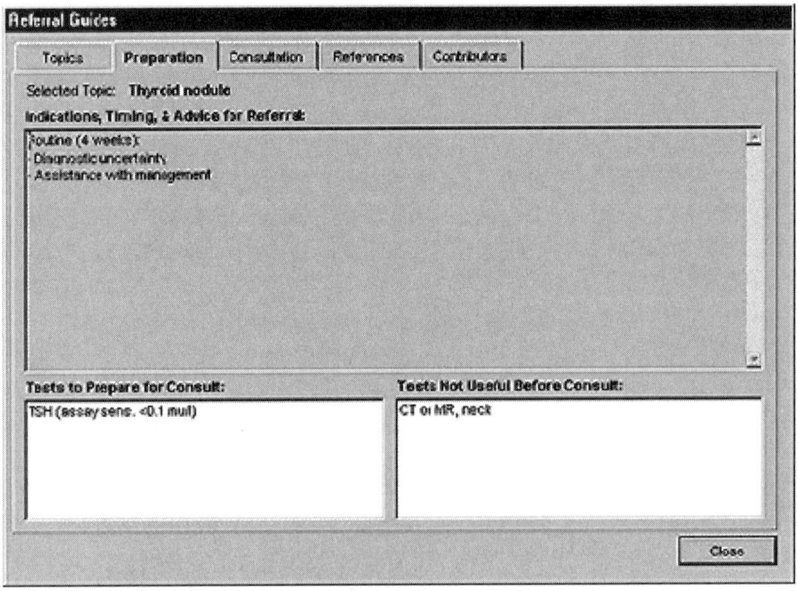

Figure 7-12 Disease guidance: referral guidelines.

dorsed by local clinical leadership before introduction into clinical practice. In addition, disease guidance solutions must be updated and refined on a regular basis. EMR vendors should provide the necessary tools, training, and support to achieve this.

Important Point. *When evaluating EMR systems, determine the capability of the system to provide on-line guidelines, reminders, and health maintenance. Evaluate both the content of the packaged guidelines as well as the ease of customization and implementation of locally derived evidence-based guidelines.*

Checklist. The EMR's method of disease guidance should provide

✓ Less time-consuming care for the clinician

✓ Better diagnosis

✓ Better therapy

✓ Better clinician knowledge

✓ Less expensive care

✓ Higher quality care

Data Analysis and Report Generation

This chapter has discussed how the EMR can assist in the day-to-day delivery of clinical care. The emphasis has been on how the clinician uses the EMR for on-line transaction processing (OLTP). The success of OLTP relies on the true integration of the EMR into clinical care. However, benefits also include enhanced analytical capabilities. Transactional EMR data can be analyzed on a retrospective basis, known as on-line analytical processing (OLAP). The generation of reports based on OLAP can provide valuable information to clinicians, including the opportunity to evaluate their own practice patterns and benchmark against colleagues and external standards. It also allows clinicians to gain powerful insight into population-wide health conditions and trends. Lists of patients requiring interventions, such as those who have missed their annual flu vaccines, can be easily generated and reminder letters sent. Examples of generated reports are shown in Figures 7-13 and 7-14.

Data analyses designed to assist clinicians in the identification of opportunities for clinical care improvement require access to a large amount of diverse data that often reside in multiple databases. Unfortunately, merging these data is often difficult and complicated. If the data are not stored electronically and reside only on paper, then OLAP is not possible. It is therefore important to determine before EMR selection not only how it will be used for transaction processing but what data are critical for retrospective analysis and report generation. Table 7-8 lists some of the key clinical data required for this purpose. In most organizations, electronic data will be stored in numerous databases. This requires the creation of a data warehouse that stores and provides access to all the required data and allows analyses to be performed using standard analytical and data mining

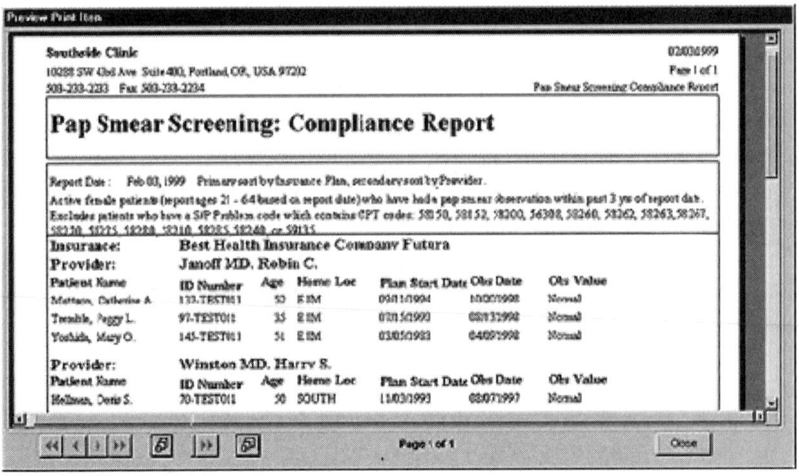

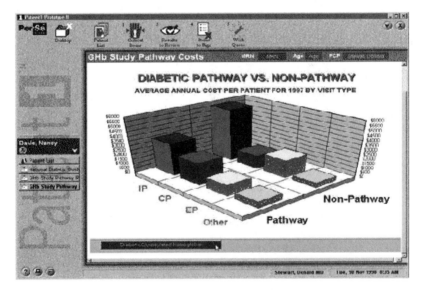

Figure 7-13 Data analysis and report generation: compliance report.

Figure 7-14 Data analysis and report generation: benchmarking.

tools. A few examples of such tools are provided in Table 7-9. Technical infrastructure requirements for data warehousing solutions are complex and have been described elsewhere (26).

Table 7- 8   Key Clinical Data Required for OLAP.

Data Element	Examples
Master patient index	Patient demographics
Admit discharge transfer (ADT)	Encounter data including length of stay and attending physician
Claims data	ICD-9, CPT-4, DRGs
Medication data	Drug, dose, route, duration of therapy
Diagnostic test utilization	Labs, diagnostic imaging, echos, PFTs
Procedures	Surgeries, endoscopies
Nursing and allied health	Workload
Outcomes	Morbidity, mortality, readmissions, quality of life
Costs	Diagnostics, therapeutics, physician, nursing

Table 7-9   Examples of Analytical and Data Mining Software.

Product	Category
Microsoft Access	SQL queries
SAS/SPSS	Statistical analysis and data mining
Intelligent Miner (IBM)	Data mining
PowerPlay (Cognos)	Data mining (OLAP)
Business Miner (Business Objects)	Data mining (OLAP)
Oracle	Data mining (OLAP)

At University Health Network, a large integrated delivery system in Toronto, five steps were used to convert EMR OLTP data to OLAP data (27). First, methods of accessing data in the EMR were assessed. Second, the scope of clinical data to be retrieved was defined. Third, a conversion method to allow clinical data to be imported into a functional OLAP system was determined. Fourth, the storage format of imported data was decided upon. Fifth, data for analysis were checked to ensure accuracy. We initially focused on areas where the data could assist, confirm, and enhance clinical decision support. Analysis of a clinical alert designed to warn clinicians about inappropriate test ordering at the time-of-order entry revealed that the "clinical alert" was able to change test-ordering practice. Analysis of residents' utilization patterns of commonly ordered laboratory tests identified several opportunities for improvement in clinicians' use of diagnostic tests. Finally, in support of laboratory re-engineering, the OLAP data warehouse identified opportunities to improve specimen turn-around times.

Important Point. *It is necessary to determine the organization's OLAP requirements before EMR selection. EMR vendors should demonstrate how retrospective data analysis and report generation can be achieved and whether their solutions are proprietary or provide an open solution such as analytical relational databases in which commercially available analytical software can be utilized.*

Checklist. The EMR's method of data analysis and report generation should provide

✓ Better diagnosis
✓ Better therapy
✓ Better clinician knowledge
✓ Less expensive care
✓ Higher quality care

Patient Education

An essential component of clinical care is ensuring that decisions respect patient autonomy and are the result of informed and shared decision-making. Patient educational interventions take time, and time is a precious resource for both clinicians and patients. A recent literature review suggested that computer-based approaches to patient education not only improve patients' knowledge and more actively involve them in decision-making but may also lead to better health outcomes (28). These approaches should be integrated into EMR systems.

Patient education handouts can be viewed on-line within the EMR and discussed with the patient and printed or saved to a disk for take-home review. Some EMR vendors have created libraries of professionally written patient handouts that assist in making information easier to understand; these handouts cover a variety of conditions and procedures (Figure 7-15).

Prescription writing can be accompanied by the automatic printing of medication information sheets that provide important educational

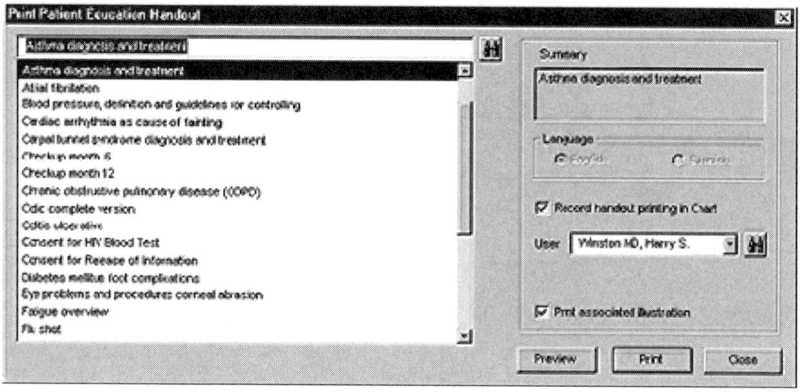

Figure 7-15 Patient education material.

information such as administration details, drug interactions, and possible side effects. In addition, patient educational interventions can be documented and tracked within the EMR for later review and assistance with reimbursement. EMR systems may also provide access to multimedia patient educational material such as audio-video files and on-line decision aids.

The ability to easily launch Internet applications and the WWW from within the EMR allows clinicians access to a wealth of patient educational material. High-quality sites can be bookmarked for later reference. Details on evaluating medical Web sites for quality have been published to assist clinicians and patients (29). In addition, many "super" medical Web sites are now available, serving as portals to a wide range of patient and clinician information management resources (see Appendix B).

Important Point. *When evaluating EMR systems determine what patient educational materials are provided and whether it is possible to integrate additional patient multimedia educational material into the EMR.*

Checklist. The EMR's method of patient education should provide
- ✓ Less time-consuming care for the clinician
- ✓ Less time-consuming care for the patient
- ✓ Better patient compliance
- ✓ Improved communication between clinician and patient
- ✓ Better patient knowledge
- ✓ Higher quality care

The Future

Computer processing power continues to increase, and costs of data storage continue to fall. As a result, emerging technologies will offer exciting advances for EMR systems.

Voice Recognition

Until recently voice recognition was severely limited in its ability to assist in clinical care processing. However, over the last two years, significant advances have occurred that make voice recognition a main contender to replace expensive dictation and transcription services and to provide EMR systems with a new modality for efficient and effective clinical documentation. The major advance in voice recognition has been the ability to understand continuous speech, while operating on industry-standard PCs in real-time with accurate results (30). A recent technical review of continuous speech recognition for clinicians showed impressive results. Clinicians were able to obtain greater than 97% accuracy with minimal training using an off-the-shelf continuous speech recognition system supplemented by a medical dictionary (31).

Handheld Computing

Handheld computing is an emerging technology that promises to become an important component of the clinician's black bag. At present, handhelds or palm computers are most useful as an electronic organizer, allowing clinicians to organize their time, schedule appointments, enter to-do lists, and recall important phone numbers and e-mail addresses. As the amount of data that can be stored has increased, handheld computers can now hold reference material such as textbooks and medication manuals. However, the ultimate goal of the handheld is to replace the clinician's pen and paper, allowing easy documentation of patient information and many of the other clinical care processes described in this chapter. Before that goal can be achieved, several technical challenges must be overcome, including faster processing speeds, longer battery life, and greater disk space, as well as the development of communication standards and secure, reliable, and accurate wireless synchronization methods between handhelds and EMR systems.*

---

*A helpful Web site is *handheldmed.com*.

Web-Based EMR Systems

In a recent report Clement McDonald and others envision EMR systems that take advantage of the WWW and evolving standards to provide clinicians with the "tools needed for seamless and secure access to their patients' data and to medical information, when and where they need it" (32). The new era envisioned by these pioneers is thought-provoking, pragmatic, and achievable. Web-based solutions to the EMR may provide more affordable, standardized, and widely applicable options to present-day EMR systems. EMR developers have recognized this and are investing heavily to capitalize on a growing need for Web-based EMR systems.

Intelligent Graphic User Interfaces

The improved design of graphic user interfaces (GUI) is a major advance over former character-based user interfaces. However, for the most part, EMR GUIs require clinicians to actively search for and "pull" the clinical data for viewing. The introduction of e-mail in-boxes and the ability to "push" critical data automatically to pagers, fax machines, and e-mail addresses represent the first stage of push technology in clinical practice. Future advances will see the introduction of intelligent agents that will be able to anticipate clinicians' information management needs and push information to clinicians based on predefined choices, scheduled patient encounters, and other clinical care requirements. For example, intelligent GUIs will recognize that the core clinical data set for a follow-up chemotherapy patient visit is different than the core clinical data set for a patient with an emergency ruptured aortic aneurysm, pushing to the clinician the right information at the right time. These intelligent agents will not only be disease specific but clinician and patient specific, and will result in significant efficiency gains for clinical care processes.

Electronic Health Records

A life-long record for every patient is the object of the electronic health record (EHR). *One patient, one record* is an appropriate motto. Such a vision covers the entire spectrum of health care delivery and the entire spectrum of a patient's life. In addition to all the features and data that constitute the EMR, an EHR supports comprehensive patient information management needs and patients actively interact with it to provide valuable health data that is stored as part of the record and accessed, reviewed, and discussed together by clinicians and patients. EHR is truly patient cen-

tered and if realized will result in significant improvements to health outcomes. Major obstacles to realizing EHR include the lack of widely available standards for the electronic communication of health data, concern
about possible breeches in patient confidentiality and privacy, unwillingness to share patient data between health care systems, and the lack of pro-
gressive policies and laws that support this vision. However, integrated
delivery systems that have the commitment and investment to realize an
EHR system are pursuing it with vigor. Besides the multitude of clinical
care benefit, the EHR will provide health consumers with greater access to
health information and knowledge. The result will be a significant competitive advantage over competing systems.

Summary

Successful EMR implementation requires a thorough understanding of the
everyday activities and work habits of those providing care. This chapter
has provided the reader with a practical approach to identify and analyze
clinical care processes for the ultimate purpose of selecting and implementing an EMR system to support clinicians, patients and health care delivery.
Regardless of the approach the reader ultimately uses, the most important
decision is whether to begin. In theory and in real-world clinical practice
there is growing evidence that EMR systems can improve clinical care. Although the growing number of successes is encouraging, there continue to
be many EMR failures. The reader should be reminded of this, not to dis-
courage his beginning, for not beginning has the potential to ultimately
cost more, but rather to emphasize critical success factors for EMR selection
and implementation. These factors include

1. Ensuring clinicians play leading roles in the EMR selection, implementation, and evaluation processes.
2. Identifying and prioritizing clinical care processes within the organization that could be positively affected by the implementation of an EMR system.
3. Setting realistic expectations given the organization's technical
   infrastructure, ability to learn, leadership, and commitment to
   the EMR system.
4. Evaluating EMR systems from a clinical care process perspective
   as well as an administrative and financial perspective. EMR systems must first and foremost support clinicians, not administrators.
5. A willingness of clinicians and, in particular, physicians to

change current practices and utilize the computer in all aspects of clinical care, including order entry and documentation.

Throughout the evaluation phase of an EMR selection process it is important to constantly revisit the checklist given in Table 7-1. If you cannot convince yourself that an EMR will have a positive impact on clinical practice, the likelihood of successful implementation is extremely remote. EMR systems are of no benefit if they are not being used. Whether they are used will depend on their value as determined by you and your clinical colleagues. A careful evaluation of the clinical care processes and both the positive and potential negative consequences that an EMR system might have is an essential exercise in the decision-making process. EMR systems promise to change the way medicine is practiced by providing clinicians with powerful new tools to assist in the delivery of high-quality cost-effective care. Understanding the impact of these systems on clinical care processes is an essential step in realizing those promises.

ACKNOWLEDGMENTS

The figures in this chapter have been provided through the courtesy of Per-Se Technologies and Medscape, Inc.

REFERENCES

1. **Forbes J.** In: Laennec RTH. A Treatise on the Diseases of the Chest. New York: Hafner Publishing, 1962, p. xix.

2. **Kohane IS.** Synopsis: Computer-Based Patient Records, Yearbook of Medical Informatics, 1998: Health Informatics and the Internet. IMIA, pp. 227-9.

3. **Tange HJ, Hasman A, deVriesRobbe PF, Schouten HC.** Medical Narratives in Electronic Medical Records, 1998: Yearbook of Medical Informatics, pp. 230-52.

4. **The Institute of Medicine.** The Computer-Based Patient Record: An Essential Technology for Health Care. Washington, DC: National Academy Press, 1991.

5. **Dick RS, Andrew WF.** Where we've been and where we're headed. Healthcare Informatics. Feb. 1997, pp. 52-6.

6. **The Institute of Medicine.** The Computer-Based Patient Record: An Essential Technology for Health Care. Rev ed. Washington, DC: National Academy Press, 1997.

7. **Williams LS.** Microchips versus stethoscopes: Calgary hospital MDs face-off over controversial computer system. CMAJ. 1992;147:1534-47.

8. **Rose JS, Gapinski M, Lum A, et al.** The Colorado Kaiser Permanente Clinical Information System: a comprehensive review. Proceedings of the CPR Recognition Symposium, Fifth Annual Nicholas E. Davies Award, CPRI; 1999:13-75.

9. **Finley SW.** The electronic medical record as a tool to improve patient care: hypothetical and practical opportunities. Journal of the Healthcare Information and Management Systems Society. 1997;11:5-11.

10. **Tonks A, Smith R.** Information in practice. BMJ. 1996;313:438.

11. **McDonald CJ, Tierney WM.** Computer-stored medical records: their future role in medical practice. JAMA. 1988;259:3433-40.

12. **Overhage M, McDonald CJ.** Medical records systems for office practice. Computers in Clinical Practice. Philadelphia: American College of Physicians; 1995:19-36.

13. **Teich JM, Wrinn MM.** Clinical decision support systems come of age. MD Computing. 2000;17:43-8.

14. **Evans RS, Pestotnik SL, Classen DC, et al.** A computer-assisted management program for antibiotics and other antiinfective agents. N Eng J Med. 1998;338:232-8.

15. **Lazarou J, Pomeranz BH, Corey PN.** Incidence of adverse drug reactions in hospitalized patients. JAMA. 1998;279:1200-5.

16. **Schiff GD, Rucker TD.** Computer prescribing: building the electronic infrastructure for better medication usage. JAMA. 1998;279:1024-9.

17. **Bates DW, Leape LL, Cullen DJ, et al.** Effect of computerized physician order entry and a team intervention on prevention of serious medication errors. JAMA. 1998;280:1311-6.

18. **Davis DD, Moriyama R, Tiwanak G, et al.** Clinical performance improvement with an advanced clinical information system at the Queen's Medical Center. Proceedings of the CPR Recognition Symposium, Fifth Annual Nicholas E. Davies Award, CPRI; 1999:77-120.

19. **Perreault LE, Metzger JB.** A pragmatic framework for understanding clinical decision support. The Journal of the Healthcare Information and Management Systems Society. 1999;13:5-21.

20. **Randolph A, Haynes RB, Wyatt JC, et al.** Users' guides to the medical literature: XVIII. How to use an article evaluating the clinical impact of a computer-based clinical decision support system. JAMA. 1999;282:67-74

21. **Hunt DL, Haynes RB, Hanna SE, Smith K.** Effects of computer-based clinical decision support systems on physician performance and patient outcomes. JAMA. 1998;280:1339-46.

22. **Miller RA, Geissbuhler A.** Clinical decision support systems: an overview. In: Berner ES (editor). Clinical Decision Support Systems: Theory and Practice. New York: Springer-Verlag, 1998.

23. **Broverman CA.** Standards for clinical decision support systems. Journal of the Healthcare Information and Management Systems Society. 1999;13:23-31.

24. **Teich JM, Kuperman GJ, Bates DW.** Clinical decision support: making the transition from the hospital to the community network. Journal of the Healthcare Information and Management Systems Society. 1997;11:27-37.

25. **Hayward RS, Guyatt GH, Moore KA, et al.** Canadian physicians' attitudes about and preferences regarding clinical practice guidelines. CMAJ. 1997;156:1715-23.

26. **Nussbaum GM, Ault SP.** The best little data warehouse. Journal of the Healthcare Information and Management Systems Society. 1998;12:79-93.

27. **Ebidia A, Mulder C, Tripp B, Morgan MW.** Getting data out of the electronic patient record: critical steps in building a data warehouse for decision support. Proceedings of 1999 Annual Symposium, American Medical Informatics Association, p. 745.

28. **Lewis D.** Computer-based approaches to patient education: a review of the literature. Journal of the American Medical Informatics Association. 1999;6:272-82.

29. **Silberg WM, Lundberg GD, Musacchio RA.** Accessing, controlling, and assuring the quality of medical information on the internet: caveat lector et viewor - let the reader and viewer beware. JAMA. 1997;227:1244-5.

30. Speech recognition: finding its voice. PC Magazine. 20 Oct 1998.

31. **Zafar A, Overhage M, McDonald CJ.** Continuous speech recognition for clinicians. JAMIA. 1999;6:195-204.

32. **McDonald CJ, Overhage JM, Dexter PR, et al.** Canopy computing: using the Web in clinical practice. JAMA. 1998;280:1325-9.

8 / The Electronic Medical Record as a Tool for Research and Patient Care

Jerome H. Carter

Electronic medical record (EMR) systems have the potential to significantly affect all aspects of health care delivery. A well-designed EMR system provides all of the documentation functions found in paper records while offering sophisticated decision support capabilities previously unavailable to most clinicians and administrators. In fact, access to new decision support capabilities is perhaps the most important justification for enduring the cost and troubles associated with an EMR implementation. Of course, using these new capabilities requires a full understanding of the information management needs that are part of the practice environment.

Managed Care

Managed care is perhaps the most influential factor affecting health care information needs. Managed care, with its emphasis on capitated payments, makes cost control essential. However, as the recent spate of medical business failures attests, cost control is much easier said than done. It is especially difficult in health care where the "product" is patient care. How does one lower the cost of care without negatively affecting quality or patient satisfaction? The answer is simple: have more and better information.

Cost-control attempts usually follow a fairly predictable pattern. First, basic services are pared (food services, facilities management, etc.). Next, nonclinical patient contact (front office) positions are scaled back. Then care-related costs come under fire. The problem here is that it is not easy to determine what is "nonessential" and simple belt-tightening may result in adverse clinical outcomes. Ethically lowering the cost of care requires that one know the "best" way to handle a case from initial diagnosis to final resolution. The attempts at understanding clinical care processes well enough to identify interventions that may be eliminated without affecting care quality have resulted in a number of additions to the vocabulary of health care: *disease management, clinical pathways, best practices,* and *outcomes analysis* to name a few (1-4). Each of these activities is based upon a few basic principles: 1) variances in care affect final outcomes; 2) data collection will aid in identifying why and where in the care process variances occur; and 3) analyzing captured data may offer information as to which interventions are helpful or harmful.

Although understanding the effects of interventions on clinical outcomes is perhaps the most significant information quest resulting from managed care, questions and issues related to operational matters are also attracting attention (5, 6). Operational efficiency and resource management obviously have a significant impact on the bottom-line, making data of this type as desirable as clinical outcomes information. Fortunately, EMRs may help with each of these tasks. The questions that an EMR is expected to aid in answering span the entire health care delivery organization and therefore must meet the information needs of a wide variety of personnel.

Evidenced-Based Medicine

A more recent player in the information needs arena is evidenced-based medicine (EBM) (7). The goal of evidenced-based medicine is to assure that the latest high-quality information from basic sciences and patient-centered clinical studies is used when making clinical decisions. The foundation of EBM is empirical clinical data. These data cover the complete range of clinical activities, from diagnostic studies to therapeutic interventions, addressing matters of efficacy, safety, and effectiveness. A basic precept of EBM is that if well-trained clinicians have access to objective information concerning the efficacy, safety, and effectiveness of clinical interventions, better decisions will be made and care quality will be optimum. Thus, although EBM advocates and those trying to "manage" care may have very different initial motives, each group has nearly identical information needs. Each wants to know what clinical interventions work best and under which conditions. This need for outcomes data along with infor-

mation on operational efficiency, costs, and resource management is helping to fuel the demand for EMR systems.

Information Needs and Electronic Medical Records

Are EMR systems the solution to our information management problems?
As with most things in life, the devil is in the details and, in the case of
EMR systems, the details are particularly devilish. Understanding the difficult issues in EMR design and functioning requires understanding the information needs of potential users. Fortunately, this task has been addressed
quite well in the *Computer-Based Patient Record: An Essential Technology for
Patient Care* (8), which analyzes the users and uses of paper medical records.
Two groups are identified: primary and secondary users/uses. Primary users
of the paper record are those who use it to provide clinical care. This group
includes all clinicians, nurses, pharmacists, and other clinical personnel.
Secondary users are identified as those who analyze information found in
the record. Typical secondary users are administrators, researchers, regulatory agencies, and third-party payers. Unfortunately, features that optimize
the EMR for one group may provide little for the other, making EMR selection and implementation a highly charged issue in many organizations. A
closer look at features important to each group will help in illustrating the
source of problems for EMR selection committees.

Information Needs of Primary Users

Doctors and nurses form the bulk of primary users. Each group devotes a
significant amount of time to direct patient care and have similar information requirements. Each needs access to laboratory results, radiology reports, results of consultations, medication lists, and progress notes. Note
that primary users are usually concerned with the status of only one patient
at a time. Rarely does a doctor want to know the average mammography
rate for all patients seen in the past two years. Likewise, few nurses monitor
the average time period that a pain medication is effective in post-op patients. Often, in clinical practice, decisions cannot be postponed until
more information is obtained. Primary users want information about a single patient and they want it *now*. Since primary users rely on rapid information retrieval for decision making, presentation and response times are

---

Table 8-1   Key EMR Features for Primary Users.

Easy-to-use interface

Rapid response time

Ease of entering progress note/orders

Clearly presented:

  Medication list

  Problem list

  Radiology reports

  Progress notes

  Laboratory values

---

important aspects of EMR systems for them. Typical primary user concerns are listed in Table 8-1.

Information Needs of Secondary Users

In most health care organizations, administrators and researchers comprise most secondary users. However, third-party payers and regulatory bodies are increasingly demanding access to formerly off-limits data. Secondary users analyze groups of patients or interventions looking for significant patterns or trends. Secondary users would be quite interested in mammography rates, patient satisfaction, which drug controls pain best with the fewest doses, and the average length of stay for community-acquired pneumonia. Secondary users insist on complete, validated data sets with few missing values, across large numbers of patients. However, time from request to presentation is rarely an issue. Many reports are required no more often than weekly, and monthly or even longer intervals are common. Typical secondary issues are listed in Table 8-2.

Information Needs and EMR Design

The needs of primary and secondary users must be taken into account during EMR design. Failure to do so will quite easily doom its implementation. Primary users require easy-to-use data entry and retrieval, rapid system re-

Table 8-2   Typical Secondary User Concerns.

Complete, valid data for each patient

Ability to ask questions across entire patient population

Ability to export data to external systems for analysis

Access to cost data

Adherence to guidelines/ protocols

Ability to conduct complex queries

sponse, and access to common clinical data. Secondary users need complete, valid data sets across the entire patient population with sophisticated query and export capability. How one meets the design criteria of each group is the focus of intense research in the medical informatics and health care information systems communities (9-11). We have modern database tools, graphical user interfaces, and access to the Internet - so what is the problem? Creating systems that address primary users is relatively easy, and most clinical systems to-date have addressed this area with some degree of success. Secondary uses are quite a different matter. Most currently available clinical information systems, including EMR systems, were designed more than three years ago when secondary issues were not so important. In addition, it takes quite a while to go from blueprint to commercially available system (at least three to four years). Companies wishing to add features to their products must not only design and add the new features but also iron-out problems introduced into older system components. Finally, secondary uses require more complex designs at lower levels in the system. The progress note and practice guidelines are perfect examples of how systems that work well for primary users may be very difficult to adapt for secondary users.

Creating a progress note in the paper chart is quite simple. Pick up a pen, find a clean area on the page, and write. In an EMR, it may be almost as simple (especially if you are a touch typist). Pull up the progress note screen and type away. More demanding primary users may request templates or drop-down menus to aid data-entry. Some may even ask for voice recognition or pen-based input options. However, no matter what input method is used, the point is simply to capture accurate data about the patient. The clinician entering the data is concerned with its readability, conformance to a standard organizational format (SOAP), and completeness.

The next clinician to access the note is concerned only about those same issues. A typical search in this setting would be finding all progress notes for this patient for the last few visits.

Looking at this progress note from a lower, more technical level, it is no different from a word-processing file: a simple collection of characters grouped under a specific file name (e.g., medical record number). Assuming that all elements of the system work well, most caregivers will be quite satisfied with it.

Now consider the plight of a researcher wishing to determine the response of a group of diabetic patients to a new medication that may help to limit long-term complications. She logs onto the system and asks for all diabetic patients taking medication X. Assuming that all goes well, she will receive in response a list of those patients. How will she determine each patient's response to medication X? She will have to read through the note just as if it were on paper! Why? Because each note was stored as a block of text. There is no index of words in the note to provide a hint of its contents, because primary users rarely want to know about all diabetic patients, just the one that they are currently seeing. Even if we assume that some search capability is possible, users have not been required to use a standard vocabulary. As a result, some notes will refer to diabetic nephropathy as "diabetic kidney disease" or "diabetic renal disease". Others will state that 2+ proteinuria is present or that the patient has renal insufficiency. All may well refer to the same pathological entity; however, there is no way to be certain. So our researcher must read through each note to determine the actual health state of the patient. The lack of a controlled, standard vocabulary makes it difficult to conduct useful queries. Controlled vocabularies are not a feature of paper-based notes, and few clinicians would insist on one as part of a new EMR system. They are absolutely essential for secondary users. However, a controlled vocabulary alone will not help our researcher.

Let us assume that the system has now been configured to include a controlled vocabulary and indexes for the progress notes. Our researcher can now easily find all diabetic patients who match her search criteria. If she wishes only to identify patients who may be subjects for further study, then she will be successful. However, what if she wants to then compare the complication rates between those who received the drug and those who did not? How do we know that the patients are comparable? How do we account for co-morbid states, affects of other medications, compliance rates, severity of the initial diabetic state? Even with a controlled vocabulary, this information may not be recorded properly or accurately. A controlled vocabulary assures that all uses of the same term have the same meaning. Information regarding health state, illness severity, and medical problems are still under the control of the user and will vary from note to note. We may solve the problem of data capture via use of a structured input monitor, or, as they may be more commonly referred to, a protocol/guideline. Simple protocols are easily implemented in a system (e.g., reminders for flu shots). Complex protocols, useful for comparing populations of patients, are much more difficult to implement and are the subject of a good deal of research (12-14). If we somehow managed to implement a protocol for managing patients with diabetes, would it be sufficient to make our researcher's work less labor-intensive? Yes, but there is still the problem of efficient queries.

Protocols assure that standard data are captured in a particular fashion. In our current system this means that we have complete data sets and well-defined terms. The progress note now exists in two forms: as a block of text and as an indexed list of terms that may be rapidly searched. Searching for terms within each block is now much easier, but remember our hypothetical researcher wishes to search rapidly across hundreds of patients. Also, we wish to maintain the temporal relationships that exist between terms. The Clinical Data Repository (CDR) (see Chapter 4 for a detailed discussion) provides a solution to this problem. CDRs are specialized databases that integrate data from a number of different systems for retrieval (usually by primary users). CDRs contain "live" data such as the most recent CBC and serum glucose level. In small installations a CDR may be sufficient to support primary and secondary users simultaneously. However, in larger installations, a separate, even more specialized database is required to support secondary users without disturbing the access and retrieval times of primary users; this is called the *data warehouse* (see Chapter 4). Information in data warehouses is aggregated as a prelude to performing complex queries. Data warehouses do not contain "live" data (i.e., this is not where you go to find the CBC from last night). Also, they rarely contain patient-specific identifiers. They exist solely to answer questions that concern entire populations and to make complex searches easier and more efficient to conduct than a CDR or similar clinical database. A well-designed data warehouse would very likely make for a very happy researcher.

However, this is unlikely to be the end the matter. What has been the effect on primary users of adding all these new features? They now must use only the terms approved by some committee, and their progress note formats are now influenced to some degree by protocols. All of the issues raised in this example are real and will be encountered by anyone attempting to implement an EMR system. However, they are not insurmountable.

Awareness is the key. Remember that it is easy to design a system that works well for one group of users and not at all for others.

Using EMR To Help Decision Making

If you are considering an EMR as an aid to decision making, the first issue which must be addressed is the type of support that you desire. For the purposes of this discussion, EMR-based decision support will be divided into three levels—basic, intermediate, and advanced—based upon their level of direct interaction with patient data. Shortliffe (15) provides a more detailed taxonomy of decision support systems for those who have a more technical interest in this area.

Access to static reference materials (electronic textbooks and journals, drug monographs, practice guidelines, etc.) is the essential feature of basic EMR decision support. These materials are simple electronic versions of paper-based products. They provide little in the way of interactivity, except basic search functions. Basic-level decision support may be an integrated component of the EMR or a simple add-on. The ultimate utility of these types of materials is limited by the fact that they are passive. They cannot affect patient care unless providers seek them out. The Internet provides a very simple mechanism for offering basic decision support services to any EMR workstation capable of supporting a standard Web browser.

Intermediate level decision support tools provide information as well as some modicum of interactivity. Two good examples of intermediate-level decision support functions are automatic alerts for abnormal laboratory results or reminders of required interventions (e.g., flu shots). Both are examples of background functions that do not require the clinician to initiate use in order to benefit from the service. A number of studies (16, 17) have demonstrated the positive effects on alerts and reminders on quality of care. Table 8-3 offers a list of typical intermediate-level decision support functions.

Because intermediate-level decision support functions offer active support, they must have access to patients' demographic and clinical information. Intelligent use of patient information requires a good deal of planning on the part of systems designers. Systems that offer this type of decision support usually support a standard architecture for encoding rules for the manipulation of patient information; the ARDEN Syntax is an example (18). In most situations encoded rules, regardless of architecture, trigger or are related to a single action or intervention. Even though limited to the

Table 8-3   Common Intermediate-Level Decision Support Functions.

Allergy/drug interaction checks

Alerts for critical/abnormal laboratory values

Reminders for standard preventive medicine interventions

monitoring of a single event, ruled-based decision support may be quite sophisticated and offer valuable assistance. For example, a system that alerts for low K+ levels for patients taking digoxin requires access to pharmacy and laboratory data and to rules that determine when a critical event has occurred. Intermediate-level decision support is available, to some degree, in commercially available EMR systems.

Advanced decision support functions are highly interactive, make extensive use of patient information, and are capable of managing the relationship between multiple interventions over time. These are essential functions for implementing complex practice guidelines or clinical protocols. There is no standard architecture for implementing these functions, though a good deal of research is being done in this area (19, 20). There are many unresolved issues. Tierney et al (21) provide useful insights into the problems inherent in computerizing complex guidelines, such as the vagueness of the wording of many guidelines ("If the patient has renal insufficency, use medication B"). What level of renal insufficiency? Computerization requires a specific value or range be given to designate the presence of renal insufficiency.

Assuming that an architecture is created that permits implementation of complex guidelines, analysis of the resulting data will not be a simple task. Musen and Shahar (22-24) at Stanford have researched problems that arise during attempts to analyze clinical trends that are temporally dependent. They found it necessary to create an entirely new set of concepts and data types that could be used as the basis for performing temporally dependent clinical queries (e.g., how many patients developed rashes due to taking medication B). This query is not as simple as it seems. Remember computers have no concept of "before", "while", or "after"; the programmer has to create them within the context of the query itself (or take the approach of Musen and Shahar). To answer this query several steps must be taken:

1. Find all patients who have ever taken medication B.
2. Determine if the patient had a rash.
3. If a rash is present *and* the patient has taken medication B:

a) Was the rash present before taking medication B?
b) Was the rash present after medication B was initiated? Before cessation?
c) If the rash ended after cessation of medication B, what was the time interval (days)?

Let us take a closer look at the matter of "Was the rash present before taking medication B?" Remember that in our database we may have thousands of patients who have taken medication B and each would have begun taking the medicine at a different point in time. Therefore, we cannot do a query for all patients taking B before a specific date. Instead, for each patient we have to find the start date for B, compare that with the start date of the rash, and note which took place earlier. Now, taking only those patients whose rash start date is after the B start date, we must determine if stopping B coincides with the disappearance of the rash. To accomplish this we must find the start and stop dates for B, then compare the rash start and stop dates. Since it is reasonable to expect that there will be a lag between cessation of B and the resolution of the rash, if B is the culprit we must set a reasonable interval to account for this lag time. Assuming that we settle on three days as a reasonable interval for the disappearance of the rash, we must now determine, for each patient, if the stop date of the rash was within three days of the stop date of B. Having done this calculation, we must do one more: "All patients who were taking B who developed a rash *and* whose rash resolved without stopping B." We must remove this group from our final set if we assume that the rash should not resolve if the patient is still taking the medication. What began as a simple question has become a very complex database query. Keep in mind that no one knows the correct answer and, if thousands of patients are involved, it will be difficult to check the results. However, it is just these types of questions that are fueling the drive toward EMRs. And few EMR systems offer support for complex guidelines or protocols.

Meeting Information Needs

Thus far, we have looked at types of users, levels of decision support, and the two major forces behind the push for EMR systems. Now let us see if we can merge all of these factors into a coherent information management strategy. At this point it should be clear that the information needs of the secondary users will be the most difficult to address. Primary users generally will be quite satisfied with basic and intermediate decision support capability. Most of this functionality is already present in many EMR packages. Using EMR successfully is usually a matter of health care providers adjusting their practice habits to a new way of doing things. The response, assuming an uneventful implementation, is almost always enthusiastic. Secondary users, on the other hand, desire access to intermediate and advanced decision support and, unfortunately, the level of support for these functions varies greatly among EMR packages. When attempting to provide for the information needs of secondary uses there are two quite separate issues that must be addressed. First, evaluation of EMR systems is much more difficult than for primary users due to the lack of a standard set of secondary use features and the wide variation in implementation quality among systems. Next, expert use of EMR features aimed at secondary users requires a good deal of planning and, very likely, significant changes in clinical care processes and financial and operational activities.

Preparing for Secondary User and Uses

Access to valid, complete data sets suitable for analysis is the ultimate goal of secondary users. Of course, capturing and maintaining a data set with these characteristics is neither simple nor straightforward. A complete data set is one that contains a value for all variables slated for capture and analysis. In a computer system designed to capture and maintain data on every patient encounter for an arbitrary number of years and encounters, a number of mechanisms must be put in place to ensure that all desired data are captured. At the software level this may be accomplished via use of specially designed input screens (forms), field-level constraints within the database, or other well-known practices.

Another, slightly different, problem is that of assuring that the data captured are done so in a manner that will permit cross-patient comparisons. This is a higher level issue and one that must be solved by those who wish to perform the analyses. This problem is much the same as those that occur during clinical trails when it is necessary to create inclusion/exclusion criteria so that the final data analysis is not confounded by variables extraneous to the study. Of course, in an open environment such as EMR in a regular medical practice clinical trial type exclusion/inclusion criteria make no sense. Yet some mechanism must be in place to assure that, if one is comparing data on the outcome of an intervention, all subjects were treated in a similar manner. The solution to this problem comes in two slightly different forms: clinical pathways and practice guidelines.

Clinical pathways are management protocols that originated in inpatient settings and are often procedure oriented (e.g., hip replacement). However, they may be disease specific. Clinical (critical) pathways usually are based upon a day-to-day scheme and offer detailed specifications concerning which interventions (diagnostic and therapeutic) should be performed in accordance with a formal, agreed-upon plan. A clinical pathway serves two very important functions. First, it decreases unnecessary doctor-doctor variations in care for the same ailment. Second, it provides a mechanism for standardizing data capture and removing common sources of variations in measuring clinical variables. For example, a pathway may state that all pain medication requests should be followed at 2 and 4 hours with a standardized pain-scale survey done by the Registered Nurse. This would allow researchers interested in post-op pain levels to compare responses of various patient groups to specific pain medications.

Practice guidelines are very similar in form and function to clinical pathways. Perhaps the most important differences, and these are by no means set in stone, are that guidelines are more prevalent in ambulatory settings and are usually intended for direct use by clinicians. Guidelines may be procedure or disease specific and seek, as do pathways, to standardize care. Since they are intended for use by clinicians, they also tend to leave more leeway for deviations on the part of the provider. If outcomes analyses are an important goal, the flexibility permitted in these guidelines represents a major barrier to assuring comparability of the collected data. This becomes a major issue with EMR implementation. If one wants to determine the value, in a specific practice setting, of a particular intervention, variations in care not dictated by the illness must be reduced as much as possible. Putting this into practice will result in less freedom on the part of providers for selecting diagnostic and therapeutic interventions, but this is essential if useful outcomes studies are to be done.

Assuring that captured data are valid is an entirely different problem. Here the issue is one of accuracy. Are all blood pressure readings captured correctly (e.g., are some clinic staff better at this than others)? This is very difficult to correct at the software level. However, it is possible to prevent temperatures of 120°F from being entered via use of field-level validity checks. A less obvious validity problem is that of laboratory results passed between two computers being matched to the correct patient. Are the computer interfaces involved in these transactions 100% reliable? Patients with multiple medical record numbers present equally troublesome challenges. Robust error-checking is an absolute must for all EMR systems and should be a major portion of the evaluation of any system. Once you have cleared the validity/completeness obstacle, useful outcomes analysis are possible.

Outcomes Analyses

Outcomes analyses come in many flavors; in fact, as many as one has questions. They may be clinical, financial, or operational in scope.

Clinical outcomes measures are probably the most widely known analyses. They may be disease specific (e.g., change in ejection fraction with use of ACE inhibitors) or patient centered (e.g., quality-of-life for those with osteoarthritis on ibuprofen vs. COX-2 inhibitors, or satisfaction with time required to schedule an appointment). Clinical outcomes analyses have the potential to most directly affect patient care quality. The evidence for what works and what is harmful should be fairly obvious once outcomes data across millions of patients becomes readily available. Locally, such information will help clinicians make better decisions and offer patients more useful advice. Managed care and evidenced-based medicine both require detailed, valid outcomes data.

Financial outcomes, which are at present less dependent upon clinical data, would be greatly enriched by access to good clinical information. Common financially oriented outcomes measures (cost-benefit, cost-effectiveness) are often not expressed in terms which the average clinician can relate to his or her daily practice. However, the ability to relate costs to interventions and outcomes may change that. For example, knowing which pain medication resulted in the most hours of relief with the fewest side effects for a specific patient population might lower the cost of care while improving the quality.

Operational issues such as lag time between request for a consultation and receipt of the completed report may affect quality-of-care and patient satisfaction. This could easily be monitored with EMR while being too labor-intensive manually. Other issues such as optimum staffing, use of resources (e.g., procedure suites), and spotting patterns in missed appointments may possibly be improved via use of outcomes data.

One area of particular concern to clinicians, provider profiling (25), is certainly amenable to analysis if one uses an EMR. Provider profiling is a very simple type of outcome measure. Data for all targeted interventions (diagnostic tests, medications, etc.) are reviewed for each physician, then compared with data from their peers with similar patient populations. Reports indicate whether services are being overutilized or underutilized compared with the norm. Third-party payers make use of this information when determining provider panels. Regulatory groups may want similar information when reviewing use of preventive health interventions. These functions should be standard in all commercially available EMR systems.

Performing Outcomes Analyses

Although an EMR can greatly enhance one's outcome analyses capabilities, what can be accomplished is very much a function of the sophistication of the research and information systems capability of the site. Some outcomes analyses are easily performed and well within the reach of any practice site. Performance reviews fall into this category.

Performance reviews, as the name implies, determine the level of utilization of a designated (desirable) intervention (e.g., the rate of vaccination for influenza and pneumococcal pneumonia in targeted populations). Assuming an EMR system has the ability to identify patients by specific traits (age, gender, diagnosis, etc.), it is possible to create guidelines for the use of a number of interventions known to improve the health status of targeted groups. An EMR then can alert the provider when interventions are due and provide useful feedback on their usage rate, reasons for rejection, and so on. For example, many patients complain of becoming sick after receiving a flu shot. An EMR would permit a simple study to determine how often this happens and in what type of patient. The HEDIS report, under the aegis of the NCQA, is an example of a nationally recognized performance review (26). Chapter 9 addresses performance reviews and quality improvement in detail.

Previously we discussed the idea of performing outcomes analyses based upon the use of detailed practice guidelines and clinical pathways. The technical issues involved in conducting these types of analyses are much more difficult. In particular, the statistical analyses required to adjust for risk factors and possible sources of bias are far beyond the capability of all but the most sophisticated practice sites.

The difficulty of the required statistical analyses is not the only issue. Most EMRs provide very little in the way of statistical functions. Therefore complicated analyses require exportation of the data. If the data in an EMR are sufficiently complete, data export may consist of a relatively simple movement of information from the EMR to the statistical analysis system. However, if data from multiple sources (EMR, laboratory, accounting department) must be pooled and validated before analysis, data export itself becomes complex. At large practice sites where data from multiple computers are aggregated to form a working EMR (clinical data repository), the management of the data pool alone becomes quite a chore. The issues of computer-computer communications (interfaces), file formats, and data types become sufficiently troublesome in such situations as to require medical informatics, information systems, and statisticians in order to assure valid data are available for analyses.

Summary

The process of managing and practicing medicine based upon evidence of what works becomes more likely if an EMR system is in place. The average practitioner can, with very little help, see immediate benefits in terms of practice efficiency, review of practice habits, and adherence to commonly accepted preventive medicine guidelines as a result of EMR use. However, an EMR system alone is not sufficient when more sophisticated analyses of the effects of interventions on patient populations is the goal. In such cases access to specialists in informatics, biostatistics, and information systems is absolutely essential.

REFERENCES

1. **Epstein RS, Sherwood LM.** From outcomes research to disease management: a guide for the perplexed. Ann Intern Med. 1996;124:832-7.

2. **Coffey RJ, Othman JE, Walters JI.** An introduction to critical paths. Quality Management in Health Care. 1992;1:45-54.

3. **Ellwood PM.** Shattuck Lecture. Outcomes management: technology of patient experiences. N Engl J Med. 1988;318:1549-56.

4. **Kibbe DC, Smith PP, LaVallee R, et al.** A guide to finding and evaluating best practices health care information on the Internet: the truth is out there? Joint Commission Journal on Quality Improvement. 1997;3:678-89.

5. **Dennis L.** Using IT to compete in managed care. Advance for Health Information Executives. 1997;1:38-44.

6. **Wess BP.** Health care: the next generation. Advance for Health Information Executives. 1999;3:27-31.

7. **Taylor DK, Buterakos J.** Evidence-based medicine: not as simple as it seems. Acad Med. 1998;73:1221-2.

8. **Dick RS, Steen EB, Detmer DE.** The Computer-Based Patient Record: An Essential Technology for Health Care. The Institute of Medicine; 1991.

9. **Zuber RF.** Electronic clinical records: what do regulators want? Home Care Manager. 1998;2:16-8.

10. **Grams RR, Morgan G.** Medical record innovations that can improve physician productivity. J

Med Syst. 1999;23:133-44.

11. **Frenot S, Laforest F.** Medical record management systems: criticisms and new perspectives. Methods Inf Med. 1999;38:89-95.

12. **Zielstorff RD.** Online practice guidelines: issues, obstacles, and future prospects. J Am Med Inform Assoc. 1998;5:227-36.

13. **Miller PL, Frawley SJ, Sayward FG, et al.** Combining tabular, rule-based, and procedural knowledge in computer-based guidelines for childhood immunization. Comput Biomed Res. 1997;30:211-31.

14. **McDonald CJ.** The barriers to electronic medical record systems and how to overcome them. J Am Med Inform Assoc. 1997;4:213-21.

15. **Shortliffe EH.** Clinical decision-support systems. In: Shortliffe EH, Perreault LE, Wiederhold G, Fagan LM, Eds. Medical Informatics: Computer Applications in Health Care. Reading, MA: Addision-Wesley, 1990.

16. **Tang PC, LaRosa MP, Newcomb C, Gorden SM.** Measuring the effects of reminders for outpatient influenza immunizations at the point of clinical opportunity. J Am Med Inform Assoc. 1999;6:115-21.

17. **McDonald CJ, Hui SL, Smith DM, et al.** Reminders to physicians from an introspective computer medical record: a two-year randomized trial. Ann Intern Med. 1984;100:130-8.

18. **Hripcsak G, Ludemann P, Pryor TA, et al.** Rationale for the Arden Syntax. Comp Biomed Res. 1994;27:291-324.

19. **Patel VL, Allen VG, Arocha JF, Shortliffe EH.** Representing clinical guidelines in GLIF: individual and collaborative expertise. J Am Med Inform Assoc. 1998;5:467-83.

20. **Ohno-Machado L, Gennari JH, Murphy SN, et al.** The guideline interchange format: a model for representing guidelines. J Am Med Inform Assoc. 1998;5:357-72.

21. **Tierney WM, Overhage JM, Takesue BY, et al.** Computerizing guidelines to improve care and patient outcomes: the example of heart failure. J Am Med Inform Assoc. 1995;2:316-22.

22. **Shahar Y, Musen MA.** RESUME: a temporal-abstraction system for patient monitoring. Comp Biomed Res. 1993;26:255-73.

23. **Shahar Y, Musen MA.** A temporal-abstraction system for patient monitoring. In: Proceedings of the Annual Symposium on Computer Applications in Medical Care. 1992:121-7.

24. **Shahar Y, Tu SW, Musen MA.** Temporal-abstraction mechanisms in management of clinical protocols. In: Proceedings of the Annual Symposium on Computer Applications in Medical Care. 1991:629-33.

25. **Shapiro DW, Lasker RD, Bindman AB, Lee PR.** Containing costs while improving quality of care: the roles of profiling and practice guidelines. Annu Rev Public Health. 1993;14:219-41.

26. http://www.ncqa.org.

9 / Quality Improvement: Concepts and Technical Issues

Jeroan J. Allison and J. Michael Hardin

n 1968, Larry Weed put forth his conception of the ideal "automated" medical record and how this automated record could be optimally configured to promote quality improvement in patient care (1, 2). Years later, the Institute of Medicine recognized that an electronic medical record (EMR) offers unique opportunities for assessing and improving the quality of health care delivered to individual patients and to populations of patients (3). This chapter presents the basic concepts of quality improvement theory as applied to health care. We move next to more technical concepts that allow optimal use of EMRs in achieving continuous improvement in health care quality. Our goal is to equip the reader to evaluate an EMR package for suitability in a broad range of quality improvement settings.

Introduction to Quality Improvement

The Quality Improvement (QI) movement gained momentum in the manufacturing industry around the middle of this century and has been assuming growing importance in health care over the past decade (4). A well-chosen EMR will assist with the application of QI principles to the daily practice of medicine, improve patient care, and help meet additional demands of quality documentation superimposed by the current health care milieu (5).

Some of the most important forces shaping health care include the development of quality measures for a wide array of diseases and the publication of performance based on these measures (6). Quality measures frequently form the basis for certification of health care organizations (7-11). Managed care organizations (MCOs) frequently tie performance on quality improvement measures to physician compensation and certification (12). Documentation of high-quality care offers leverage in the negotiation of managed care contracts (13-15).

The Health Employers Data and Information Set (HEDIS), sponsored by the National Committee on Quality Assurance (NCQA), is one of the most visible quality data sets. The NCQA describes HEDIS as a "standardized set of performance measures designed to ensure that purchasers and consumers have the information they need to reliably compare the performance of managed health care plans" (16). HEDIS measures quality of health care in the domains of effectiveness, access/availability, patient satisfaction, health plan stability, use of services, and cost of care. Certain aspects of care measured by HEDIS are strongly influenced by factors such as severity of illness, compliance, and other health behaviors that are beyond the direct control of the health plan and the individual physician. The assumption that improvement on these measures leads to improvement in patient-based outcomes (e.g., depressive symptoms, general distress, health status, satisfaction with care) is left for empiric evaluation (17). However, HEDIS has been put forth as a "gold standard", and physicians are being asked to focus more and more on their performance across these measures (18).

Somewhat analogous to the HEDIS measures developed by NCQA, The Health Care Financing Administration (HCFA) currently uses "quality indicators" in national quality improvement projects for the Medicare population. In the sixth scope of work for Medicare quality improvement, HCFA is mandating that the peer review organizations of each state demonstrate substantial improvement across a broad array of chronic disease quality measures (19). For example, the Ambulatory Care Quality Improvement Project (ACQIP) for diabetic Medicare patients is being modified and generalized to a national level (20, 21). With ACQIP, physician performance is measured on several items such as periodic monitoring of glycemic control, lipid status, and renal status. ACQIP also considers such preventive interventions as administration of influenza vaccine and receipt of yearly ophthalmologic exams.

Basic Quality Improvement Concepts

The implementation of EMR does not automatically lead to effective QI. The most effective use of EMR demands at least a working knowledge of QI philosophy and methodology. Although many QI principles follow from the basic concepts of outcomes research (see Chapter 8), QI consists of more than the rote application of the methodology and findings of outcomes research. Examples of successful implementation of a computer-based patient record include the work of the Department of Informatics at the University of Utah and the Department of Family Medicine at the University of South Carolina (22-25).

Perhaps the most important basis of QI is that it focuses on the system, not the individual (26). Berwick summarizes the QI method as three steps: (1) define the aim to be accomplished; (2) measure process and outcome to know that a change is an improvement; and (3) ascertain what changes will produce improvement (27). Step 2, which holds that improvement comes from data, is where an EMR offers the most benefit by supplying data for use with standard QI tools such as automated prompts, performance feedback reports, control charts, and instrument panels (28, 29).

Change comes through a cyclic process of planning, doing, and studying the results. Improvement, not perfection, is the goal. QI teams often are multidisciplinary and break traditional barriers, because those who actually do the work are best qualified to make the changes. QI activities usually do not involve resource-intensive scientific methodology such as the randomized controlled trial. Instead, the emphasis is on the application to the day-to-day practice of medicine of what such rigorous research has previously revealed. Although the investigation of the efficacy of QI methods is also the object of rigorous research, this research is not usually the emphasis of QI activities.

The QI team may focus on any one particular component of quality: structure, process, and outcome. Interventions (processes of care) are delivered to patients in a given health care environment (structure) to mediate changes in health status (30, 31). Examples of structural measures include hospital characteristics, such as location (rural versus urban), teaching status, availability of various procedures, and patient-to-bed ratios; medical staff characteristics, such as degree of training, supervisory hierarchy, and nursing-to-bed ratios; and characteristics of physician group practices, such as representation of medical subspecialties.

Although structural measures are important and implementing an EMR is an important structural change, we focus below on process and outcome. Process and outcome each have their advantages and disadvantages as a focus of QI activities (32, 33). Although process measures are more sensitive to changes or disparities in quality of care, outcome measures are more specific. For example, it may take many episodes of poor operative technique to produce one adverse outcome. As a corollary, the lack of bad outcomes does not necessarily guarantee quality of care because an insufficient number of observations may circumvent the detection of an adverse outcome that would ultimately occur as more patients were treated.

Outcome measures require risk adjustment, and all methods developed to date have been less than perfect (34, 35). Multiple factors extraneous to the control of a particular provider impinge on outcomes, and these factors may not be amenable to risk adjustment. In addition, Palmer explains why risk-adjustment assumes less importance for process measures (32). Because "process measures match patients to specific health care processes that are indicated for given conditions," they, in effect, contain "built-in" risk adjustment. Here, additional risk adjustment may obscure important findings. For example, consider the process-based indicator that measures compliance with screening mammography for women between ages 50 and 70. Adjusting for age will obscure any differences in use due to age. However, screening mammography should be performed for most women in this age group, and health plans with lower screening rates because they have an older population should change their practices rather than be evaluated on an age-adjusted basis.

Risk adjustment provides a unique perspective on the epidemiological concept of confounding. Outcome measures provide indirect measures of quality of care because so many factors in addition to quality of care influence outcomes. This mandates the application of risk adjustment, which is usually done with epidemiological tools that address confounding. In contrast, process measures provide more direct measures of quality. When quality of care is measured by the proportion of a population receiving appropriate care, confounding is much less important because important exclusionary factors are reflected in the denominator of eligible patients.

Process-of-care measures may be gamed, leading some to question whether they produce better "quality of measurement or quality of medicine" (36). In this spirit, the provider might design an intervention for increasing adherence to a process without influencing outcomes. Epstein notes that report cards may lead to "focusing on the components of care that are assessed in the report card and ignoring others" (37). Other literature suggest specific approaches to improving process measures without necessarily improving quality of care (38, 39).

In addition to the traditional process measures, the importance of patient-based measures is being recognized. Clancy and Eisenberg note that only recently have we started to gather the scientific evidence necessary for making the most important health care decisions (40). These outcomes, or the "end results of health care," center upon health perceptions, functional ability, preference-based measures of health states, and patient satisfaction. In contrast, quality improvement efforts often focus on process of care, and health care report cards often focus on physiologic endpoints or mortality

(41-46). Such an evaluation that fails to consider preferences or perceptions forces physicians away from a patient-centered focus to an illness-centered focus.

Health services researchers are closely studying the factors that lead to beneficial changes in physician practice patterns (47-54). Although many methods are applicable depending upon the circumstances (e.g., use of computerized reminders for immunization [55-57]), one generic method of improving process of care involves feedback of peer-based comparisons to physicians (58-60). The link between measurement of quality and change in process relies implicitly on performance feedback to providers, with the assumption that knowledge of one's own performance, together with the ability to compare this performance against a given reference level (internal or external), will facilitate improvement (61). Finally, this improvement will be reflected in better performance as measured by process and outcome indicators.

The concept of benchmarking is frequently used to operationalize the transition from measurement to performance improvement (62-65). Benchmarking begins with the identification of superior performance followed by analysis of the process of care that lead to "best-in-class" status so that the performance can be emulated.

Feedback profiles are usually based on "quality indicators". For our purposes, quality indicators capture the frequency with which a given intervention was *appropriately* given or withheld (66-69). In making the determination of appropriateness, quality indicators often rely on practice guidelines (70-72). The following criteria, presented in priority order, guide indicator selection: (1) strength of supportive evidence that the measure will improve clinical outcomes (evidence obtained from randomized controlled trials given greatest emphasis), (2) ability to capture the recommendation reliably and reproducibly during data collection, and (3) the expected frequency of the condition in the target population. The Agency for Healthcare Research and Quality (AHRQ) maintains a large repository of quality indicators along with documentation of their operating characteristics in the CONQUEST database. CONQUEST is available on the Internet at the AHRQ Web site (*www.ahrq.gov*).

Electronic Medical Records and Quality Improvement

Using an EMR to supply QI data offers several advantages over other modes of data collection and management (25, 73). First, with an EMR clinicians can more easily process large amounts of data from many different sources. Second, an EMR avoids duplication of effort by partially freeing the QI team from primary data collection. Third, with minor modifications, an EMR can automate data presentation in a specified format for a variety of projects. Fourth, an EMR can greatly increase the immediacy of the data compilation. Fifth, an EMR enables the QI team to implement online applications that perform such functions as the generation of reminders and the provision of real-time decision support. An EMR system may have Internet hyperlinks to practice guidelines, quality measures, and decision-support tools (74-80).

The Computer-Based Patient Record Institute (CBPRI) has defined the characteristics of optimal EMR, and compliance with CBPRI standards greatly facilitates QI work (81-83). For example, an optimal EMR allows the QI team to accomplish sophisticated searches. Searches may be stratified by almost any element contained in the EMR such as age, sex, diagnosis, functional status, quality-of-life measurements, medications, procedures, test results, and health maintenance. The QI team may need to search textual entries in the progress notes. Use of a structured language with a defined vocabulary mitigates the difficulty with text-based searches (e.g., use of synonyms), and medical language processing may offer a better solution in the future (84-87). The QI team may also need to examine data at the level of the patient or the practice.

Several examples demonstrate the importance of linking the EMR with external local, regional, and national sources of information. For example, in following the outcome of a group of patients, the QI team may wish to track the patients as they move through the health care system (e.g., offices of primary care and specialist physicians, hospital, emergency department, or skilled nursing facility). A QI project designed to minimize waiting time and decrease "no-shows" might benefit from linkage with local administrative data. Likewise, a project designed to increase compliance with the complicated and ever-changing Medicare documentation standards might benefit from linkage with billing data. A QI project may use real-time clinical decision support systems based on an EMR to improve processes of care.

Often, linkage of a local EMR with data from a MCO will be advantageous. MCOs often maintain a "data warehouse" that contains excerpted data drawn from disparate sources (88). The data warehouse may provide access to almost every aspect of the patient encounter with the health care system and, by using the data warehouse, the QI team may make regional and national comparisons. The data warehouse allows the QI team to longitudinally track items such as (1) visits to multiple physicians, hospitals, and emergency departments, (2) diagnostic codes assigned by multiple providers, (3) procedures and specific services from multiple providers, and (4) prescription refills at multiple pharmacies. With the data warehouse, time lag may be appreciable, and it may take between three and six months to be certain that most of the data have been processed and are present. Also, encounter data from fee-for-service plans may be more reliable than claims data from capitated plans because there is a direct financial incentive for filing a claim in a fee-for-service system but not in a capitated system where payment is already set.

The QI team must remember that the implementation of projects based on data from the EMR involves secondary data analysis, where data are collected for one purpose and analyzed for another (89, 90). Secondary data analysis offers certain strengths and limitations when compared with primary data collection, and many of these considerations are important to the QI team (91-96). The advantages of secondary analysis using administrative data, which have long been recognized by health services researchers, include lower cost, less intrusiveness to patients, broader population-based representation conveying increased statistical power, ability to perform longitudinal studies with a high proportion of follow-up, ability to link with other data sets, lack of bias introduced by selective presentation of patients to certain providers, and lack of bias introduced by the researchers' influence upon data collection. Much of the controversy about the use of claims data to answer clinical questions centers on quality, lack of clinical detail, and the inability to perform adequate risk adjustment due to the under-reporting of chronic diseases.

Given these caveats, data from EMRs should be adequate for most QI projects. Resources are often better spent working with data that are reasonably accurate and useful rather than striving to meet rigorous scientific standards such as those required for a randomized clinical trial (97, 98). This principle holds as long as the data are used internally to examine processes of care rather than for other purposes where the consequences of poor-quality data may be severe (e.g., evaluating physician credentials, comparing health plans, making population-wide policy decisions, conducting clinical trials). From this perspective, QI data provide a starting point for subsequent iterative cycles of improvement.

Technical Issues

The preceding sections have provided an overview of QI philosophy and methodology; we now turn to more technical issues involved in the optimal use of EMRs toward these ends. Before proceeding, some basic definitions are in order. For the sake of clarity in the technical discussion, we will take as our example an EMR system that includes not only images of the documents with "basic lists of noncodified information that is available across time, such as past histories, free text, and medications" but a "clinical data dictionary, standard technology, standard codes, and reports" (73). Thus, in order to provide this required level of functionality, EMRs will be implemented through a standard database methodology. The most common methodology is the relational database, although other methodologies, such as the hierarchical and network models, are possible.

Database Models

The relational database has proven to be extremely effective for developing operational systems. First proposed by E.F. Codd in a foundational paper in 1970 (99), relational databases gained widespread commercial acceptance during the 1980s. To better appreciate the relational model, a short description of both the network and hierarchical models is given. Both of these later models have been used for clinical systems and, in particular, the hierarchical model underlies the MUMPS system.

The *hierarchical model* was developed by IBM during the mid-1960s as an outgrowth of the data processing needs of the aerospace industry (100). The Information Management System (IMS), marketed by IBM, was the leading system employing this methodology, and it is still in use today. A hierarchical database system consists of a nested structure of ordered "trees", where a tree consists of a single "root" record type together with an ordered set of zero or more lower-level dependent "subtrees" (101). Subtrees consist of a single record and again an ordered set of zero or more lower-level dependent trees. Thus, the overall structure is nested, hierarchical, and recursive. Note records are made up of fields in the usual sense.

The *network model* is best conceptualized as a linked-list set of records. A given record may be associated with many other records, and the given record may also be the object of a relationship from many other records. Relationships between records, such as many-to-many, are represented as ones in which one item may be linked to any other item. This model was first developed in 1957 by the U.S. Department of Defense and the Database Task Force Group (DBTG) and was standardized by DTBG in 1971 (100).

Each of these models for database systems suffers from major disadvantages that the relational model was created to address. For example, three major disadvantages are (1) access to data is difficult and must be performed on a record-to-record basis; (2) data and programs are not insulated from each other (i.e., they are not independent) so that changes to data formats may affect programs; and (3) no theoretical model serves as the foundation for either of these models and hence no consistent data manipulation language, such as Structured Query Language (SQL), is possible (102).

The relational model uses four basic components: entities, attributes, values, and relationships (103). These components are represented as tables made of rows. Entities are most commonly composed of objects, although relationships, which are described below, may function as objects. Objects are those things, such as people and equipment, which are of interest to be captured in the database. Relationships specify how objects are linked to one another. This is accomplished through "tokens", often called "primary keys" or "foreign keys" depending on usage.

Attributes contribute to the definition of entities. If an entity is thought of as a noun, then attributes are the adjectives for the noun. That is, attributes belong to entities and describe the essential features of the object being represented by the entity. Attributes will appear as columns in the tables associated with the entities. Values are associated with an attribute and are the particular occurrences of the attribute for a given row of the table. Values are members of the domain of possible occurrences for the attribute. For example, an entity may represent a patient, and one attribute of this patient is age. A value for the attribute might be 62, which is one element from the domain of the attribute. In this case the domain is the set of all possible patient ages.

Relational database systems achieve high levels of efficiency in data storage through their use of entity relationship modeling and normalization. Because the relational model is derived from a rigorous mathematical foundation, data extraction and manipulation can be achieved in a very systematic manner using a standard language such as SQL. These capabilities lead to a database system that can be optimized for high performance in transaction processing environments.

Because many vendors and developers often attempt to build EMRs using an existing system, it is important that the purchaser and final implementers be aware of all advantages and disadvantages. From the perspective of the QI team a key component of the system must be data access and manipulation; hence the relational model may well be the most appropriate.

System Architecture

It is well documented that systems providing the operational capabilities for an enterprise should not be taxed with queries and data extractions for analyses and reporting (104-106). Viewed from a database perspective, an

EMR will be an operational (or transactional) system. It will provide the essential data and information needed by clinicians for patient care. Thus the available data must be current, and access to data must occur in near real-time. Demands on the system that degrade this level of performance will not be acceptable. To accomplish the goals of QI, however, data queries and extraction for analyses are exactly what is required. How can both goals be attained?

Many implementations of EMRs are centered about a single, central clinical repository (107). The central repository is best built with a relational database management system and functions as the on-line transaction processing system for the healthcare facility. Various terms are used to refer to this central database: *clinical data repository, clinical data warehouse, data warehouse,* and *operational data store.* Here, we use the term *clinical data repository* (CDR).

The CDR will obviously be an integral component of the EMR system. The CDR will facilitate the integration of physician-entered data with data derived from laboratory systems, radiology systems, pharmacy, admissions, etc. It will also provide the operational functionality to support patient care. The difficulties with using only a single, central repository model, however, are numerous. Gilbreath describes the following problems: (1) degradation of the operational functionality of the system takes place when decision support or QI analysis occurs, especially for mission critical functions such as order entry and results reporting; (2) overhead in terms of database indexing becomes large; (3) maintenance of the system is inefficient; and (4) time horizon of transaction must be extended to support the decision or QI queries (106).

The use of a data warehouse offers an alternative architecture to realize the query and analysis needs of QI and decision support (108). William H. Inmon first coined the term *data warehouse* in 1993, although many others were using the idea several years earlier. Inmon defines a data warehouse as a "subject oriented, integrated, non-volatile, and time variant collection of data" (104). Chapter 4 discusses the data warehouse and related ideas in greater detail, and the reader is referred to that chapter for more information. Briefly, as a tool to facilitate the needs of QI the data warehouse is a key component in an overall EMR information system. The warehouse should serve as a location in which to integrate both the clinical data and other data of interest in QI (e.g., financial data and external data sources such as were mentioned previously).

The data warehouse should be modeled with the constructs of multidimensional model (105, 106, 109). Dimensional modeling involves conceptualizing the data as a cube in which the key data of interest lie in the cells of the cube, and the dimensions of the cube represent key dimensions of the data (intuitive constructs within the business setting) as understood within the organization. For example, date of admission, diagnosis, and physician might be three dimensions of interest, and the data might be patient length of stay, total cost of patient stay, etc. This data model can easily be constructed as a multidimensional database against which query and analysis tools such as OLAP (Online Analytic Processing) can be implemented. Tools such as OLAP provide rapid "drill-down" capabilities into the data and are more efficient than traditional SQL-type queries (110). Many analyses and queries that will be of use to QI can be effectively and efficiently implemented in this manner.

It may be helpful to note that dimensional modeling attempts to achieve different objectives from those in entity-relational modeling. Relational database models are developed to optimize storage, so they are highly normalized. That is, they use many, small tables, with the data being represented through these tables and relationships between them, thereby eliminating data redundancy. Such an arrangement, however, is very inefficient for queries because many tables may have to be traversed and/or joined in order to retrieve the desired data. The multidimensional model, however, allows some redundancy of data within its central fact and dimension tables. The goal of the model is not to optimize storage space but to optimize query speed.

Summary

Electronic medical records offer many opportunities and advantages for the QI efforts within healthcare. However, these opportunities can not be realized simply by an EMR system itself. Instead, the EMR must be seen within the context of a more encompassing information system, allowing the integration of various data sources and providing data query and analysis support. An information system incorporating a data warehouse in addition to the clinical data repository associated with the EMR offers the best solution for meeting these needs and for assessing the needs of the QI team.

REFERENCES

1. **Weed LL.** Medical records that guide and teach [Part 1]. N Engl J Med. 1968;278:593-600.
2. **Weed LL.** Medical records that guide and teach [Conclusion]. N Engl J Med. 1968;278:652-7.

3. **Dick RS, Steen EB, Detmer DE.** The Computer-Based Patient Record: An Essential Technology for Health Care. The Institute of Medicine; 1997.

4. **Deming WE.** Out of the Crisis. Cambridge, MA: Massachusetts Institute of Technology, Center for Advanced Engineering Study; 1992.

5. **Anderson EG.** Making the grade: an MD's report card. Postgrad Med. 1995;98:12-3.

6. **Jencks SF.** Changing health care practices in Medicare's Health Care Quality Improvement Program. Jt Comm J Qual Improv. 1995;21:343-7.

7. **Landis NT.** NCQA draft accreditation standards for 2000 address formularies: National Committee for Quality Assurance [News]. Am J Health System Pharm. 1999;56:846.

8. **Kaegi L.** Medical Outcomes Trust Conference presents dramatic advances in patient-based outcomes assessment and potential applications in accreditation. Jt Comm J Qual Improv. 1999;25:207-18.

9. **Bohigas L, Brooks T, Donahue T, et al.** A comparative analysis of surveyors from six hospital accreditation programmes and a consideration of the related management issues. Int J Qual Health Care. 1998;10:7-13.

10. **Arce HE.** Hospital accreditation as a means of achieving international quality standards in health. Int J Qual Health Care. 1998;10:469-72.

11. **O'Malley C.** Quality measurement for health systems: accreditation and report cards. Am J Health System Pharm. 1997;54:1528-35.

12. **Hanchak NA, Schlackman N.** The measurement of physician performance. Quality Management in Health Care. 1995;4:1-12.

13. **Tinsley R.** Negotiating or renegotiating managed care contracts. Medical Group Management Journal. 1998;45:70-1.

14. **Rosenbaum S.** Negotiating the new health system: purchasing publicly accountable managed care. Am J Prev Med. 1998;14(3 Suppl):67-71.

15. **Caesar N.** How you can get the most out of contract negotiations. Managed Care. 1998;7:68-9.

16. Quality Compass. Annapolis Junction, MD: National Committee for Quality Assurance Publication Center; 1999.

17. **Wilson IB, Kaplan S.** Clinical practice and patients' health status: how are the two related? Medical Care. 1995;33(4 Suppl):AS209-14.

18. **Stout NJ.** Understanding HEDIS (Health Employer Data Information Set) can help providers attract health plan contracts. Health Care Strategic Management. 1994;12(8).

19. **Frankenfield DL, Marciniak TA, Drass JA, Jencks S.** Quality improvement activity directed at the national level: examples from the Health Care Financing Administration. Quality Management in Health Care. 1997;5:12-8.

20. **Weiner JP, Parente ST, Garnick DW, et al.** Variation in office-based quality: a claims-based profile of care provided to Medicare patients with diabetes. JAMA. 1995;273:1503-8.

21. **Pemberton JK, Kiefe C, Weissman NW.** Physician perspectives on clinical performance feedback with achievable benchmarks of care. Abstract Book/Association for Health Services Research;15:202-3.

22. **Ekstrom MK, Orthner HF, Warner HR.** Capturing clinical reports in a large academic medical center: feeding a central patient data repository. Proceedings of AMIA Annual Fall Symposium. 1997:2-6.

23. **Warner HR, Guo D, Mason C, et al.** En route toward a computer based patient record: the ACIS Project. Proceedings of the Annual Symposium on Computer Applications in Medical Care. 1995:152-6.

24. **Haug PJ, Gardner RM, Tate KE, et al.** Decision support in medicine: examples from the HELP system. Comput Biomed Res. 1994;27:396-418.

25. **Ornstein SM, Oates RB, Fox GN.** The computer-based medical record: current status. J Fam Pract. 1992;35:556-65.

26. **Nolan TW.** Understanding medical systems. Ann Intern Med. 1998;128:293-8.

27. **Berwick DM, Nolan TW.** Physicians as leaders in improving health care: a new series. Ann Intern Med. 1998;128:289-92.

28. **Nelson EC, Splaine ME, Batalden PB, Plume SK.** Building measurement and data collection into medical practice. Ann Intern Med. 1998;128:460-6.

29. **Nelson EC, Batalden PB, Plume SK, et al.** Report cards or instrument panels: who needs what? Jt Comm J Qual Improv. 1995;21:155-66.

30. **Donabedian A.** The Definition of Quality and Approaches to Its Assessment: Explorations in Quality Assessment and Monitoring, Vol. 1. Ann Arbor, MI: Health Administration Press; 1980.

31. **Donabedian A.** Evaluating the quality of care. Milbank Mem Fund Q. 1996;44:166-203.

32. **Palmer RH.** Process-based measures of quality: the need for detailed clinical data in large health care databases. Ann Intern Med. 1997;127:733-8.

33. **Palmer H.** Measuring clinical performance to provide information for quality improvement. Quality Management in Health Care. 1996;4:1-6.

34. **Kuttner R.** The risk-adjustment debate. N Engl J Med. 1998;339:1952-6.

35. **Iezzoni LA.** Risk Adjustment for Measuring Health Care Outcomes. Ann Arbor, MI: Health Administration Press; 1994.

36. **Nash DB.** Quality of measurement or quality of medicine? JAMA. 1995;273:1537-8.

37. **Epstein A.** Performance reports on quality: prototypes, problems, and prospects. N Engl J Med. 1995;333:57-61.

38. **Parisi LL, Sulfaro M.** Six steps to maximizing HEDIS results. J Nurs Care Qual. 1996;11:8.

39. **Clarke A, McKee M, Appleby J, Sheldon T.** Efficient purchasing. BMJ. 1993;307:1436-7.

40. **Clancy CM, Eisenberg JM.** Outcomes research: measuring the end results of health care. Science. 1998;282:245-6.

41. **Brook RH, McGlynn EA, Cleary PD.** Quality of health care. Part 2: measuring quality of care. N Engl J Med. 1996;335:966-70.

42. **Ash A.** Identifying poor-quality hospitals with mortality rates: often there's more noise than signal. Med Care. 1996;34:735-6.

43. **Localio AR, Hamory BH.** A report card for report cards. Ann Intern Med. 1995;123:802-3.

44. **Montague J.** Report card daze. Hosp Health Netw. 1996;70:33-6.

45. **Rainwater JA, Romano PS, Antonius DM.** The California Hospital Outcomes Project: how useful is California's report card for quality improvement? Jt Comm J Qual Improv. 1998;24:31-9.

46. **Schneider P.** How do you measure success? Healthcare Informatics. 1998(March):45-56.

47. **Davis DA, Thomson MA, Oxman AD, Haynes RB.** Changing physician performance: a systematic review of the effect of continuing medical education strategies. JAMA. 1995;274:700-5.

48. **Bero LA, Grilli R, Grimshaw JM, et al.** Closing the gap between research and practice: an overview of systematic reviews of interventions to promote the implementation of research findings. The Cochrane Effective Practice and Organization of Care Review Group. BMJ (Clinical Research Ed.). 1998;317:465-8.

49. **Thomas MA, Oxman AD, Haynes RB, Davis DA.** Local opinion leaders to improve health professional practice and health care outcomes. The Cochrane Library; 1998.

50. **Oxman AD, Thomson MA, Davis DA, Haynes RB.** No magic bullets: a systematic review of 102 trials of interventions to improve professional practice. JAMA. 1995;153:1423-31.

51. **Soumerai SB.** Principles and uses of academic detailing to improve the management of psychiatric disorders. Int J Psychiatry Med. 1998;28:81-96.

52. **Soumerai SB, Avorn J.** Principles of educational outreach ('academic detailing') to improve clinical decision making. JAMA. 1990;263:549-56.

53. **Horowitz CR, Goldberg HI, Martin DP, et al.** Conducting a randomized controlled trial of CQI and academic detailing to implement clinical guidelines. Jt Comm J Qual Improv. 1996;22:734-50.

54. **Greco PJ, Eisenberg JM.** Changing physicians' practices. N Engl J Med. 1993;329:1271-3.

55. **Litzelman DK, Tierney WM.** Physicians' reasons for failing to comply with computerized preventive care guidelines. J Gen Intern Med. 1996;11:497-9.

56. **Litzelman DK, Dittus RS, Miller ME, Tierney WM.** Requiring physicians to respond to computerized reminders improves their compliance with preventive care protocols. J Gen Intern Med. 1993;8:311-7.

57. **McDonald CJ, Hui SL, Tierney WM.** Effects of computer reminders for influenza vaccination on morbidity during influenza epidemics. MD Comput. 1992;9:304-12.

58. **Hayes RP, Ballard DJ.** Review: feedback about practice patterns for measurable improvements in quality of care: a challenge for PROs under the Health Care Quality Improvement Program. Clinical Performance & Quality Health Care. 1995;3:15-22.

59. **Thomas MA, Oxman AD, Davis DA, Haynes RB.** Audit and feedback to improve health professional practice and health care outcomes (Part I). The Cochrane Library; 1998.

60. **Thomas MA, Oxman AD, Davis DA, Haynes RB.** Audit and feedback to improve health professional practice and health care outcomes (Part II). The Cochrane Library; 1998.

61. **Donabedian A.** The role of outcomes in quality assessment and assurance. QRB Qual Rev Bull. 1992;18:356-60.

62. **Camp R.** Benchmarking: Finding and Implementing Best Practices Milwaukee: ASQC Press; 1994.

63. **Camp RC, Tweet AG.** Benchmarking applied to health care. Jt Comm J Qual Improv. 1994;20:229-38.

64. **Berkey T.** Benchmarking in health care: turning challenges into success. Jt Comm J Qual Improv. 1994;20:277-284.

65. **Kiefe CI, Weissman NW, Allison JJ.** Identifying achievable benchmarks of care (ABCs): concepts and methodology. Int J Qual Improv. 1998;10:443-7.

66. **Harr DS, Balas EA, Mitchell J.** Developing quality indicators as educational tools to measure the implementation of clinical practice guidelines. Am J Med Qual. 1996;11:179-85.

67. **Hofer TP, Bernstein SJ, Hayward RA, DeMonner S.** Validating quality indicators for hospital care. Jt Comm J Qual Improv. 1997;23:455-67.

68. **Turpin RS, Darcy LA, Koss R, et al.** A model to assess the usefulness of performance indicators. Int J Qual Health Care. 1996;8:321-9.

69. **Barak N, Margolis CZ, Gottlieb LK.** Text-to-algorithm conversion to facilitate comparison of competing clinical guidelines. Med Decis Making. 1998;18:304-10.

70. **Dans PE.** Credibility, cookbook medicine, and common sense: guidelines and the college. Ann Intern Med. 1994;120:966-8.

71. **Farquhar DR.** Recipes or roadmaps? Instead of rejecting clinical practice guidelines as "cook-book" solutions, could physicians use them as roadmaps for the journey of patient care? CMAJ. 1997;157:403-4.

72. **Tierney WM, Overhage JM, McDonald CJ.** Computerizing guidelines: factors for success. Proceedings/AMIA Annual Fall Symposium. 1996:459-62.

73. **Mohr DN.** Benefits of an electronic clinical information system. Healthcare Information Management. 1997;11:49-57.

74. **Vissers MC, Hasman A.** Building a flexible protocol information system with ready-for-use Web technology. Int J Med Informatics. 1999;53:163-74.

75. **Kindler H, Baranov AE, Fliedner TM, et al.** Internet-based physician's workbench as user interface for a central medical case repository. Methods Inf Med. 1999;38:194-9.

76. **Shortliffe EH.** The evolution of health-care records in the era of the Internet. Med Inf. 1998;9(Pt 1):8-14.

77. **Wang DJ, Harkness KB, Allshouse C, et al.** Development of a Web based electronic pa-tient record extending accessibility to clinical information and integrating ancillary applica-tions. Proceedings of the AMIA Annual Symposium. 1998:131-4.

78. **Middleton B, Anderson J, Fletcher J, et al.** Use of the WWW for distributed knowledge en-gineering for an EMR: the KnowledgeBank concept. Proceedings / AMIA Annual Sympo-sium. 1998:126-30.

79. **Lovis C, Baud RH, Scherrer JR.** Internet integrated in the daily medical practice within an electronic patient record. Comput Biol Med. 1998;28:567-79.

80. **Quaglini S, Dazzi L, Gatti L, et al.** Supporting tools for guideline development and dissemi-nation. Artif Intell Med. 1998;14:119-37.

81. **Miller RA, Gardner RM.** Recommendations for responsible monitoring and regulation of clinical software systems. American Medical Informatics Association, Computer-based Pa-tient Record Institute, Medical Library Association, Association of Academic Health Sci-ence Libraries, American Health Information Management Association, American Nurses Association. J Am Med Inform Assoc. 1997;4:442-57.

82. **Miller RA, Gardner RM.** Summary recommendations for responsible monitoring and regu-lation of clinical software systems. American Medical Informatics Association, The Com-puter-based Patient Record Institute, The Medical Library Association, The Association of Academic Health Science Libraries, The American Health Information Management Asso-ciation, and The American Nurses Association [see comments]. Ann Intern Med. 1997;127:842-5.

83. **Elliott J.** CPRI (Computer-based Patient Record Institute) seeks industry-wide standards compliance. Healthcare Informatics. 1997;14.

84. **Elkin PL, Mohr DN, Tuttle MS, et al.** Standardized problem list generation utilizing the Mayo canonical vocabulary embedded within the Unified Medical Language System. Pro-ceedings of the AMIA Annual Fall Symposium. p. 1997.

85. **Friedman C.** Towards a comprehensive medical language processing system: methods and is-sues. Proceedings of the AMIA Annual Fall Symposium. 1997:595-9.

86. **Spyns P.** Natural language processing in medicine: an overview. Methods   Inf Med. 1996;35:285-301.

87. **Sager N, Lyman M, Nhan NT, Tick LJ.** Medical language processing: applications to pa-tient data representation and automatic encoding. Methods Inf Med. 1995;34:140-6.

88. **Hanchak NA, Murray JF, Hirsch A, et al.** USQA Health Profile Database as a tool for health plan quality improvement. Managed Care Quarterly. 1996;4:58-69.

89. **Nicoll LH, Beyea SC.** Using secondary data analysis for nursing research. AORN Journal. 1999;69(2).

90. **Mainous AG 3rd, Hueston WJ.** Using other people's data: the ins and outs of secondary data analysis. Fam Med. 1997;29:568-71.

91. **Hannan E Jr, Lindsey M, Lewis R.** Clinical versus administrative data bases for CABG surgery: does it matter? Med Care. 1992;30:892-907.

92. **Jollis J, Ancukiewicz M, DeLong E, et al.** Discordance of databases designed for claims payment versus clinical information systems: implications for outcomes research. Ann Intern Med. 1993;119:844-50.

93. **Kahn L, Blustein J, Arons R, et al.** The validity of hospital administrative data in monitoring variations in breast cancer surgery. Am J Public Health. 1996;86:243-5.

94. **Roos L, Sharp S, Cohen M.** Comparing clinical information with claims data: some similarities and differences. J Clin Epidemiol. 1991;44:881-8.

95. **Romano P, Roos L, Luft H, et al.** A comparison of administrative versus clinical data: coronary artery bypass surgery as an example. J Clin Epidemiol. 1994;47:249-60.

96. **Iezzoni LI.** Using administrative diagnostic data to assess the quality of hospital care: pitfalls and potential of ICD-9-CM. Int J Tech Assess Health Care. 1990;6:272-81.

97. **Pellegrin KL, Carek D, Edwards J.** Use of experimental and quasi-experimental methods for data-based decisions in QI. Jt Comm J Qual Improv. 1995;21:683-91.

98. **Berwick DM.** Quality comes home. Ann Intern Med. 1996;125:839-43.

99. **Codd EF.** A Relational Model of Data for Large Relational Databases. Commun ACM.1970;10:377-87.

100. **Kroenke DM.** Database Processing: Fundamentals, Design, and Implementation. Upper Saddle River, NJ: Prentice-Hall; 1998.

101. **Date CJ.** An Introduction to Database Systems. Vol. 1. Reading, MA: Addison Welsey; 1991.

102. **McFadden F, Hoffer, JA, Prescott, MB.** Modern Database Management, 5th ed. Reading, MA: Addison Welsey; 1999.

103. **Celko J.** Data & Databases: Concepts in Practice San Francisco: Morgan Kaufmann Publishers; 1999.

104. **Inmon WH.** Building the Data Warehouse, 2nd ed. New York: John Wiley; 1996.

105. **Kimball R.** The Data Warehouse Toolkit. New York: John Wiley; 1996.

106. **Gilbreath R, Schilp J, Pickton R.** Toward an Outcomes Management Informational Processing Architecture. Journal of Healthcare Information and Management Systems Society. 1996;10:83-97.

107. **Gilbreath R.** Health Care Data Repositories: Components and a Model. Journal of Healthcare Information and Management Systems Society. 1995;9:63-73.

108. **Nussbaum G, Ault SP.** The Best Little Data Warehouse. Journal of Healthcare Information and Management Systems Society. 1998;12:79-93.

109. **Devlin B.** Data Warehouse: From Architecture to Implementation Reading, MA: Addison Welsey; 1997.

110. **Thomsen E.** OLAP Solutions: Building Multidimensional Information Systems. New York: John Wiley; 1997.

SECTION III

Preparation

10 / Physician Adoption Strategies

Lyle L. Berkowitz

There are many compelling reasons to believe that electronic medical record (EMR) systems will become an integral part of improving our health care system. They have the potential to improve the quality of care, increase efficiency, decrease costs, and strengthen relationships between physicians and patients. Additionally, data repositories created by their use will help create the framework by which we can improve disease management, physician profiling, and quality improvement systems. However, these potential benefits will never be fully realized unless there is significant physician involvement and adoption of these systems. Instead, we will see feature-rich systems that fail because they are unable to achieve a critical mass of users.

This chapter discusses several strategies and tools to help a health care system improve acceptance and use of an EMR system. Specific strategies include how to induce a cultural shift, how to manage expectations, and how to work with different types of physicians.

Background

Many attempts at computerizing medical records have experienced trouble (and sometimes even revolt) because of poor physician adoption strategies (1, 2). One group of authors (3) superbly analyzed and described how their institution's EMR system failed because it did not offer the advantages touted at the beginning of the process but instead "resulted in information overload and standardization, clerical task load increase, work organization rigidity, and expert autonomy negation". Furthermore, they noted that because a unilateral vision was chosen for the system, the EMR project team could not benefit from the potential benefit of process innovation and instead made crucial design and implementation errors that resulted directly from the rigid vision that was used. In another paper, the same authors recognized that the failure of their EMR project was due to "profound misunderstandings, largely spread within the project team, that led to fatal decisions which resulted in the failure of the CPR experiment. These misunderstandings were of a dual nature: the true nature of the CPR on the one hand, and the reality of medical practice and informational needs of the experts on the other hand" (4). However, from these and other failures, we can learn how to improve the likelihood of success in future systems.

Laying the Groundwork

Cultural Shift: Moving Physicians Towards Computers

Infrastructure: Hardware, Software, and Connectivity
A critical first step in establishing any clinical information system is to build a reliable computing infrastructure that starts a "cultural shift" towards computerization. All physicians should become comfortable using computers in their office well before an EMR system is installed. A physician should therefore have easy access to a computer that has standard applications (e.g., e-mail, word processing, Internet access), basic clinical software (e.g., patient education handouts, medical books online), and an enterprise-wide Intranet suite that contains information such as hospital policies, paging directories, and local disease management guidelines. This computer network should be fast, reliable, and easy to use. If the Information Systems (IS) Department can successfully initiate this infrastructure, it can gain significant credibility with the physicians while concurrently laying the physical and cultural groundwork for future projects.

A Head Start: Practice Management Systems
Another strategy for a large health care system is to first install an enterprise-wide practice management system in all physician offices. A major benefit from this strategy is that it will be significantly easier to choose and install an EMR system when there is a stable administrative system operating because there will be more infrastructure in place and fewer interfaces required. Additionally, the experience the IS Department receives will make it more comfortable working on large projects in an ambulatory set-

ting. The main caveat is to choose a practice management system that is scaleable and interfaces well with EMR systems. In fact, the choice of a practice management system may be made in parallel with the EMR system (and may even be from the same vendor). That way, when the vendor initiates the practice management system, it can quickly follow in certain offices with a staged installation of the EMR system, even before the practice management system roll-out is completed in every clinic.

Executive Level Support

Physicians at every institution know that new programs and policies must be well supported by both the administrative and clinical executive levels to achieve success. The executive level must not only support the EMR project philosophically and financially but also vocalize that support to the medical staff. They should make it clear that they understand and accept that an EMR project may be a slow and costly process, but that it will eventually result in happier doctors, healthier patients, and a more financially fit enterprise. Another way for executive level officers to show their support is to become involved with educational processes and committee meetings when appropriate. Lastly, executive level officers must be tough negotiators with vendors to ensure that there is support and integration whichever EMR product is chosen.

Expectation Management

Some physicians believe that an EMR can solve all of their problems, others that an EMR can only hurt them, and many are in between. It is important to identify these expectations early on so they can be managed appropriately. Identification of these expectations comes about by personal experiences, committee input, and workflow and needs analysis studies.

Managing these expectations will involve both formal and informal education. Formal education may include newsletters, lectures, and other forms of communication that focus on explaining the potential benefits and processes involved with an EMR system. Informal education relates to the inclusion of EMR strategies in other discussions that do not focus on the EMR system itself. For example, a Grand Rounds lecture on the increasing problem of drug-to-drug interactions may include a study that shows how an EMR system can help to significantly decrease those occurrences. An important caveat is to be very careful not to "oversell" the system. One should try and provide realistic expectations that can be enhanced by descriptions of case studies involving institutions that have gone through a similar process.

Education

Formal education of physicians and their staff should include discussion of problems with the current system, potential future benefits, and explanation of the processes that will be involved in moving forward. A powerful strategic vision should clearly define the reasoning behind having an EMR system in a particular institution and should include both immediate and long-range benefits. This vision should include the high-level goals or mission of the enterprise as well as specific benefits for individual physicians. If possible, it should also describe the return on investment for both physicians and the enterprise.

One of the difficulties in educating physicians on this topic is the number of anecdotal reports that can bias their beliefs. While these reports and case studies can be beneficial at times, it is also important to describe some more scientific reports. The following paragraphs list some important studies that can be used to help educate physicians about the problems with today's paper-based systems, and thus the potential benefits of computerizing patient records. These studies can help physicians realize that there is often both a high demand and an alarming deficiency involving basic pieces of data such as lab results and medications.

1. *Physicians greatly underestimate their informational needs.* In a classic study of practicing internists in an ambulatory clinic, researchers found that physicians believed that they needed patient information about once a week to assist in decision making when in fact they had two questions for every three patients seen and were only able to find answers to 30% of those questions. It was estimated that four management decisions in a typical half-day might have been altered if needed information was available (5).

2. *Patient data can be difficult to find.* A 1994 report observed that physicians in an academic internal medicine clinic could not find at least one piece of patient data in 81% of their cases. The data were either missing from the chart or could not be found in a reasonable period of time (e.g., a poorly organized medical record). The three main categories of deficiency were labs and procedures (36%), history (31%), and medications and treat-

ment (26%). Overall, 5% of the charts were completely un-available, accounting for almost 20% of the missing data (6).

3. *Access to historical data is important.* One study examined physician use of historical laboratory data, which was defined as being greater than 12 months old. During a 1-month period, 38% of providers looked for these older data to use in their clinical decision making (7).

4. *Chart documentation may not always reflect the patient's complete history.* One study found that only 59% of information obtained in a medical interview was actually entered into the patient's chart. A second study found that resident physicians were worse, recording only about 50% of the visit information in their charts (8, 9).

5. *Chart documentation may not fully reflect a patient's medication list.* One study, done in an HMO setting, found that the prescription of a commonly used nonsteroidal anti-inflammatory (NSAID) drug was not documented in over 10% of charts. An earlier study, done in a VA setting, found that 21% of the charts omitted the name of one or more drugs prescribed by the physicians and that 62% of the charts contained inaccuracies regarding dosage or directions. And, unfortunately, the documentation of potentially toxic drugs was not significantly different from that of less toxic drugs (10, 11).

6. *Medication errors may be as high as 100 errors per 1000 cases but often go unrecorded.* At the national Forum on Quality Improvement in Health Care in December 1998, Lucian Leape, MD, reported that, depending upon the procedure used to identify medication errors, error rates can vary widely. Per 1000 cases, self-reported incidents resulted in an error rate of two, and retrospective chart review produced an error rate of seven. Using Intermountain Health Care's computer screening method gave a rate of 38 and a daily chart review yielded a rate of 65. Combining daily chart review with computer screening showed 100 errors per 1000 cases. According to Leape, "If you are relying on incident reports, you are missing 95% of them [medication errors]" (12).

7. *Drug-related illness is a significant health problem.* Drug-related illness accounts for 5% to 23% of hospitalization, 1.75% of ambulatory visits, and 1 in 1000 deaths. Errors in prescribing account for 19% to 36% of hospital admissions from drug-related events and up to 72% of drug-related events occurring in the hospital setting. Physician prescribing habits can increase the risk of ad-

verse drug effects through two mechanisms: 1) the prescription of drugs that are unnecessary for the treatment of ailments that might be better managed nonpharmacologically and 2) the inappropriate prescription of drugs that are either contraindicated or prescribed in combination with other drugs that produce potential drug interaction (13).

8. *Physicians do not always ensure that they receive the results of all ordered tests, that they report those results to patients, or that they document this notification.* A survey found that 17% to 32% of physicians reported having no reliable method to make sure that the results of all tests ordered are received, and over 30% of physicians do not always notify patients of abnormal results. Additionally, residents were significantly less likely to document their notification to patients about abnormal results. Finally, almost 80% of physicians reported having no reliable method for identifying patients overdue for follow-up. The conclusion was that these problems could lead to both suboptimal patient care and an increased risk of malpractice litigation (14).

Physician Involvement: Definitions and Strategies

It is crucial to involve physicians and their staff throughout the process of choosing, implementing, and maintaining an EMR system. As noted in the previous section, education and expectation management are important ways to involve the majority of stakeholders. However, a health care system should also plan to identify, provide incentives, and define roles for physician leaders in their organization. The level of physician involvement can range from an active Physician Champion, to a Physician EMR Committee, to general communications with any physician who is part of the system. The following definitions and strategies will help to clarify the different characteristics and roles for the physicians most involved in the EMR process.

The Physician Champion

In small medical groups that have successfully implemented an EMR system, there is always at least one physician who leads the charge in getting the system into place. In larger systems, it is vital to have a physician who is primarily devoted to doing the same job for the whole organization. This may be the Medical Director of the IS Department or an individual who concentrates only on the EMR project. Hospitals or groups with an EMR project in place have usually created and funded a full-time or part-time EMR supervisory position.

Ideally, this person will have a background in and understanding of computers and medical informatics and at least three years of clinical experience. Characteristics of these physicians usually include a person who can communicate well and bridge the gap between the technologists in the IS Department, administrators in the organization, and physicians in the clinics. This person must be a leader who is "willing to learn about the nature of systems, how to control them, and how to improve them" and who must also "look beyond [his] own professional or organizational identities and see [himself] as part of the larger system" (15). In other words, this person needs to be able to analyze and improve the clinical workflow, understand that the benefits from an EMR system will only result if the system is adequately used by a majority of physicians, and feel comfortable representing all of the various types of physicians found in the organization. Lastly, this physician needs to be committed, as this role may take between 50% and 100% of his time and resources.

Beware of the "Techno-Geek" as Leader

Unfortunately, a common mistake has been to choose a physician who is a highly charged "techno-geek", often more enamored with the technology than the processes. This person often has a very good understanding of computers but believes that all physicians have (or should have) the same computer understanding. This physician may thus be most interested in helping to write EMR software and in changing everyone else's workflow to conform to the EMR system. Rather, he should be interested in understanding how to shift the culture towards an EMR system, while bringing the EMR and the physician workflow together synergistically. Additionally, this individual may want to choose a vendor with an ultra-sophisticated EMR system that is perfect for his individual practice but which is much too difficult for the normal physicians in the system to use. Although these computer-savvy physicians can be helpful in other ways, it is unlikely they will perform well as the clinical leader of an EMR project.

The Anti-Champion

An important point about physician involvement is that not everyone will want to join in. There will never be an EMR system that satisfies absolutely everyone from the very beginning. Physicians with negative viewpoints should certainly be heard, but do not get too involved in trying to respond to a vocal minority. Do not try to force these negative physicians to use a system they do not like. This will not only prove unsuccessful but will very likely produce angry clinicians who may create negative feelings across the whole institution. Instead, listen to their opinions, identify their fears and needs, and realize that the success of the EMR system in their colleagues' offices may eventually win them over.

The Physician EMR Committee

The physician champion attempts to represent most physicians in the organization, but other forms of physician involvement are crucial as well. A Physician EMR Committee should include a group of physicians who are well-respected in the institution, are knowledgeable about the different types of clinicians and workflow in their organization, and are interested in the general concept of improving quality and efficiency with the use of technology. The mandate of this committee should be to represent the organization's physicians in choosing and using EMR systems, and to disseminate information to their colleagues about how and why the system can benefit them and their organization. This committee should try to meet every month, more often if there are many decisions to make. However, care must be taken that the physicians' time and workload are respected. For example, all meetings should have a clear agenda and the committee should have the power to make appropriate decisions. It also may be important to give incentives to these physicians. Depending on the organizational structure and the time of involvement, this may vary from a nice meal during meetings to a partial subsidy of their salaries.

Superusers

Superusers are computer-literate physicians who are willing to become early adopters and high-volume users of the EMR system. Their offices may be used as pilot sites, and their success often helps to break through barriers of resistance. Therefore, it is very important to identify these users and expend extra resources to make sure their use of the system is successful.

Office Staff

A physician's office staff can provide invaluable information and support to an EMR project. Make sure to include them in the evaluation, implementation, and continued management of any EMR system.

Other Physician Support

Support Desk

An important element from the beginning is to have a reliable Help Desk in place. Physicians feel that time is their most important commodity and will want a single phone number for immediate assistance on whatever they are working. Though this initially may be for basic computer applications, physicians will remember how IS handled those calls when they consider whether to use an EMR system controlled by the same department. It is thus crucial to acquire a great support staff that understands the technology and knows how to talk with clinicians.

Clinical Liaisons

An IS Department attempting an EMR project should try to increase its staff of clinical liaisons. These are usually nurses or other clinical staff who have a good understanding of information systems and an excellent ability to understand and communicate with physicians. This group will act as a vital link between IS and the physicians. Besides serving as the main educators and trainers, they will help to define problems, create solutions, overcome barriers, and serve on the front-line in improving physician use and acceptance of EMR systems. To achieve the highest amount of acceptance, most of this interaction should be done at one-on-one sessions with physicians.

EMR Assistants

One of the major problems with physician adoption has been the issue of data entry. In many cases, the process of entering data in a computerized system takes longer than traditional methods. Even if there are long-term benefits to entering these data, there are few immediate benefits to do so, thus creating a large barrier to using the system.

Physicians have been using "provider extenders" to help them with similar tasks in their daily workflow for years. These extenders range from medical assistants to nurses to physician assistants. It is therefore no surprise that there has been discussion about informatics assistants (personal discussion with Robert Spena, ACP-ASIM Informatics, 1999). One author has discussed a new kind of medical support person, whom he called the "Physician's Information Assistant", or PIA (16). These assistants would be responsible for using the EMR system to retrieve and input information for the physician. Alternatively, there may be a middle ground, in which the typical physician extenders take on some of the responsibilities of retrieving or entering data for their physicians. An increasingly attractive option is for patients to input some of their own data on-line, possibly via the Internet.

Choosing a Successful EMR System

This section describes some strategies and tools to help ensure the choice of an EMR system that will be most successfully accepted and used by physicians.

The FIRST Principles

Physicians can be very demanding about their expectations. Therefore an EMR system should try to adhere to the following guidelines, called the FIRST principles:

1. *Flexible*—Physicians need to be able to practice the way they feel is best. Therefore an EMR system should allow physicians to individualize screens and order sets. Additionally, it should allow multiple ways to document a visit, including writing, typing, templates, and dictation (whether for voice recognition and/or transcription).
2. *Intuitive*—The system should be so easy to use that only minimal training time is needed to get started (e.g., under an hour). In-depth training should be offered for advanced features.
3. *Reliable*—There should be essentially no down-time during active hours; this can be accomplished with hardware and software redundancy. Additionally, there should be effective backup plans if a problem occurs.
4. *Speedy*—Screen changes should be under 1 to 2 seconds, and signing in and out must be quick. Data entry should be kept to a minimum. Doctors should be able to document by any means available, including writing notes, checking off templates, or dictating. The system must be at the least time-neutral.
5. *Topical*—The EMR system needs to address the physician's issues, not the administrator's. For a physician to use an EMR system, there must be obvious benefits. For example, many physicians expect EMR systems to make them more efficient. It therefore makes sense to identify some particularly inefficient workflow patterns and see if the EMR system can immediately help with that. These small wins will help build up confidence and use of the system.

Interfaces

Physicians will expect that the EMR system be connected to all the other computerized systems in the organization. To help deal with this important expectation, real-time interfaces should be a crucial feature in all EMR systems. Specifically, physicians will be more likely to use an EMR system if it interfaces with their practice management system, their transcription service, their lab information system, and their hospital's clinical data repository (CDR). With these interfaces, they can retrieve demographics, schedules, dictated notes, lab results, and any other result held in the CDR. Additionally, they can order lab tests and perform billing electronically via the EMR system. These features help to quickly overcome the barrier that would be encountered by starting an EMR project with no information populating its database.

Advice for Site Visits

Before choosing an EMR vendor, it will be important to perform site visits to at least two or three institutions using EMR in similar practices. It is equally important to involve physicians in these evaluations. Additionally, one should attempt to bring along others who will be using the system, such as nurses, clinical assistants, front-office staff, transcriptionists, and billing administrators.

Define Active Clinical Users

When vendors describe how many users they have at their "busy sites", be sure to clarify what that means. Some vendors will include every potential user (including physicians, clinical staff, and administrative staff), whereas others might just count the clinicians. However, it is more important to define "active clinical users", and to further define exactly which functions are being used. An EMR system can have a "great feature", but there may be a problem if clinicians are not using that feature routinely. For example, if a vendor describes a formulary feature as a key component of his system, he should clarify how many physicians are using the EMR to electronically write prescriptions at the point of care and how many of those are actively using the formulary function. A feature is only beneficial if used.

Site Visit Questions

At the sites themselves, physicians should have the opportunity to talk with their peers about the specific EMR system. It will be important for them to talk with a cross-section of physicians at the site, not simply the superusers that the vendor wants them to meet. Specifically, this means that they should talk to those physicians who use the system only occasionally or only use parts of the system. If physicians use the system differently, it is important to determine why that is the case.

Understanding Physicians

To best understand how to improve physician adoption of an EMR system, it is important to understand how physicians work, think, and feel, and how computers can affect their lives. It is also useful to identify the bottlenecks in information flow that cause physician pressure and frustration. Equally important is to identify where individual physicians are on the Information Technology continuum and how they feel about and respond to technology.

Workflow and Needs Analyses

Workflow and needs analyses can help a health care system better understand how to identify and satisfy the major requirements of physicians. The chances for successful adoption of an EMR system will therefore increase if the EMR can fulfill the specific needs that have been identified by the physicians themselves. For example, a needs analysis might reveal that physicians want to access clinic notes from home, and furthermore that they want to document their review of those notes. The project team should thus ensure that their EMR allow off-site access to physicians and permit them to use an electronic attestation feature to confirm their viewing of the note.

Workflow Analysis
Workflow studies should define how physicians access, use, and document information. Specifically, they should identify current systems of information flow and clarify how physicians are dealing with this flow. For example, a workflow analysis can study how physicians retrieve and document a patient's lab results, how they exchange data with a colleague (e.g., phone, letters, fax, e-mail), and how they document their visits (e.g., dictation, hand-written notes). Specific workflow issues to study include

1. *Documentation*—How is a patient visit documented? How is a telephone encounter documented? Describe the timing and modality, including free-form written notes, structured templates, and dictation.

2. *Chart Dynamics*—In how many physical locations can the chart potentially be found? For what circumstances is the chart pulled? Detail the physical flow of the chart in each of those circumstances.

3. *Chart Organization*—Describe how the chart is organized with respect to demographics, problem list, allergy list, medication list, history, flow sheets, visit notes, phone encounters, lab results, other test results, clinical correspondence (e.g., referral letters), administrative correspondence, etc.

4. How do physicians use the chart when they see or telephone a patient? Look at the summary sheet? Leaf through old notes?

5. Describe the ordering process for the following: lab tests, hospital-based studies, referrals, and billing. Include the timing and modality (e.g., paper-based, verbal, electronic).

6. How are test and referral results obtained? Is there a process to ensure that all orders were done? Describe the process that ensures a physician has seen the results and documents its review and any action taken.

7. How do physicians find useful clinical information such as drug dosages, formularies, and treatment options?

8. How do physicians find useful administrative information such as specialist phone numbers and billing information?

9. How do physicians use their computers in the office, hospital, or home? Describe both medical and nonmedical applications.

10. How do physicians communicate with their office staff, with each other in the same office, and with physicians in other offices?

11. Where in the physician's office can a computer physically fit? Specifically, is there space in the exam rooms for any type of computer system?

12. Detail a typical day for a physician, from seeing patients, to returning phone calls, to filling out paperwork. Look for obvious inefficiencies and problems that can be automated or improved with a computerized system.

Needs Analysis

Needs studies further define what informational needs are most important to physicians and how those needs can best be met. This is usually done by a survey or a face-to-face meeting. Some of the specific questions to include in a needs analysis study are

1. Describe the most important pieces of information you would want to have about every patient. Rank the following in order of importance: demographics, problem list, allergy list, medication list, visit notes, phone encounter notes, lab results, other test results, and referral letters.
2. How often do you believe the patient chart is not available when needed?
3. How often do you believe certain test results are not in the patient chart when needed?
4. Do you find it difficult to effectively communicate with your staff or other physicians?
5. Describe other bottlenecks or sources of frustration in your daily workflow.
6. How do you envisage incorporating a computer system into your workflow in the next year? In the next five years?
7. What are your expectations about computer systems with respect to size, speed, cost, and reliability?
8. What are your expectations about EMR systems? Do you think a computer system can increase your efficiency, improve your quality of care, or increase your revenues?
9. What are your expectations about the access and security issues involved with EMR systems? How do you feel about home access, assigned passwords, hardware tokens, and audit trails?
10. How do you think your patients would react to having a computer in the exam room?
11. Do you think your patients would want to e-mail you? How do you feel about patients using e-mail for nonurgent issues? What are your thoughts about e-mail security?
12. What are the good things done by the Information Systems Department?
13. What are the bad things done by the Information Systems Department? How can they be improved?

Defining and Understanding Goals

An important part of understanding physicians is to understand their goals. While individuals in the administrative and executive level may have clear goals concerning quality and productivity, the goals of physicians may be somewhat different. To reiterate, the organizational goals will best be met if the physicians' goals are satisfied quickly.

As previously mentioned, important methods of understanding these goals are the workflow and needs analyses, in which physicians describe what goals and benefits they expect, and why those would be important to them. These goals will likely focus on improving efficiency, decreasing "busy work" (e.g., filling out forms), and improving revenues. While improved quality and research may be important by-products of fulfilling these goals, they are often not the driving force that gets most physicians to change their workflow. The sections below describe some high value and immediate features that can be used to help satisfy the goals of physicians. It will be important to consider features such as these when evaluating and choosing the EMR system.

High-Value EMR Applications

Certain EMR applications, such as results reporting, clinical messaging, and order entry, can offer high value functionality to physicians by addressing their needs for improved access to information and increased efficiency in routine tasks. A results reporting application allows physicians to access labs and other reports from computers in their office, hospital, or home. A more sophisticated results reporting system can even provide "value added" utilities such as graphing of lab data or other relevant actions (e.g., electronic attestation confirming review of data, computerized letter writing to inform patients of results). Clinical messaging is a sophisticated e-mail system that provides a secure and reliable way for physicians to communicate with staff, colleagues, or patients. Finally, order entry applications can increase efficiency by computerizing certain routine tasks (e.g., lab ordering, prescription writing, patient handouts, billing). Cost-effectiveness and quality can be improved with all of these applications by obtaining increased capture of relevant patient data in a centralized repository and by providing decision support tools at the point of care (e.g., drug-interaction checking, formulary and referral management, E&M coding evaluation). Once physicians are using certain modules, there will be less inertia to overcome for their evolutionary movement towards use of a full EMR system.

Another high-value feature involves the use of EMR data for analysis and reports for individual physicians (e.g., a monthly clinical report automatically generated about a physician's diabetic patients). An internist or endocrinologist might be more apt to use a system if he knew he would receive a monthly report about the rate of ophthalmologic referrals or glyco-hemoglobin tests in his diabetic patients, and if there was the opportunity to easily send patients personalized reminders about those tests.

Immediate Benefits

One of the main goals for physicians is to see an obvious benefit very quickly. There should thus be at least one EMR function that can improve their efficiency within the first few days of use. This will help to improve adoption and thus secure the long-term benefits that are of greater interest. To help define an immediate benefit, use information from physician advisers, as well as workflow and needs analyses, to identify "key functions" that most doctors would use on a daily basis. An obvious source for these key functions will come from close examination of normal tasks that are long and repetitive. Examples may include results reporting, prescription refills, referral forms, or patient summaries.

A specific example of an immediate benefit involves prescription management. Even on the first day of use, a physician should be able to obtain some benefits with this function. In one scenario, a doctor documents a patient's new diagnosis of hypertension and the EMR system provides a list of potential antihypertensive medications based upon physician preference, formulary restrictions, and individual patient characteristics (e.g., age, sex, race, weight, co-morbidities). After the doctor chooses the desired medication, an expert system ensures that there are no drug interactions, the prescription is printed (or sent to the patient's pharmacy), and the electronic chart documents it all. On return visits, the system can allow for easy drug refills.

The Four Types of Physicians: The EMR User Continuum

Although physicians have a number of similar characteristics, they are a very heterogeneous group due in part to their high intellectual aptitude, their strong desire for independence, and their unrelenting quest for perfection. Unfortunately, many administrative departments still assume that they are dealing with one type of individual. This assumption has meant the failure of many EMR projects because too much time and energy is wasted on trying to change physicians, when instead it is the strategies themselves that should be altered to fit the users.

With respect to EMR adoption strategies, an appropriate way to understand and work with physicians is to think of them as being in four different groups based upon their willingness to use computerized systems in the office setting. These groups, the "Four Physician Types", have been described by at least two separate authors (16, 17). Type 1 is a "Resistant User", or technophobe, who will not directly use a computer system. Type 2 is a

"Variable User", who will only use a computer in specific situations (e.g., to do a Medline search or print out a patient education handout). Type 3 is a "Consistent User", who will use an EMR system if it provides some reasonable benefits to his practice style. Type 4 is a "Technophile User", who believes so passionately in the technology and "rightness" of these systems that he is willing to use EMR even if the benefits are not always clear.

Every health care system has an assortment of these different physician types. And while the two extremes (Type 1 and 4) may be the most vocal, most physicians fall somewhere in between. Many of the strategies described in this chapter can be used for all physicians, but there are also individualized strategies that can be used for each of these four types. The general vision is to move the Type 1 and 2 physicians towards Type 3 status, while satisfying the Type 3 and 4 physicians at the same time. An example of one system that had success with this type of evolutionary approach found that by providing volunteers with basic information on computers, and gradually adding functionality over time, they were able to gain the support of most of the physicians in their enterprise (18). The following sections describe some of the strategies that can be used to move physicians along this information technology continuum.

Type 1: Resistant Users

Type 1 doctors are a difficult group with which to work. In fact, it is usually best not to expend too many resources on these physicians initially because they may cause the project team to become frustrated. Instead, start a slow "cultural shift" towards computerization (as described previously). This will involve providing these physicians with computer resources, sharing some of the benefits of computerizing parts of the medical record, and letting them see how well their colleagues are doing with the EMR system. At no point, however, should you attempt to change their workflow. Rather, you should wait and let them come to you when they are ready to advance to the next level.

Over time, there may be several opportunities to start changing the perceptions and actions of Type 1 physicians. These opportunities usually involve improved access to patient information through automation of their paper-based processes. One example is an application that automatically prints all of a patient's new test results in a physician's office, no matter the source of the data. This can reduce waiting time and improve quality by consolidating multiple sources of data. Physicians might even start asking to see flow charts of the lab data or how to obtain other clinical reports such as echocardiogram readings or discharge summaries. It is hoped that they will come to the conclusion that they can best access and analyze those reports at their offices, hospitals, or home—if they are willing to use a computer.

Type 2: Variable Users

Type 2 physicians will also benefit from the process of the cultural shift described above. Additionally, they are more willing to alter their workflow if they believe a system will help improve their efficiency or quality. They may use a single EMR function with all patients (e.g., results reporting) or they may use the full EMR application for a selected group of patients (e.g., the chronically ill). The appropriate strategy is thus to support their current use of the system, while offering them an increasingly more sophisticated set of solutions. For example, many physicians may just use the results reporting function of an EMR system. You should support and encourage this function by making sure as many pieces of data as possible are in the system. You can then try and introduce other high-value functions such as clinical messaging, patient education handouts, prescription writing, and problem list maintenance. As you begin to show physicians the vast possibilities of using computers in their workflow, you should then try to increase the demand for these products while carefully managing their expectations.

Type 3: Consistent Users

Type 3 physicians want to use an EMR because they believe in its benefits, but they will not use a system if it slows them down significantly or makes their workflow too complex. The strategy for this group is thus to ensure that you provide a truly usable EMR system (as described earlier) and support it. Their success will be one of the major factors in advancing the Type 1 and 2 physicians along the curve. Additionally, there should be strong and frequent lines of communications between these physicians and the IS Department. The requests made by them will be made by many others if they are not addressed quickly.

Because these physicians will use an EMR system with all of their patients, they can also be provided with special features that can only be used by consistent users. One of these features involves reporting capabilities that allow a physician to more easily identify high-risk patients. For example, these physicians can be sent a report that lists all heart failure patients who are not on ACE inhibitors or they can be allowed to quickly create a mailing that reminds all appropriate individuals to get an annual flu vaccine. A more complicated report could attempt to predict which patients are sickest, thus allowing disease management protocols to be used more effectively. Another example is drug recalls. Noncomputerized physicians will have to look through their charts, take calls from upset patients, or simply wait for the patient to show up at their next visit. Physicians using an EMR, however, can easily get a list of all patients on a recalled drug, and the computer can even print out a letter to be mailed to all of them. Ideally, this would cause the demand for an EMR system to increase quickly in the Type 1 and 2 groups.

Type 4: Technophile Users

Type 4 doctors enthusiastically use computers and fully accept the vision of the EMR. The strategy for them is similar to that for Type 3 users: provide a good EMR system, support the physicians, and listen closely to their advice and comments. These physicians are often at the forefront of new technology use, and they should help plan information technology in their organization.

Be careful, however, of basing the results of a clinical computing project on the success of Type 4 physicians alone. Although it is important that they use the EMR system, their success will not readily translate to the other physician types in the organization. Because they are so knowledgeable about computer systems in general, they will likely perform at a much higher level than any of the other physicians. Alternatively, they may have unrealistic expectations about what an EMR system can do, and they can even be disruptive to your project if they become too demanding. One expert who has dealt with this problem suggests that you assign these individuals to a special EMR developmental task force, where they can have an advanced forum to provide their input (19).

Top Ten Tips for Implementing EMR Systems

1. Create a cultural shift towards computerization.
2. Ensure there is adequate support from the executive level.
3. Educate physicians and their staffs about the advantages of an EMR system.
4. Correctly define and manage both high and low expectations.

5. Identify, provide incentives, and define roles for physician leaders and participants.
6. Provide excellent support, including quick and personalized training.
7. Choose a system that is fast, flexible, easy to use, reliable, and physician oriented.
8. Use workflow and needs analyses to improve understanding of physicians.
9. Identify immediate benefits for physicians who use the EMR system.
10. Understand how to work with the different types of physicians that will be encountered.

Conclusion

An EMR system has the potential to help physicians, patients, and administrators practice health care with a higher quality and greater efficiency than ever before. However, one of the main barriers to achieving this goal is ensuring physician acceptance and use of these systems. This may be difficult due to ingrained practice styles, expensive systems, and difficulty in creating immediate value for physicians. This chapter has explained how to increase involvement and improve understanding of physicians so that an EMR system has the best chance to be successfully accepted and used in your organization.

REFERENCES

1. Dambro MR, Weiss BD, McClure CL, Vuturo AF. An unsuccessful experience with computerized medical records in an academic medical center. J Med Educ. 1988;638:617-23.
2. Massaro TA. Introducing physician order entry at a major medical center. I: Impact on organizational culture and behavior. Acad Med. 1993;681:20-5.
3. Sicotte C, Denis JL, Lehou P. The computer-based patient record: a strategic issue in process innovation. J Med Syst. 1998;226:431-43.
4. Sicotte C, Denis JL, Lehou P, Champagne F. The computer-based patient record: challenges towards timeless and spaceless medical practice. J Med Syst. 1998;224:237-56.
5. Covell DG, Umann GC, Manning PR. Information needs in office practice: are they being met. Ann Intern Med. 1985;1034:596-9.
6. Tang PC, Fafchamps D, Shortliffe EH. Traditional medical records as a source of clinical data in the outpatient setting. In: Proc Annu Symp Comput Appl Med Care. 1994:575-9.
7. Mathews M, Gleser M. Value of a long-term clinical database. MD Comput. 1994;113:178-81.
8. Romm F, Putnam S. The validity of the medical record. Med Care. 1981;193:310-5.

9. **Moran MT, Wiser TH, Nanda J, Gross HJ.** Measuring medical residents' chart documentation practices. Med Educ. 1988;63:859-65.

10. **West SL, Strom BL, Freundlich B, et al.** Completeness of prescription recording in outpatient medical records from a health maintenance organization. J Clin Epidemiol. 1994;47:165-71.

11. **Monson RA, Bond CA.** The accuracy of the medical record as an index of outpatient drug therapy. JAMA. 1978;240:2182-4.

12. NewBytes. MD Comput. 1999;16:9.

13. **Tamblyn R.** Medication use in seniors: challenges and solutions. Therapie. 1996;51:269-82.

14. **Boohaker EA, Ward RE, Uman JE, McCarthy BD.** Patient notification and follow-up of abnormal test results: a physician survey. Arch Intern Med. 1996;156:327-31.

15. **Nolan TW.** Understanding medical systems. Ann Intern Med. 1998;128:293-8.

16. **Sachs R.** Ten predictions of the future of electronic medical records. In: 1999 HIMSS Proceedings. 1999;2:99-105.

17. **Berkowitz LL.** Diagnosing doctors: four types of physicians require four approaches to promote clinical computing acceptance. Healthcare Inform. 1998;15:93-6.

18. **Dewey JB, Manning P, Brandt S.** Acceptance of direct physician access to a computer-based patient record in a managed care setting. In: Proc Ann Symp Comput Appl Med Care. 1993:79-83.

19. **Bria WF, Rydell RL.** The Physician-Computer Connection. American Hospital Publishing; 1996:28.

SUGGESTED READING

Anderson JD. Increasing the acceptance of clinical information. MD Comput. 1999; 161:62-5.

Berkowitz LL. Breaking down the barriers: improving physician buy-in of CPR systems. Healthcare Inform. 1997;14:73-6.

Bria WF, Berkowitz LL, Gaillour FR, Wald J. Physician adoption strategies for CPR systems. In: 1999 HIMSS Proceedings. 1999;3:11-20.

Bria WF, Rydell RL. The Physician-Computer Connection. Revised edition. American Hospital Publishing; 1997.

Moore, GM. Crossing the Chasm. New York: HarperCollins; 1995.

Weaver MJ. Improving Physician Participation and Satisfaction with Information Systems and Technology. In: 1999 HIMSS Proceedings. 1999;4:39-48.

11 / Legal Issues

Terri Thompson Mallett

Key Terms

Electronic Medical Records—Electronic patient records that reside in a system specifically designed to support users through availability of complete and accurate data, alerts and reminders, clinical decision support systems, links to bodies of medical knowledge, and other aids. The EMR system is envisioned as a patient's longitudinal health record.

Health Information—Any information, whether oral or recorded in any form or medium, that

1. Is created or received by a health care provider, health plan, public health authority, employer life insurer, school or university, or health care clearinghouse, and
2. Relates to the past, present, or future physical or mental health or condition of an individual, the provision of health care to an individual, or the past, present, or future payment for the provision of health care to an individual.

Individually Identifiable Health Information—Any information, including demographic information collected from an individual, that

1. Is created or received by a health care provider, health plan, employer, or health care clearinghouse, and
2. Relates to the past, present, or future physical or mental health or condition of an individual, the provision of health care to an individual, or the past, present, or future payment for the provision of health care to an individual, and

a) Identifies the individual, or
b) With respect to which there is a reasonable basis to believe that the information can be used to identify the individual.

Health Care Clearinghouse—A public or private entity that posesses or facilitates the processing of nonstandard data elements of health information into standard data elements. The preamble to the proposed electronic transaction standards adds the following sentence to the statutory definition of *health care clearinghouse:* "The entity receives transactions from health care providers, health plans, other entities, or other clearhouses, translates the data from a given format into one acceptable to the intended recipient, and forwards the processed transaction to the appropriate recipient." Billing services, repricing companies, community health management information systems, communication health management information systems, communication heath information systems, and "value-added" networks and switches are considered to be health care clearinghouses for purposes of the Health Insurance Portability and Accountability Act (HIPAA).

Health Plan—An individual or group plan that provides, or pays the cost of, medical care (as such term is defined in Section 2791 of the Public Health Service Act). The term *health plan* includes the following and any combination thereof:

1. A group health plan as defined in Section 2791(a) of the Public Health Service Act, but only if the plan
   a) Has 50 or more participants (as defined in Section 3(7) of the Employee Retirement Income Security Act of 1974, or
   b) Is administered by an entity other than the employer who established and maintains the plan;
2. A health insurance insurer as defined in Section 2791(b) of the Public Health Service Act;
3. A health maintenance organization as defined in Section 2791(b) of the Public Health Service Act;
4. Part A or Part B of the Medicare program under Title XVIII;
5. The Medicaid program under Title XIX;
6. A Medicare supplemental policy;
7. A long-term care policy, including a nursing-home fixed indemnity policy (unless the Secretary determines that such a policy does not provide sufficiently comprehensive coverage of a benefit so that the policy should be treated as a health plan);

8. An employee welfare benefit plan or any other arrangement which is established or maintained for the purpose of offering or providing health benefits to the employer of two or more employees;

9. The health care program for active military personnel under Title 10, United States Code;

10. The Veterans health care program under Chapter 17, Title 38 of the United States Code;

11. The Civilian Health and Medical Program of the Uniformed Services (CHAMPUS), as defined in Section 1072(4) of Title 10, United States Code;

12. The Indian Service Program under the Indian Health Care Improvement Act (25 U.S.C. 1601 et seq.);

13. The Federal Employee Health Benefit Plan under Chapter 89 of Title 5, Unites States Code.

Introduction

Historically, paper-based medical record systems have been largely provider-centered, each health care provider who delivered care to a patient maintaining a separate medical record on the patient. As increasing numbers of health care providers and provider networks, managed care organizations, and payers establish information linkages to acquire and disseminate patient data electronically, there will be a paradigm shift towards patient-centered medical records. Electronic medical records (EMR) have the ability to capture in a single longitudinal patient record clinical information concerning each encounter that a patient has with practitioners who are geographically and often organizationally dispersed. A patient-centered medical record makes possible improvements in the quality, continuity, and cost-effectiveness of health care that are not achievable if each provider treating a patient maintains a separate record.

As providers continue to make the transition from a hospital-based organization model to an integrated health care delivery system (IDS), patient clinical information must travel throughout the system quickly and efficiently over increasing distances, particularly with the emergence of widely dispersed referral networks, and be available to practitioners along the continuum of care. It is increasingly common for all providers within an IDS to have access to patient information (including medical records information) maintained by every other provider within the IDS. For example, master patient indexes are being established to identify each patient uniquely and to facilitate linking patient data across numerous care settings. In addition, clinical data repositories and other shared clinical databases permit participating providers to capture all of the clinical data recorded about a patient at any point of care within an IDS over time.

An electronic or fully computer-based medical record is created on a computer (i.e., optical, digital, or magnetic media), authenticated by computer (i.e., by computer key or computer code), and stored on media readable and retrievable by computer. The fact that the law is trailing advances in health information technology means that there often is an uncomfortable fit between law developed in an era of paper records and the manner in which providers now share patient information electronically in integrated delivery environments. The use of an EMR system thus raises myriad legal issues not generally of concern in the context of paper-based medical records including regulatory compliance, identification of acceptable media to store patient records, the validity of electronic signatures, ensuring the accuracy and reliability of patient records, maintaining the confidentiality and security of patient records accessible by computer, ownership of patient data, and contracting with vendors. Indeed, the Code of Medical Ethics of the American Medical Association now contains extensive guidance on protecting computerized medical records (1). Successful implementation of an EMR system requires a re-engineering of traditional medical record methodologies and an analysis of the corresponding legal issues in this new context.

Ownership of Health Information

In the Information Age, it is increasingly difficult to determine who controls or should control health information and who should control the value of the information that is shared or integrated. The issue of information ownership in the health care industry is even more complex because of special privacy and security laws and regulations that apply to the often sensitive information involved, based on traditional concerns for patient confidentiality. Another trend in health information law—that of stronger protection of patients' rights to access their medical information—further complicates the analysis of who owns health information.

In many respects, the traditional concept of ownership is not a useful construct when applied to patient-identified information. If what is meant by ownership of patient information is the right to exercise complete sovereignty over information, it cannot be said that any one person or entity "owns" the information. A discussion of the various classes of persons' rights and responsibilities with respect to patient information is a more useful way to consider what is often the real question being asked when the question, "Who owns health information?" arises—namely, "Who can do what to which data under what circumstances?"

The classic statement of the rule concerning ownership of medical records is that the provider owns the medical records maintained by the provider, subject to the patient's rights in the information contained in the record (2). This statement of the rule was developed in the era of paper records, when rights in the physical medical record and rights in the information contained in the record were more easily separated. Even under the traditional rule, however, no one person or entity can be truly said to "own" patient-identifiable information (in which the identity of the patient may be derived or inferred from data), if what is meant by ownership is the ability to exercise complete sovereignty over the information—to disclose, sell, destroy, alter, or determine who shall have access to it at will.

Although some state statutes and regulations state that providers own medical records, many states also grant patients rights to their medical information. These rights may be viewed as "ownership" rights. Patient rights to medical information generally fall into three categories: 1) the right to access or obtain copies of the information, 2) the right to request correction of such information, and 3) the right to confidentiality.

Ownership of Masked and Aggregated Data

When medical record information is cleansed of identifiers, the law generally places few restrictions on the use of this information and generally terminates patient rights. Most statutes and regulations protecting the confidentiality of personal health information apply only if the information is linked to, or can be linked to, the identity of the patient.

If the identity of individuals cannot be determined from the data, whether by itself or combined or crossmatched with other data or databases, the general rule is that anyone who has acquired a legitimate right in the data can own it. This rule is implied by statutory definitions of the medical information protected by confidentiality statutes. For example, the California Confidentiality of Medical Information Act defines protected "medical information" as "any individually identifiable information in possession of or derived from a provider of health care regarding an individual's medical history, mental or physical condition, or treatment" (3). From this definition, it is apparent that this act does not protect such information if it is not individually identifiable. Likewise, the California statute providing civil and criminal penalties for wrongful disclosure of HIV test results provides those penalties for a variety of unauthorized disclosures of HIV test results to a third party "in a manner that identifies or provides identifying characteristics of the person to whom the test results apply" (4). From this statute, it can be inferred that an individual's rights with respect to disclosure of the individual's HIV test results terminate when such results no longer identify or provide identifying characteristics of the individual.

In evaluating whether the identity of a patient can be determined from data, two concepts are useful, those of patient-identified and patient-identifiable data. Data are patient-identified if the subject of the information is disclosed by the data. Patient-identifiable data need not explicitly identify the patient; rather, if the identity of the patient can be derived or inferred from the data, with or without the assistance of computers and artificial intelligence, data are patient identifiable (5).

Masking the identity of individuals in the information age may require more than merely stripping the data of common identifiers such as name, address, and Social Security number. Because of computers, inference engines, and the existence of nonmedical databases that link individual identities to demographic and other information concerning an individual's identity, it is possible to associate information with the identity of an individual even when the information has been stripped of obvious identifying data elements. Thus, masking the obvious identifiers in individual records may not always be sufficient to make the information truly anonymous.

Multiprovider Systems Integration Arrangements

It is not uncommon for a primary organization within an integrated delivery system to insist during negotiations that the contract provide that it is the owner of the information maintained in the shared or integrated system. Such a provision should be avoided. First, the provision may be unenforceable, because it conflicts with the originating provider's responsibilities with respect to the data and will often also conflict with patients' rights in the data. In addition, a provision purporting to transfer ownership of shared or integrated clinical data may provide a platform for lawyers for the plaintiff in a malpractice case or others to argue that the infomation should be discoverable (or is discoverable if the data are not patient identified) and that the purported "owner" of the data should be forced to conduct "computer peer review" to test whether the defendant provider is guilty of negligent credentialing or has pervasive quality problems of a type present in the alleged malpractice at issue in the case. For this reason, it is advisable for the contract between participants in the systems integration initiative to state that, among the parties, each party shall be deemed to own the data it originates. In some instances it may be advisable to tag certain data, such as laboratory results, to multiple "owners" to mirror what would be included in the medical records maintained by participating providers in a paper record environment.

To address the problems that can rise when one provider participating in a shared clinical information system relies on data originating with another provider to provide care to a patient who suffers a therapeutic misadventure, a contract among participating providers should grant the entity operating the shared or integrated system a perpetual license to maintain the data in the system. This license should be subject to a continuing obligation to comply with security and confidentiality obligations and should survive termination of the contract as well as termination or withdrawal of any participating provider.

Additionally, the rights to the data in the event one provider within the network withdraws or is otherwise terminated should be addressed by the provisions of the contract. At a minimum, the systems integration or network agreement should provide that, upon termination or withdrawal, a participating provider is entitled to copy the data originated by such provider and documentation of the chain of copying. This provision should be drafted so as not to compromise the agreement of the parties with respect to rights in aggregated/anonymous data.

Information Systems Vendors and Clearinghouses

All agreements between health care providers' external computer service or data organizations should address whether the outside entity will be permitted to use patient information or create comparative databases or other proprietary information products for distribution to third parties. Permitting a vendor to include patient-identifiable data of a provider or an integrated delivery system in a database or other information product will result in the provider or integrated system losing an important degree of control over patient data. The vendor's manipulation of such data for purposes of conducting statitistical analysis or for constructing comparative databases will be substantially different from the way the vendor processes data for purposes of performing its obligations under its contract with the provider or the integrated delivery system. Permitting vendors to process patient data in this manner may expose participating providers to potentially serious liability for the vendor's improper disclosure of patient-identifiable information. This increased liability exposure may be sufficient to prevent providers and integrated delivery systems from agreeing to permit vendors to use patient-identifiable data in this manner. Such use should be permitted by contract only if the contract includes detailed vendor confidentiality obligations also applicable to the vendor's agents, employees, and subcontractors, and provides for the protection of patient-identifiable data and information identified as proprietary information of the provider, system, or network.

Electronic Medical Records

Computerization of medical records permits more accurate, timely, legible, and complete record-keeping than is possible with paper records. In emergency situations an EMR permits physicians easy and quick access, because the records can be retrieved from remote locations more quickly and because search engines permit a physician to find the needed data without leafing through volumes of paper. In addition, proper back-ups can ensure that EMR will be easily restorable, whereas the restoration of misplaced or destroyed paper records is often impossible. An EMR will eventually be easier to transport than paper records, and this may result in greater mobility of patients, which in turn could increase competition among physicians and other health care providers. An EMR may be accessed simultaneously by multiple users in different locations. Computerized medical data can be displayed in different formats and manipulated by computer-based tools so that records can be turned into interactive diagnostic devices. Finally, an EMR may actually increase privacy through the utilization of "audit trails", which make unauthorized access easier to detect and trace, and limited access, which makes only that portion of a record that is pertinent available to a particular user (e.g., a radiology file clerk has access only to radiology records in a patient's medical file, whereas a patient's primary care physician has access to the entire file).

Electronic records, however, are also susceptible to risks inherent in the use of computer technology. Records not properly backed-up may be lost or destroyed, because computerized records are subject to programming errors, spikes and other discontinuities in electricity, and other events to which paper records are impervious. "Cybermicrobes" or viruses can infect and damage a system without notice. Finally, computerization of medical records creates a risk of inaccessibility to the record when there is a computer malfunction or the media or operating system used for creation of the records is no longer useable.

Human activities may also pose a threat to an EMR system. Whereas paper records can be locked in a file room or safe, controlling access to computer records is not as easily accomplished; the concept of locking computerized information is complex and controversial. Disgruntled employees may seek to retaliate against their employer by destroying or rendering inaccessible medical records. Dishonest employees may disseminate confidential information for personal gain. Computer "hackers" may seek unauthorized access to information and may be able to recover records that have been deleted. Even honest users can cause problems. Programming errors can cripple a system, and those who do not know how to use a system properly may crash the system or otherwise misuse it in a harmful way.

Prompted by privacy concerns of this nature, the Health Care Financing Administration (HCFA) recently required that all Region II HMOs and CMPs cease using the Internet to transmit or store any information that identifies patients. In a letter explaining this policy, HCFA stated that "acceptable encryption mechanisms are not currently available for Internet use to insure the degree of privacy HCFA, plans, and contractors are required to maintain". Other agencies and legislatures have addressed privacy concerns by promulgating ethical guidelines, enacting privacy laws, and establishing policies for ensuring the confidentiality of patient records. The following three sections outline these developments in detail.

Federal Law

In light of recent and ongoing technological developments, it is important for hospitals and health care professionals to understand the regulatory requirements that apply to the use of these computerized systems. The most significant and effective federal legislation related to EMR is the Health Insurance Portability and Accountability Act (HIPAA) (6), signed by President Clinton on August 21, 1996.* HIPAA requires the Secretary of Health and Human Services (HHS) to adopt standards for health care financial and administrative transactions and data elements for transactions to enable health information to be exchanged electronically. Any health plan, health care clearinghouse, or health care provider who transmits any

---

*As this book went to press (February 2001) significant changes in the HIPAA rules were announced. Therefore the discussion which follows may not entirely reflect the content of the final guidelines. [Editor]

health information in electronic form in connection with a transaction covered by HIPAA is required to maintain reasonable and appropriate administrative, technical, and physical safeguards to 1) ensure the integrity and confidentiality of the information, 2) protect against any reasonably anticipated threats or hazards to the security or integrity of the information, and 3) prevent unauthorized use or disclosure of the information (7). HIPAA does not require health care providers to conduct transactions electronically. If they do, however, they must comply with HIPAA standards, which they may do either directly or by contracting with a clearinghouse or third-party administrator (TPA) to conduct standard transactions for them (8). All health plans, payers, and clearinghouses must comply with HIPAA standards.

Under HIPAA, the Secretary promulgated proposed rules for the electronic transfer of medical records on August 12, 1998 (see 63 Fed. Reg. 43242 (1998)). Several of these rules, which are published by HHS to implement the administrative simplification provisions of HIPAA, outline the requirements that a health care provider would need to address "in order to safeguard the integrity, confidentiality, and availability of its electronic data". The rules would add Part 142 to Title 45 of the Code of Federal Regulations and provide for 1) a unique health identifier for each individual, employer, health plan, and health care provider for use in the health care system; 2) the transfer of information among health care providers; and 3) electronic signatures. In promulgating these rules, HIPAA directs the Secretary to take into account 1) the technical capabilities of record systems used to maintain health information, 2) the costs of security measures, 3) the need for training persons who have access to health information, 4) the value of audit trails in computerized record systems, and 5) the needs and capabilities of small and rural health care providers.

As a condition of participation in the Medicare program, hospitals must meet certain record-keeping requirements (9). Hospitals must 1) keep records that are accurately written, promptly completed, properly filed and retained, and accessible; 2) use a system of author identification and record maintenance that ensures the integrity and security of the records; 3) have a system of coding and indexing for its records; and 4) implement a procedure for ensuring the confidentiality of patient records. All entries must be legible, complete, and authenticated and dated by the person responsible for the entry.

Records must document evidence of a physical examination, the admitting diagnosis, results of all consultative evaluations, documentation of complications, properly executed informed consent forms, all orders and other information necessary to monitor the patient's condition, and a discharge summary and final diagnosis, if appropriate. Other record-keeping requirements are imposed depending on the nature of the medical services provided (10). For example, a long-term care facility may not participate in the Medicare program if the facility does not keep the clinical records of residents confidential (11).

Two federal statutes protect the identities and records of patients seeking treatment for drug or alcohol addiction at federally funded or regulated facilities. The statutes make some exceptions: if the patient has consented to the disclosure, if the disclosure is made for research purposes and does not identify the patient, if the disclosure is made to medical personnel to meet a bona fide medical emergency, or the disclosure is made by order of a competent court.

The Privacy Act of 1974 (the "Act"), which applies only to federal agencies and health care facilities and which expressly covers medical records, restricts disclosure of records by federal agencies, guarantees individuals access to records that concern them, and requires agencies to make annual disclosures of the existence of identifiable personal information in the Federal Register. The Act extends to health care facilities operated by the federal government as well as to medical records systems operated under contract to the federal government. The Act does not extend to private entities and therefore has no direct impact on the private health care industry.

A person commits the federal offense of wrongful disclosure of individually identifiable health information if the person knowingly, and in violation of the statute(s), 1) uses or causes to be used a unique health identifier, 2) obtains individually identifiable health information relating to an individual, or 3) discloses individually identifiable health information to another person. The penalties for each offense are as follows:

1. A fine of not more than $50,000, imprisonment of not more than 1 year, or both;
2. If the offense is committed under false pretenses, a fine of not more than $100,000, imprisonment of not more than 5 years, or both;
3. If the offense is committed with intent to sell, transfer, or use individually identifiable health information for commercial advantage, personal gain, or malicious harm, a fine of not more than $250,000, imprisonment of not more than 10 years, or both.

Except for violations of the provisions concerning wrongful disclosure of individually identifiable health information, violations of the administrative simplification requirements of HIPAA carry a penalty of not more than $100 for each such violation, except that the total amount imposed upon the person for all violations of an identical requirement or prohibition during a calendar year may not exceed $25,000. The procedures for imposition of such penalties follow the procedures for imposition of civil monetary penalties under Section 1128A of the Social Security Act, with certain defined exceptions (subsections (a) and (b) and the second sentence of subsection (f)). Except for violations of the provisions concerning wrongful disclosure of individually identifiable health information, a penalty may not be imposed with respect to violation of an administrative simplification provision if it is established to the satisfaction of the Secretary that the person liable for the penalty did not know, and by excercising reasonable diligence would not have known, that such person violated the provision.

A penalty may not be imposed for a violation of an administrative simplification provision, except for violations of the provisions concerning wrongful disclosure of individually identifiable health information, if 1) the failure to comply was due to reasonable cause and not to willful neglect, and 2) the failure to comply is corrected during the 30-day period beginning on the first date the person liable for the penalty knew, or by exercising reasonable diligence would have known, that the failure to comply occurred. The period referenced in the latter may be extended as determined appropriate by the Secretary based on the nature and extent of the failure to comply. If the Secretary determines that a person failed to comply because the person was unable to comply, the Secetary may provide technical assistance to the person during the aforementioned period. Such assistance shall be provided in any manner determined appropriate by the Secretary.

In the case of a failure to comply that is due to reasonable cause and not to willful neglect, the penalty may be waived to the extent the payment of such penalty would be excessive relative to the compliance failure involved.

State Law

In general, a provision or requirement under the Act or a standard or implementation specification adopted or established as required by the Act for the transactions will supersede any contrary provision of State law. This includes a provision of State law that requires medical or health plan records (including billing information) to be maintained or transmitted in written rather than electronic form. A provision of requirement under the

Act, or a standard or implementation standard adopted or established as required by the Act, for financial and administrative transactions shall not supersede any contrary provision of State law, if the provision of State law is a provision the Secretary determines

1. Is necessary to prevent fraud and abuse, to ensure appropriate State regulation of insurance and health plans, for State reporting on health care delivery or costs or for other purposes, or addresses controlled substances; or
2. Subject to the health information privacy preemption provision of HIPAA relates to the privacy of individually identifiable health information.

HIPPA does not invalidate or limit the authority, power, or procedures established under any law providing for the reporting of disease or injury, child abuse, birth or death, public health surveillance, or public health investigation or intervention. Further, it does not limit the ability of a State to require a health plan to report, or to provide access to, information for management audits, financial audits, program monitoring and evaluation, facility licensure or certification, or individual licensure or certification.

In February 1998, New York amended its medical records regulations, becoming one of the few states with well-defined requirements for the use of computerized medical records (13). A review of these regulations suggests that hospitals should keep in mind three primary goals when designing and instituting a computerized medical record system: 1) authenticity, 2) security, and 3) confidentiality. The purpose of these amendments has been to reflect the use of new and emerging technologies and to give hospitals greater flexibility in using such technologies, while also ensuring that orders are authenticated and accurate and protecting patient records from unwarranted access. These amendments require hospitals to adopt certain internal criteria and procedures for the use of computerized medical records but do not specifically dictate the details of the safeguards needed to ensure authenticity, security, and confidentiality of those records.

The majority of the newly adopted regulatory amendments are found in a new subdivision that addresses the authentication of medical records, record entries, and medical orders (14). This subdivision makes electionic signatures and computer-generated signature codes acceptable as authentication when used in accordance with hospital policy (15). In addition, the date, time, category of practitioner, mode of transmission, and point of origin must be recorded in the medical record for each electronic or computer entry, or order or authentication (16). The most detailed portion of the authentication regulations sets forth safeguards to ensure security and confidentiality of a computerized medical records system (17).

Additionally, there has been the establishment of an ongoing verification process that hospitals must implement to "ensure that electronic communications and entries are accurate" (18). The regulation includes two examples of acceptable ongoing verification processess:

1. Protocols for ensuring that incomplete entries or reports or documents are not accepted or implemented until reviewed, completed, and verified by the author; and
2. A process implemented as part of the hospital's quality assurance activites that provides for sampling of records for review to verify the accuracy and integrity of the [electronic medical records] system (19).

New Jersey hospitals using computer-generated orders with a physician's electronic signature must "develop a procedure to assure the confidentiality of each electronic signature and to prohibit the improper or unauthorized use of any computer generated signature" (20). The regulations for EMRs used by ambulatory care and long-term care facilities have been adopted in New Jersey (21).

Other states, including New Jersey, California, and Florida, have state regulations that contemplate the use of EMR, but such regulations lack the detailed guidance provided by the New York regulations. These statutes and/or regulations reinforce, however, the importance of safeguarding the authenticity, security, and confidentiality of computerized medical records. In some states that lack any meaningful statutory or regulatory guidance on the use of EMRs, such as Wisconsin, case law authority has begun to define what state legislatures and health departments have not. In these states, hospitals should determine whether, and to what extent, the state courts have interpreted existing statutory or regulatory law to apply to EMRs. Hospitals in New York that have, or intend to have, EMRs should carefully review these new amendments. For hospitals in other states, it may be prudent to look for guidance to the standards set forth in New York's medical records amendments. Since there are a number of ways for a hospital to customize such a system, each hospital should consider designing its own system with the proper safeguards for authenticity, security, and confidentiality.

In states lacking statutes and regulations that directly relate to EMR use, hospitals may need to determine whether existing law has been interpreted by the courts to apply to electronic systems. In Wisconsin, for example, a court recently ruled that the existing statute requiring written prescription orders to be signed by the prescribing physician could be interpreted to allow the use of computer-transmitted prescriptions Recognizing that the existing statute did not contemplate the use of computers to transmit prescriptions electronically from physician to pharmacy, the Wisconsin Court of Appeals held that such transmissions were similar to prescriptions transmitted orally by telephone, which the statute expressly allowed to be filled without being signed by the physician (22).

In addition to institutional guidelines, the New Jersey Board of Medical Examiners and Board of Physical Therapy require their respective licensees, when using EMRs, to have systems that are designed to protect the integrity, authenticity, and confidentiality of the patient records maintained on these systems (23).

Medicare and Medicaid Requirements

Storage requirements under federal regulations are found in the Conditions of Participation for providers. Although the regulations provide varying degrees of specificity, they place the burden of safe storage on the provider. For example, hospitals participating in Medicare and/or Medicaid are required to have a system of "coding and indexing medical records" that allows for "timely retrieval by diagnosis and procedure in order to support medical care evaluation studies" (24).

The Joint Commission for Accreditation of Health Care Organizations' (JCAHO) Hospital Accreditation Standards holds the hospital responsible for ensuring that it has a mechanism "designed to safeguard records and information against loss, destruction, taping and unauthorized access or use" (25). The Secretary of HHS recommended that providers and payers "maintain reasonable and appropriate administrative, technical and physical safeguards to assure the integrity and confidentiality of health information as to protect against any reasonably anticipated threats or hazards to the security or integrity of the information and unauthorized uses or disclosures of the information" (26).

Critical Information Technology Feasibility Issues

If the EMR system is to be used by more than one organization, it is important to determine whether the parties' information systems are compatible and if not whether they can be made so. In determining compatibility, it is important to look at different versions of the same software (or software that has been customized for each party) as well as at structures of key databases. It is important that realistic financial projections be developed for integrating systems, system acquisitions, and system conversions and that these numbers be incorporated into the parties' financial feasibility analysis and projections. These projections should include the cost of new systems and/or of additional licenses for existing technology. These projections should also include the cost of development and installation, training services, and any additional staff.

REFERENCES

1. American Medical Association. Code of Medical Ethics, 1998-99 ed., E-5.07, Confidentiality: Computers.

2. See, e.g., Waller AA, Alcantara OL. Ownership of health information in the information age. Journal of AHIMA. 1998; 69(3); Position statement: confidentiality of patient health information. Journal of the American Medical Record Association. 1985;56(12); Roach WH Jr and Aspen Health Law Center. Medical Records and the Law. Gaithersburg, MD: Aspen Publishing, 1994.

3. Cal. Civ. Code § 56.05(b) (1996).

4. Cal. Health & Safety Code § 120980 (1996).

5. Adele A, Waller MD, Alcantara OL. Ownership of health information in the information age. Journal of AHIMA. 1998; 69(3).

6. Public Law 104-191; 110 Stat 1936 (1996).

7. Section 1172 of Health Insurance Portability and Accountability Act (HIPAA).

8. Section 1173 of HIPAA defines "health care provider" as a provider of services, as defined in Section 1861(u) of the Social Security Act, a provider of medical or other health services, as defined in Section 1861(s) of the Social Security Act, and any other person furnishing health care services or supplies. The rule concerning provider identifiers clarifies that the definition of health care provider is limited to entities that furnish, or bill and are paid for, health care services in the normal course of business and that all individuals and entities who are health care providers for purposes of HIPAA.

9. 24 CFR § 482.24.

10. 42 CFR §§ 405, 482-85, 492.

11. 42 CFR § 483.10(e).

12. Reference deleted in proof.

13. 10 NYCRR §§ 405.4(c)(10); 405.5 (c)(1); 405.10(a), (c).

14. 10 NYCRR § 405.10(c). See also N.J. Admin. Code tit. 8, § 8:43G-15.2(b) (1998).

15. 10 NYCRR § 405.10(c)(2).

16. 10NYCRR § 405.10(c)(3).

17. 10 NYCRR §§ 405.10(c)(4)(i) through (v).

18. 10 NYCRR § 405.10(c)(5).

19. 10 NYCRR § 405.10(c)(5)(i),(ii).

20. NJ Admin. Code tit. § 8:43G-15.2(b)(1) (1998).

21. NJ Admin. Code tit. § 8:43G-13.4(b)and 8:39-35.2(g) (1998).

22. Walgreen Co. v. Wisconsin Pharmacy Examining Board, No. 97-1513, 217 Wis.2d 290, 577 N.W.2d 387, 1998 WL 65551 at 4 (Wis. App. Feb. 19, 1998) Eich, J.

23. NJ Admin. Code tit. § 13:35-6.5 and 13:39A-3.2 (1998).

24. 42 CFR § 482.24(b). The hospital must have a procedure for ensuring the confidentiality of patient records. Information from or copies of records may be released only to authorized individuals, and the hospital must ensure that unauthorized individuals cannot gain access to or alter patient records. Original medical records must be released by the hospital only in accordance with federal or state laws, court orders, or subpoenas.

25. Hospital Accreditation Standards, I.M. 2.3 (1998).

26. Recommendation, at p. 23.

12 / Security and Confidentiality

Merida L. Johns

During the past two decades phenomenal changes have occurred in the collection and use of health information. Environmental forces coupled with technological advances have played primary roles in these changes. As a result we are experiencing an unparalleled growth in the depth and breadth of the collection and use of personal health information. The extent of primary and secondary uses of health information has widened tremendously. Primary uses of patient specific information have traditionally included patient care delivery, support, and management as well as billing and reimbursement. This information is usually collected and maintained by the provider in the course of delivering health care services to the patient. However, there are other secondary users not directly involved with the care of the patient who collect and maintain health care information. Among these are educational institutions, civil and criminal justice systems, pharmaceutical companies, health and life insurers, credit agencies, banking centers, and medical and social researchers (1). In addition, some secondary users and other private companies have "begun to act on the commercial incentive to collect health care data" (2) by gathering and selling aggregate data without the patient's knowledge.

The patient medical record includes some of the most sensitive, private, and intimate information about an individual's life. It is also the primary source of information to health care providers in the delivery of direct patient care. The Institute of Medicine's report, *The Computer-Based Patient Record: An Essential Technology for Health Care*, envisioned that computerization of health information would play an increasingly important role in the health care environment by providing opportunities for improving quality of care, reducing administrative costs, and capturing relevant data necessary for provider and consumer education, technology assessment, and health services and outcomes research (3). Computerization of health information has the potential, if appropriately implemented, to provide support for streamlining and improving the health care delivery system. It also, however, heightens concerns surrounding the protection of individual privacy and the provision of adequate data security. The implementation of technology solutions for the capture, storage, and use of health information must be coupled with strong institutional data security programs and legislative initiatives that protect privacy interests.

Privacy, Confidentiality, and Security of Health Information

The importance of privacy and confidentiality has been acknowledged for over 2000 years, having its roots in the Hippocratic Oath which compels physicians to keep confidential any information obtained during the attendance of the sick. Other health-related professions have acknowledged the confidential nature of information obtained during the course of health care delivery and have adopted similar oaths (4). In 1994, the Computer-Based Patient Record Institute (CPRI) prepared a position paper on "Access to Patient Data" that advocated the establishment of a national regulatory framework to protect patients' informational privacy (5). Several recent governmental reports have recommended that an environment must be maintained in which the patient who discloses personal information in the course of health care delivery is free of fear of improper redisclosure of this information (1, 6).

Confusion between the terms *privacy, confidentiality,* and *security* results in their misuse. *Privacy,* also called *informational privacy,* is usually understood in the health care context to mean the right of individuals to limit access to information about their person (7). Informational privacy includes the right of individuals to determine at what time, in what way, and to what extent information about them is shared with others. *Confidentiality,* on the other hand, refers to the expectation that information shared by an individual with a health care provider during the course of care will be used only for its intended purpose. Disclosure of information beyond its intended purpose would not be accomplished without the patient's knowledge and consent.

The Center for Democracy and Technology (CDT) has defined the terms *personal information, information privacy, data confidentiality,* and *security* in an attempt to clarify the terminology associated with privacy and security issues in health information (8). The CPRI has also published a glossary of terms related to information security (9). *Personal information* is health information that contains data that identifies or can reasonably identify an individual. Examples of such data include name, Social Security number, and date of birth. Personally identifiable information may also include data that together contain a sufficient number of variables to allow identification of an individual.

Privacy as defined by the CPRI is "the right of individuals to keep information about themselves from being disclosed to anyone" (10). The CDT elaborates on information privacy by saying that it encompasses the individual's right to control the collection, use, and disclosure of personal information.

As opposed to *privacy*, the CPRI defines *confidentiality* as the act of limiting disclosure of private matters. Ball and Collen (11) further explain that confidentiality is a status accorded to information that is sensitive. By conferring a confidential status on data, there is an assumption that specific controls will be established to ensure against its theft, improper use, or inappropriate disclosure.

Security provides the protection measures and tools for safeguarding information and information systems. The National Research Council (12) has defined security as the protection of information systems against unauthorized access to or modification of information, denial of service to authorized users, and provision of service to unauthorized users. The American Society for Testing and Materials (ASTM) has divided security into two concepts: data security and system security (13). *Data security* encompasses protection measures that safeguard data and computer programs from undesired occurrences and exposures. This includes measures that would safeguard data against: 1) accidental or intentional disclosure of information to unauthorized users, 2) accidental or intentional alteration of data, 3) unauthorized copying, and 4) theft of data or loss of data through hardware or software failures. *System security*, as defined by ASTM, includes the totality of security safeguards associated with hardware, software, personnel, and enterprise-wide institutional policies. Table 12-1 compares CPRI, CDT, and ASTM definitions of these various terms.

Uses and Users of Health Information

With the fundamental restructuring of the U.S. health care delivery system, there has been a parallel increase in the collection and use of patient-related data. Certainly development of integrated delivery systems,

Table 12-1   Comparison of Definitions of Security Terms.

Term	CPRI	American Society for Testing and Materials (ASTM)	Center for Technology and Democracy
Information Privacy	The right of individuals to keep information about themselves from being disclosed to anyone	A state or condition of controlled access to personal information; the ability of an individual to control the use and dissemination of information that relates to himself or herself; the individual's ability to control what information is available to various users and to limit redisclosures of information	Specific right of an individual to control the collection, use, and disclosure of personal information
Confidentiality	The act of limiting disclosure of private matters	Status accorded to data or information indicating that it is sensitive for some reason and therefore needs to be protected against theft, disclosure, and improper use	Tool for protecting privacy
Security	Means to control access and protect information from accidental or intentional disclosure to unauthorized persons and from alteration, destruction, or loss.	Totality of safeguards including hardware, software, personnel policies, information practice policies, disaster preparedness, and oversight of these components	Encompasses all the safeguards in an information system

managed care programs including health maintenance organizations, and general concerns over the rising cost of health care services has stimulated the demand for more and more information. The availability of information technologies has provided the conduit for data sharing within and across organizational boundaries. Expenditures on information technology in health care have been estimated at between $10 billion and $15 billion a year and are expected to grow by 15 to 20% over the next few years (14).

There are various accounts of the number of individuals who have access to an individual's health information. Estimates range from 150 to as many as 400 individuals who may see the sensitive data that are collected in a patient's medical record (15, 16). Individuals having access to health care data fall within two categories: those classified as health care providers and those classified as non-health care providers.

To support a patient care encounter, many functions must be performed that require internal data sharing (e.g., registration and admission functions, direct patient care functions, case management and utilization review, and discharge planning). Ancillary departments whose functions support the delivery of patient care require data from the patient care areas to carry out their activities (e.g., dietary, laboratory, pharmacy, social services, physical therapy, and respiratory therapy departments). Internally, an organization also shares data to support disease registries, risk management, outcomes and quality management, and infection control. Information to support research and education is also abundantly shared internally.

Data distribution also occurs to external entities such as county and state health departments, state disease registries, state data commissions, and contract outcomes management databases. Reports to third-party payers contain patient-specific data and determine a patient's initial and continued eligibility for coverage. Although third-party payer organizations vary in their procedures, many have data-sharing relationships that are either direct or indirect with employers, third-party benefits managers, marketers and database developers, and life insurers. The American Health Information Management Association has developed a situation analysis and position paper on the Confidentiality of Medical Records that presents a schema for health information and how it is used (17).

The National Research Council in its report identified new entrants in the information-sharing market (12). The new users of health information are typically those who provide products and services to the health care industry and have significant business interests in the collection of individually identifiable health information. Examples of such companies include medical and surgical suppliers, pharmaceutical companies, reference laboratories, and companies that provide information technology services. Table 12-2 lists typical individuals and organizations that may receive personal health information related to one clinical encounter.

Table 12-2   Typical Users of Health Information.

• Patient	• Accrediting organization
• Primary care physician	• Employer
• Health insurance company	• Life insurance company
• Clinical laboratory	• Medical information bureau
• Local retail pharmacy	• Managed care company
• Pharmacy benefits manager	• Attorney
• Consulting physician	• State public health agencies
• Local hospital	• Medical researcher
• State Bureau of Vital Statistics	

From National Academy of Sciences. For the Record: Protecting Electronic Health Information. National Research Council, Washington, DC: National Academy Press, 1997.

Breaches in the protection of confidential data have become widespread as a consequence of the pressures for more information, the technology capacity to deliver such data, and the potential commercial advantage to collect health care information. In some instances these breaches occur within the parameters of present law, whereas others have been illegal. Pharmacies in some states can legally sell individual prescription records to pharmaceutical companies for use in marketing and mailing list brokers can sell the names of individuals suffering from specific conditions to those marketing specific products or services (17).

Illegal breaches in the protection of confidential data run the gamut from releasing personal medical information of politicians during campaigns, to leaking names of HIV-positive patients to newspapers, to selling patient records to lawyers soliciting malpractice plaintiffs (17). Specific privacy violations cited in the Center for Democracy and Technology report include (8)

- During the 1992 campaign of a Congresswoman from New York, confidential medical records were faxed to a local newspaper. The Congresswoman won her seat in the House only after overcoming the fallout from the unauthorized disclosure of her medical history.
- In December 1994, six pages of detailed data on HIV status and drug abuse history of volunteers in an AIDS prevention unit were faxed to another organization.

- An HMO plan recently admitted to maintaining detailed notes of psychotherapy sessions in computer records that were accessible by all clinical employees.
- In Maryland, eight Medicaid clerks were prosecuted for selling computerized record printouts of recipients' financial resources and dependents to sales representatives of managed care companies.

The corresponding social consequences of breaches in safeguarding confidential information have far-reaching results. The aftermath of inappropriate information disclosure includes the denial of employment, insurance, health care, and housing. As more information is collected at greater levels of granularity, the inappropriate dissemination of information may potentially be more devastating. This is particularly the case with genetic information. A recent article in the *Journal of the American Medical Association* (18) notes that:

> Participants in genetic testing should be informed that the genetic testing for cancer susceptibility may limit their ability to obtain health, life, or disability insurance; may lead to limitations in health insurance coverage; or may result in higher premiums for insurance products. Participants also should be informed that genetic testing might pose a risk to their present or future employment.

Growth and Impact of Information Technologies

Even a decade ago, the threat to informational privacy due to technology advance and capacity was not as enormous as it is today. Computer and network security is one of the most challenging issues facing the computer technology industry. Experts in 1985 estimated that the real cost of computer/network crime was in the area of $15 billion annually (19). Today, companies in the United States could be losing more than $250 billion annually to information thieves. Fifty-six percent of Fortune 500 companies responding to a survey conducted by the American Society for Industrial Security (ASIS) reported at least one attempted or suspected information misappropriation (20).

It is true that the application of security measures can greatly reduce the threat to informational privacy; in fact, some insist that protections in the computerized environment offer more security opportunities than in the paper world (21). Nonetheless, these opportunities can only be realized when security systems are properly designed and implemented, monitored, and managed through an appropriate security organizational infrastructure.

Several technological advances have allowed greater depth and breadth of data collection, storage, and dissemination. Certainly the computer network revolution and the development and refinement of distributed processing technology have provided greater opportunities for data access and dissemination. Such systems are remarkably complex and heterogeneous and pose some of the most confounding security concerns to ever face the information systems environment. Threats to information security are particularly heightened when networks go beyond the physical boundaries of the enterprise campus.

Maturing of information technologies that allow for the development of data repositories and warehouses also has a great impact on data access, dissemination, and potentials for security breaches. Older technology allowed for the infamous "silos" of information. While this approach hindered data access and integrity and encouraged data redundancy, it did provide some intrinsic security by separating data. Today, however, the very nature of aggregating data in one virtual space provides a breakdown of physical boundaries between records and data and those who may want to access them. In addition to greater access opportunities, the aggregation of data provides a broader range and depth for information access. Besides being useful to the organization for clinical and management decision support, the aggregation of data also provides more opportunity for intrusion into sensitive information.

The application of technologies such as data mining, neural networks, and artificial intelligence to large data stores also poses new and potentially ominous security threats. As defined above, personally identifiable information includes data that together contain a sufficient number of variables to allow identification of an individual. With the combined application of sophisticated statistical techniques, data visualization, and pattern recognition, individuals can be uniquely identified given a set of variables that may not necessarily by themselves contain personally identifiable information.

The explosion of the Internet brings immense security and law enforcement challenges. Reports indicate the growing vulnerability of information systems connected to public infrastructures such as the Internet, which have allowed interlopers a frequently easy avenue for intrusion (6). Interstate and international consumer fraud have been made significantly easier in a number of respects as a result of the Internet, and jurisdiction and identification issues have also complicated the prosecution of Internet crime (22). The exponential growth of electronic mail, a result of the Internet, also brings with it its own security problems. Electronic mail can be intercepted and read or even altered during transit by unauthorized intermediaries. Even the authenticity of an e-mail sender cannot be ensured, because e-mail headers can be easily altered or faked. The Internet and electronic mail both provide avenues for intruders into private health information.

The Imperative for Health Information Security

The imperative for health information security is greater today than ever before. Technological advances and increases in information systems capacity bring opportunities to streamline health care delivery, reduce costs, and improve quality. These advances, however, when associated with increased collection and storage of personal information, also create greater vulnerabilities in safeguarding and protecting privacy.

The traditional paper environment inherently provided some protection of privacy (8). Information on a given individual was more difficult to aggregate, access, and analyze. In today's sophisticated electronic environment the collection and storage of aggregate data on an individual is much easier. The granularity of data is greater; the number of users of health data has exploded; and database technology and networks have opened up an entirely new world for information aggregation, sharing, and access. Data mining and other analytical techniques can not only invade patient privacy but provider privacy as well. Information about corporate activities is just as vulnerable in today's world as patient-specific data.

No private practice, institution, organization, or enterprise is free from cyber-intrusion by people either inside or outside the corporate walls. The scope of the problem must be recognized and dealt with through the development of a systematic and encompassing security program. Such a program must be directed toward protecting information from insider attacks from current and former employees, on-site contractors, consultants, partners, and suppliers. The security program must also safeguard information from outsiders who may attempt to steal or corrupt information through electronic break-ins, employing surveillance technologies, or engaging in competitive intelligence. As reports cited previously indicate, the stakes and costs are too large to ignore. Protecting patient's right to privacy and respect for the confidentiality of health information has been an important underpinning in the provision of health care for over two thousand years. To continue to safeguard personal health information will require a concerted effort on the part of health care providers, health care organizations, health policy developers, the information technology industry, and the federal government.

Governmental and Legislative Protections

No uniform national standard exists that protects the confidentiality of health information. The fragmented, state-by-state approach yields little uniformity regarding the confidentiality of health information and provides no consistent or comprehensive privacy protection for health information. For example, among the states that have regulations, statutes, or case law recognizing medical records as confidential and limiting access to them, many do not recognize computerized medical records as legitimate documents under law. The range of medical privacy law does not address the practice of compiling medical information about patients, with or without their consent, or the identification of personal information for sale to businesses with a financial interest in the data (1). Existing statutes also vary in regard to allowing patients a right to access their own information. Furthermore, most statutes do not address redisclsoure of health information and lack penalties for misuse or misappropriation (23).

Although 36 states impose a general requirement for patient confidentiality upon physicians and 26 states extend that duty to other health care providers, only 4 states have legislation specifically extending the duty to insurers and only 9 states impose restrictions on employers (24). On the federal level, only the Privacy Act of 1974 provides protection of confidential information, and this is limited only to the disclosure by the government of individual health records maintained by government agencies.

The Office of Technology Assessment report (1, p. 15) concluded that

> This patchwork of State and Federal laws addressing the question of privacy in personal medical data is inadequate to guide the health care industry with respect to obligations to protect the privacy of medical information in a computerized environment. It fails to confront the reality that, in a computerized system, information will regularly cross State lines, and will therefore be subject to inconsistent legal standards with respect to privacy. The law allows development of private sector businesses dealing in computer databases and data exchanges of patient information without regulation, statutory guidance, or recourse for persons who believe they have been wronged by abuse of data. These laws do not address the questions presented by new demands for data prompted by computerization, and the obligations of secondary users in accessing and maintaining data. Lack of legislation in this area will leave the health care industry with an uneven sense of their responsibilities for maintaining privacy.

Model Legislative Language

In response to the absence of legislative statutes protecting confidential medical information, the American Health Information Management Association (AHIMA) drafted model legislative language that outlined a code of fair information practices. This language attempts to address the inadequacies in safeguards that currently exist. The language was published by the Office of Technology Assessment in its report as a model code (1) and was subsequently used in the drafting of several bills in the 103rd, 104th, and 105th Congresses. The key provisions in AHIMA's model language include the following principles of fair health information practices (23):

- *Patient's Right to Know*—The patient (or patient's representative) has the right to know that the patient's health care information is maintained by any person and to know for what purpose the health care information is used.
- *Restrictions on Health Care Information Collection*—Health care information must be collected only to the extent necessary to carry out the purpose for which it is intended.
- *Collection and Use Only for Lawful Purpose*—Health care information must only be collected and used for a necessary and lawful purpose.
- *Notification to Patient*—Each person maintaining health care information must prepare a formal, written statement of the fair information practices observed by such person and this must be provided to each patient.
- *Restriction on Use for Other Purposes*—Health care information may not be used for any purpose beyond that for which it is collected, except as otherwise provided.
- *Right to Access*—The patient (or patient's representative) may have access to health care information concerning the patient, has the right to have a copy of such health care information, and has the right to have a notation made of any amendment or correction of such health care information requested by the patient (or patient's representative).
- *Required Safeguards*—Any person maintaining, using, or disseminating health care information shall implement reasonable safeguards for the security of health care information and its storage, processing, and transmission.

- *Additional Protections*—Methods to ensure the accuracy, reliability, relevance, completeness, and timeliness of health care information should be instituted.

Recent Legislative Initiatives

During the 103rd, 104th, and 105th Congresses several bills were introduced to address privacy protection of health care information. During the 105th Congress, six bills were introduced that provide varying degrees of protection:

- Fair Health Information Practices Act of 1997 (HR52)
- Medical Privacy in the Age of New Technologies Act of 1997 (HR 1815)
- Consumer Health and Research and Technology Protection Act (HR 3900)
- Medical Information Privacy and Security Act (S1368)
- Health Care Personal Information Nondisclosure Act (S 1921)
- Medical Information Protection Act of 1998 (S 2609)

None of these bills was considered for legislative action before the end of the 105th Congress. Several issues, however, arose during the hearings. Some groups felt that many of the bills did not go far enough to safeguard confidential information. Other groups were concerned how health care information is used outside the care setting, especially in areas of law enforcement and employment. Still other groups had concerns about the restrictive nature of some federal legislation, particularly in the area of health care information use in research and evaluation of services. Federal preemption of state statutes has also been a major issue, even among groups that support federal legislation.

In the current Congress several bills have been introduced that address federal health care information privacy protection:

- Medical Information Privacy and Security Act (S 573)
- Health Care Personal Information Nondisclosure Act (S 578)
- Medical Information Protection Act (S 881)
- Medical Information Privacy and Security Act (H 1057)

With the passage of the Health Insurance Portability and Accountability Act of 1996 (HIPAA), if Congress does not meet a self-imposed deadline of August 21, 1999, to enact comprehensive standards for protecting the privacy of individually identifiable health information, the Secretary of Health and Human Services is required to promulgate security standards. In September 1997, the Secretary, pursuant to the HIPAA legislation, delivered recommendations for privacy legislation to Congress. The report recommended that Congress enact national standards that provide fundamental privacy rights for patients and define responsibilities for those who serve them. The recommendations were based on five key principles (25):

- **Boundaries.** An individual's health care information should be used for health purposes and only those purposes, subject to a few carefully defined exceptions. It should be easy to use information for those defined purposes, and very difficult to use it for other purposes. Federal health record confidentiality legislation should impose a legal duty of confidentiality on those who provide and pay for health care and on other entities that receive health information from them.
- **Security.** Organizations to which we entrust health information ought to protect it against deliberate or inadvertent misuse or disclosure. Federal law should require such security measures.
- **Consumer Control.** Patients should be able to see what is in their records, get a copy, correct errors, and find out who else has seen them. Our recommendations significantly strengthen the ability of consumers to understand and control what happens to their health care information.
- **Accountability.** Those who misuse personal health information should be punished, and those who are harmed by its misuse should have legal recourse. Federal law should provide new sanctions and new avenues for redress for consumers whose privacy rights have been violated.
- **Public Responsibility.** Individuals' claims to privacy must be balanced by their public responsibility to contribute to the common good, through use of their information for important, socially useful purposes, with the understanding that their information will be used with respect and care and will be legally protected. Federal law should identify those limited arenas in which our

public responsibilities warrant authorization of access to our medical information, and should sharply limit the uses and disclosure of information in those contexts.

Security Threats to Health Care Information

Security of health care information encompasses three basic concepts. The first of these is protection of the information. Specifically this includes the defense or safeguard of information against attack through either intentional or unintentional acts. This concept encompasses informational privacy concerns. The second concept involves data integrity. This includes assurance that quality characteristics are maintained and that data are relevant, comprehensive, appropriate, timely, current, and consistent. The third concept involves reliability (i.e., the dependability of a system to perform exactly as expected and without error). Thus, given these principles, the major goals of any security program are to provide for information privacy, integrity, and availability.

Threats to health care information can be identified in terms of threats to informational privacy, data integrity, and information availability. Table 12-3 presents a matrix of common threats that can interfere with achievement of security program goals.

Table 12-3   Common Threats to Health Care Information Security.

Goals/Threats	Information Privacy	Information Integrity	Information Reliability
	• Insider accidental disclosure	• Insider accidental errors	• Natural hazards
			• Equipment failure
	• Insider abuse of access privileges	• Insider malicious attack	• Software failure
	• Insider unauthorized access	• Intruder accidental or malicious attack	• Human error
			• Theft
	• Outsider intruders	• Equipment failure	• Malice
		• Software failure	• Strategic attack
		• Strategic attacks (e.g., virus)	

Threats to Informational Privacy

There are several common threats to informational privacy:

- *Insider Accidental Disclosures/Errors*—This is probably the most common threat to informational privacy. In this case the employee, due to lack of knowledge of organizational policy or for some other reason, releases private information to unauthorized individuals.
- *Abuse by Insiders of Their Access Privileges*—In this case individuals who have authorized access to target data violate the trust associated with that access (e.g., an employee who reviews the medical information of a colleague, family member, or friend for non-health care delivery purposes).
- *Insider Unauthorized Access*—This includes those cases where an employee may have access to the information system but targets access to unauthorized information through exploitation of system vulnerability or through other means. Frequently this type of action will be for spite or profit.
- *Outside Intruders*—These are individuals who do not have authorized access to the system but gain such access through exploitation of system vulnerabilities or other means to explore information stores or to mount attacks to damage systems or disrupt operations.

Threats to Information Integrity

Several of the threats to informational privacy also apply to those related to information integrity:

- *Insider Accidental Error*—In this case the employee inputs incorrect values or collects data inappropriately. This may be due to lack of knowledge or to poor system constraints.
- *Insider Malicious Attack*—In this case the employee purposefully corrupts data that for which there may be authorized or unauthorized access.
- *Intruder Attack*—In this case an intruder gains access to the system by exploitation of system vulnerability or other means and either accidentally or purposefully corrupts or destroys data.

- *Software Failure*—Application or system software fails to adequately protect data integrity due to nonperformance, inadequate performance, inadequate code, or other reason.
- *Strategic Attack*—This includes a purposeful attack such as launching of a computer virus that corrupts or destroys data.

Threats to Information Reliability

Threats to information reliability involve a wide spectrum of incidents ranging from natural disasters to human error. Among these are

- *Natural Hazards*—This includes such things as earthquakes, tornadoes, ice storms, fires, floods, and electrical storms.
- *Equipment and Software Failures*—This includes hardware breakdowns and software failures that cause unexpected systems suspension or shutdown.
- *Human Error*—This includes any human error that would cause hardware or software to improperly function, in turn causing unexpected system disruption or shutdown.
- *Theft, Malice, or Strategic Attack*—This includes purposeful theft or attack on any component of the information system with the intent of causing system disruption or shutdown.

Approaches for Ensuring Health Care Information Security

Various security strategies and countermeasures can be employed to help ensure information security. To be successful, however, these must be embedded within an overall enterprise-wide security program. A piecemeal approach to implementation of countermeasures, techniques, and safeguards will not ensure a robust security program that will protect the interests of the enterprise or public.

Several strategies make up the components of a strong security program. Among these are development of a formal security organization; development and implementation of administrative, physical, and technical controls including the establishment of a risk analysis program; and development of a business continuity plan.

Development of the Security Organization

The most fundamental security strategy is the establishment of a formal security organizational structure. Frequently in health care institutions security functions have been placed under the direct control of the information systems department or delegated to those who operate departmental information systems. A security program, however, because of its multifaceted purposes, is multidisciplinary and no one person or department will likely have the knowledge and skills to staff the security function adequately (4). Thus, the security organization should include the appropriate mix of personnel with skills to carry out the security function and also include a variety of individuals who function in an oversight or matrix organizational structure.

For the security function to be successful, it must have the support of executive management. Security programs require resources and delegation of appropriate authority and responsibility to individuals to carry out security management functions. The support of top management signals clear support for the security initiative and indicates that responsibility and associated accountability has been delegated.

Various organizational structures can be used to support the security function. Most importantly, though, the security function should be positioned within an organization so that it has significant authority to successfully carry out the functions of a security program. Furthermore, the security organization should be independent of those organizational units that are subject to security measures. In other words, the security function should not report to the information systems department or internal audit department. Frequently institutions will designate a chief security officer (CSO) or information security officer (ISO) with overall responsibility for the security function. The CSO may report directly to the Chief Information Officer or report to another top executive officer of the organization. The CSO will normally be responsible for the design, implementation, and evaluation of the total security program encompassing information protection, integrity, and availability. Typical functions of a CSO are listed in Table 12-4. In addition to the CSO, the formal security organization should be staffed by individuals who have both technical and managerial expertise in the area of systems security. Depending on the organization, this may include individuals with special expertise in personal computing, local area networking, access control administration, contingency planning, and training and awareness development.

Table 12-4   Typical Functions of the Chief Security Officer.

- Plan security strategy

- Develop enterprise-wide security policy for safeguarding the access, integrity, and availability of information and information systems

- Develop enterprise-wide procedures and standards for security policy implementation

- Coordinate the administration of security software

- Manage confidentiality agreements for employees, contractors, and other involved parties

- Coordinate security procedures

- Coordinate employee security training

- Monitor audit trails to identify security violations

- Conduct risk assessment of enterprise information systems

- Develop business continuity plan

In addition to staffing, the security organization must also define resource requirements; develop and manage a budget; establish job descriptions; develop mission, goals, and strategies for the security initiative; and develop and foster interdepartmental relationships. Additionally, a formal information security management committee should be established that is multidisciplinary and composed of departments that represent major computer users and those who have a significant responsibility for information security.

Administrative Controls

Administrative controls consist of management constraints, operational procedures, accountability procedures, and supplemental controls that provide an acceptable level of protection for computing resources. One of the best preventive controls is employee education and training. Security awareness training helps employees understand the importance of security practices and includes heightening awareness of general overall policies as well as training in fundamental technical techniques. For example, awareness of the destructiveness of a computer virus can help employees understand why external software or files should not be loaded on individual workstations. Understanding procedures for backing up files can save the company and the employee enormous amounts of time and cost should there be a software or equipment failure. Frequently, simple preventive measures will result in major cost and time savings.

Every organization should have appropriate recruitment and termination procedures. While this preventative measure seems simplistic, it is surprising to note how many organizations do not do an adequate job of screening individuals before hiring or employ appropriate computer security procedures at the time of termination. Regardless of the conditions of termination, all access rights should be immediately discontinued upon cessation of employment. In cases of involuntary termination, the employee should be asked to leave the premises immediately; computer rights should be discontinued; all badges, keys, or other devices should be confiscated; and all locks to computer resource areas should be changed.

Security policies and procedures should be established that are enterprise-wide. These include policies and procedures that cover the use and control of computing resources including equipment, files, and software; access to and use of organization information; protection of confidential information; security incident reporting; and potential consequences of employee noncompliance with security policy or procedures. All employees, volunteers, contractors, students, consultants, or others who may use computer resources or have access to organizational information should sign a confidentiality statement or agreement at time of employment, and this should be updated on a yearly basis. Samples of such agreements can be obtained from the CPRI (27).

Another type of administrative control is a security review or audit. Such reviews should be periodically scheduled to ensure that those policies and procedures are being followed. For example, periodic review or audit of local workstation drives may reveal the presence of unauthorized software or application programs, inappropriate use of local passwords, or other violations of security policy.

Physical Controls

Physical controls fall into two categories: preventive and detective. The use of locks, badges, and alarms helps to control access to physical computing resources. Physical controls can also provide protection to the computing resource from theft and destruction or damage from accident, fire, or natural disasters.

Some very simple and inexpensive measures can provide a wide umbrella of protection of computing resources. A fundamental strategy is storage of backup files and documentation off-site so that one incident will not destroy both active data files and software and back-up copies. Back-up copies should be afforded the same security as active data files and stored in a secure location with appropriate environmental safeguards. Backup power supply should be used to ensure that computing resources are available should there be a power outage. Backup power should be minimally available to allow for an appropriate period of time to safely shutdown the computer systems so that files and/or software are not damaged during a power outage of long duration.

Badge systems, locks, and keys should be used at all entrances to restrict access to computing resource areas. Closed-circuit television monitors may also be employed to monitor access to computing rooms and equipment. Various sensors and alarms should be used to detect dangerous changes in air or cooling systems or to detect fire or smoke.

Technical Controls

A wide variety of technical controls should be used to protect the information resource. Access control software is a fundamental technique for security protection and is used to limit access of computer data files to approved users. This type of software verifies computer users and limits their privileges to view, copy, delete, or otherwise alter files. Frequently this type of software is used in conjunction with the categorization of the degree of confidentiality, class, or security of information. For example, military organizations give access rights to classified, confidential, secret, or top secret information according to the corresponding security clearance level of the user.

Associated with access control software is the use of fixed and dynamic password protections. Passwords are used to verify that the user of identification is the owner of the identification. To be effective, *fixed passwords* must be difficult to guess and should not be composed of meaningful words or something that is associated with the user (e.g., pet's name, user birthdate). Fixed passwords should contain both alphabetic and numeric characters and be at least six characters in length. Fixed passwords should be changed on a regular basis (at least every 90 days).

Dynamic passwords are created by a token that is programmed to generate passwords randomly. Tokens are tamper-resistant plastic cards with an inset microprocessor chip that contains a stored password that automatically and frequently changes. When a token is used to access a computer, the computer reads the token's password, reads another password entered by the user, and matches these two to an identical token password generated by the computer and user's password. Tokens are expected to be rein-forced by biometric identification; that is, by unique personal characteris-tics such as fingerprints, retinal patterns, skin oils, voice variations, and keyboard-typing rhythms (28).

Encryption, another technical security control, is a method by which data are made unintelligible to those who do not have appropriate access. Usually encryption is used with network transmissions. Essentially, infor-mation is changed by encryption from readable text to ciphertext, or un-readable data. This is accomplished by scrambling data using mathematical equations and secret codes called *keys*. Two keys are usually used, one used by the sender to change the data into ciphertext and one used by the re-ceiver of a message to decode the data. Encryption is considered to be the only sure way of protecting data during network transmission (26).

In addition to the aforementioned methods, detection and intrusion systems can be used to protect data. The most commonly used detective method is the audit trail. The audit trail or log is a record of system activi-ties. The log captures various types of data. These data include a record of log-ins and log-outs; specific events that have been taken against data such as reading, writing, modification, or creation; date and time of events and identification of the user associated with the event; and success or failure of the event. Violation reports can be automatically generated that can indi-cate potential significant security violations. However, audit trails and logs are not effective unless there is a procedure in place for regular and fre-quent review of their results. Furthermore, procedures need to be activated whereby possible security violations are investigated.

Intrusion detection systems use artificial intelligence methods to iden-tify possible security breaches. Such systems track users while they are using the computer system and, based upon a unique user profile, determine whether user actions are consistent with their personal profile or an estab-lished norm. A user profile can be composed of various elements including usual CPU, input/out usage, command, compiler, or editor use. Such pro-files often contain information about what files the user usually accesses, what programs are usually executed, types of errors frequently made, and usual hours and days of use.

Computer networks pose an enormous security threat to any organiza-tion. Protection of data within a computer network is very complex and in-volves the application of a number of security services. Among these are integrity services, authentication services, access control services, confi-dentiality services, and nonrepudiation services. All of these services must be well organized, interfaced, and managed by skilled professionals. In addition to these services, networks are also protected from outside intruders through the use of firewalls and security gateways. Essentially these methods filter access to the network while still allowing users access to the outside world. Firewalls limit the types of information that can be passed to or from computers located on the internal network.

To be effective technical controls must be implemented in a deliberate and organized manner into a system of controls. Application of control techniques must be based on a systematic plan that identifies potential risk of exposure (risk analysis), levels of information security, and the degree of consequence to the organization should data become altered, destroyed, or unavailable (risk assessment).

A critical part of any security program is the management of risk. Risk management encompasses the identification, management, and control of untoward events. Conducting a risk analysis includes 1) identifying threats or risks to security, 2) determining how likely it is that any given threat may occur, and 3) estimating the impact of an untoward event. Among the threats to security are human error, such as a data entry mistake, unauthorized physical access to data, sabotage, power failures, and malfunction of software or hardware.

In addition to identifying risks, their likelihood of occurring, and their impact, informational assets must also be identified. Not all information is equal in importance or criticality to the operation of the organization. Determining the value of information is based on several factors. For example, what impact would a security breach have on quality of care, revenue, service, or organizational image?

Several different methodologies, ranging in complexity and computation, can be used to carry out a risk analysis. Calculation of risks based on unintentional occurrences, such as power failures or data entry error, is usually based on the probability of the specific event occurring. Calculation of risks based on intentional events, such as fraud or theft, is usually based on such factors as the attractiveness of a system to a perpetrator and the degree of vulnerability of the system.

Business Continuity Planning

A frequently overlooked security measure is the business continuity plan (BCP). The purpose of BCP is to ensure that an organization is able to deliver its goods and services without interruption. Frequently BCP is referred to as *the disaster plan*. However, BCP goes far beyond the response to a disaster. The goals of a BCP are to

- Identify potential disasters and their effects
- Take preventive measures to minimize the likelihood of disasters
- Develop an organized response should a disaster strike
- Ensure that business processes continue during the disaster recovery period

The business continuity plan is based on the information gathered during risk assessment and analysis: 1) identification of minimum allowable time for system disruption, 2) identification of alternatives for system continuation, 3) evaluation of cost and feasibility of each alternative, and 4) development of procedures required to activate the plan. The typical contents of BCP include

- Responsibility for development and implementation of the plan (e.g., security management team, emergency operation team, damage assessment team, coordination and implementation)
- Disaster identification (e.g., definition of disaster and its identification, notification procedures, identification of disaster cause, communication procedures)
- Recovery plan (e.g., organization and staffing, vendor contracts, backup plans, recovery plans, alternative-site contacts)
- Plan testing (e.g., method and frequency of testing the plan)

Conclusion

Protection of computerized information must be a top priority for health care enterprises. Security breaches cost American industry billions of dollars each year. For the health care industry in particular, the cost of security breaches must also be measured in relation to the degree to which informational privacy is jeopardized and the extent to which quality of patient care is threatened.

Electronic information can be protected when a combination of administrative, technical, and physical controls are developed and implemented within a framework of a total security program. Each of these controls is equally important in providing a safety net surrounding information and information systems. The National Research Council's report indicated that "health care organizations will have to work individually, collectively, and with relevant government entities to address the broad scope of concerns regarding privacy and security" (6, p. ES-4). The Council also made five overriding recommendations for improving the privacy and security of electronic health information at the level of both individual organizations and the health care system as a whole (6, p. ES5-12):

1. All organizations that handle patient-identifiable health care information, regardless of size, should adopt the set of technical and organizational policies, practices, and procedures outlined in its report.
2. Government and health care industry should take action to create the infrastructure necessary to support the privacy and security of electronic health information.
3. The federal government should work with industry to promote and encourage an informed public debate to determine an appropriate balance between the privacy concerns of patients and the information needs of various users of health information.
4. Any effort to develop a universal patient identifier should weigh the presumed advantages of such an identifier against potential privacy concerns.
5. The federal government should take steps to improve information security technologies for health care applications.

REFERENCES

1. Protecting Privacy in Computerized Medical Information, OTA-TCT-576, U.S. Congress, Office of Technology Assessment, Washington, DC: U.S. Government Printing Office, September 1993.
2. Protecting Privacy in Computerized Medical Information, OTA-TCT-576, U.S. Congress, Office of Technology Assessment, Washington, DC: U.S. Government Printing Office, September 1993, p11.
3. **Dick RS, Steen EB (Eds).** The Computer-Based Patient Record: An Essential Technology for Health Care. The Institute of Medicine. Washington, DC: National Academy Press, 1991.
4. **Johns ML.** Information Management for Health Professionals. Albany, NY: Delmar, 1997.
5. Position Paper: Access to Patient Data. Chicago: Computer-Based Patient Record Institute, April 1994.
6. National Academy of Sciences. For the Record: Protecting Electronic Health Information. National Research Council, Computer Science and Telecommunications Board, Committee on Maintaining Privacy and Security in Health Care Applications of the National Information Infrastructure, Computer Science and Telecommunications Board, Commission on Physical Sciences, Mathematics, and Applications, Washington, DC: National Academy Press, 1997.
7. **Gostin LO, Turek-Brezina J, Powers M, Kozloff R.** Privacy and security of health information in the emerging health system. Health Matrix: Journal of Law-Medicine. 1995;Winter:18.
8. The Center for Democracy and Technology. Privacy and Health Information Systems: A Guide to Protecting Patient Confidentiality. Seattle, WA: Foundation for Health Care Quality.

9. Glossary of Terms Related to Information Security. Schaumburg, IL: Computer-Based Patient Record Institute, 1996.

10. Glossary of Terms Related to Information Security. Schaumburg, IL: Computer-Based Patient Record Institute, 1996, p10.

11. **Ball MJ, Collen MF (Eds).** Aspects of the Computer-Based Patient Record. New York: Springer-Verlag, 1992.

12. Computers at Risk: Safe Computing in the Information Age. National Research Council, System Security Study Committee, Computer Science and Telecommunications Board, Commission on Physical Sciences, Mathematics, and Applications. Washington, DC: National Academy Press.

13. ASTM Standard E 1869-97. Confidentiality, Privacy, Access, and Data Security Principles for Health Information Including Computer-Based Patient Records. West Conshohocken, PA: American Society for Testing and Materials, 1997.

14. **Munro N.** Infotech reshapes health care marketplace. Washington Technology. 8 August 1996, p1.

15. **Gorman C.** Who's looking at your files? Time. 6 May 1996, p60 et seq.

16. **Ganzer D.** Community Concerns on Information Security. Presentation delivered at the 1996 Annual Meeting of the Healthcare Open Systems & Trials, 21 March 1996. Cited in: Privacy and Health Information Systems: A Guide to Protecting Patient Confidentiality. Center for Democracy and Technology, Seattle, WA: Foundation for Health Care Quality, 1996.

17. Confidentiality of Medical Records Situation Analysis and AHIMA's Position. Chicago: American Health Information Management Association.

18. **Galler R, et al.** Genetic testing for cancer. JAMA. 14 May 1997.

19. **Shaffer SL, Simon AR.** Network Security. Boston: Harcourt-Brace, 1994.

20. **Denning DE.** Who's stealing your information? Information Security. April 1999.

21. Security Features for Computer-Based Patient Record System. Schaumburg, IL: Computer-Based Patient Record Institute, 1996.

22. Statement of Robert S. Litt, Deputy Assistant Attorney General, Criminal Division, U.S. Department of Justice, before the Subcommittee on Technology, Terrorism, and Government Information. United States Senate, 19 March 1997.

23. **Frawley KA.** Federal legislation on confidentiality: possibility or insurmountable challenge? Journal of the American Health Information Management Association. 1999;70:19-22.

24. **Gosin, Lazzarinia, Flaherty.** Legislative Survey of State Confidentiality Laws. Report to U.S. Centers for Disease Control, June 1996.

25. Confidentiality of Individually Identifiable Health Information. Report to the Senate Committee on Labor and Human Relations, Recommendation of the Secretary of Health and Human Services, pursuant to Section 264 of the Health Insurance Portability and Accountability Act of 1996, 11 September 1997.

26. **Ruthberg A, Tipton H (Eds).** Handbook of Information Security Management. Boston: Auerbach, 1993.

27. Sample Confidentiality Statements and Agreements for Organizations Using Computer-Based Patient Record Systems. Washington, DC: Computer-Based Patient Record Institute, 1996.

28. **Parker DB.** Computer Security. Microsoft Encarta Encyclopedia. http://encarta.msn.com/encarta

29. **Levitt AM.** Disaster Planning and Recovery: A Guide for Facility Professionals. New York: John Wiley & Sons, 1997.

PART TWO

ELECTRONIC MEDICAL RECORD IMPLEMENTATION (WORKBOOK)

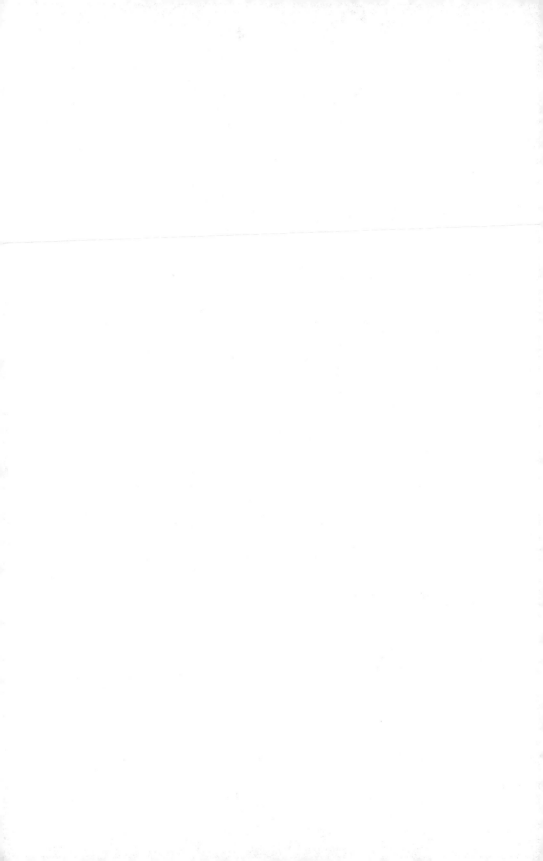

13 / Beginning the Selection Process

Jerome H. Carter

The fact that you are reading this book indicates that you are interested in an electronic medical record (EMR) and in buying an EMR system. This can be a very costly undertaking. Depending upon whom you consult, the cost of computerizing a three-physician practice can easily be $50,000 to $75,000. Others estimate the cost at between $8000 and $20,000 per provider. Aside from the dollar cost, there is a price to be paid in lost income, low morale, and simple frustration when an implementation goes sour. So I offer a simple plan and a few words of advice. The advice first.

1. *Take the time to study your practice.* There is no rush. You do not have to worry about being the last on your block to have a shiny new EMR system. Prudence dictates that you assess your short-term and long-term practice goals, economic situation, employee skills and attitudes, and ability to deal with fear, uncertainty, and doubt. Talk to your accountant to determine how much you can afford to spend and what overall economic benefits you might expect from an EMR. Increased productivity does not necessarily mean fewer full-time employees (FTEs). Along the same lines, can you afford the slow-down that frequently occurs after a new system is installed? How do your employees feel about an EMR? Will their fears of being replaced lead to destabilizing resignations? Finally, do you have the patience to see this through to the end? Take your time.

2. *What worked in a friend's practice will not automatically work in yours.*

Electronic medical record systems are not "one size fits all". Your practice environment (patient mix, employee skills, specialty) will play a substantial role in determining the type of EMR product that best meets your needs. What works for surgeons may not work for family practitioners, and what works for a solo practitioner may not work for a large multi-specialty group. Remember, when viewing demonstrations or conducting site visits, "your mileage may vary". Keep this mind. When comparing your practice to another, always match as many practice variables as possible to assure that the respective practices are similar. Your colleague may be a touch typist; are you?

3. *On the surface most products are similar; the differences are small but significant.* EMR products have come a long way over the last five years. Most are technically sound and offer similar features. However, the way the features are implemented may lead to significant differences in ease-of-use or utility. Consider a feature as basic as automatic drug interaction checking. Most EMR systems offer this feature. However, all do not allow you to turn off the feature easily, adjust the number or type of interactions that are flagged, or check for food-drug interactions. You may be surprised to find how much the ability to adjust any of these features affects your comfort in using a product.

4. *The vendor is as important as the product.* Quality, service, and continued existence count whether you are buying an EMR or an automobile. New vendors may have great products, but will they be around next year? Vendors may tout the fact that they have been in business for ten years, but how often have they updated their products? Does the vendor offer interfaces to other important types of software found in medical offices (e.g., practice management systems, outside labs)? How do they handle upgrades? Do they have a local office? Can they provide service during the hours that your site operates?

After pondering these points, if you still feel that you are ready to plunge ahead, the next step is to draw up a plan. Take planning seriously. Success depends upon your willingness to create a plan and stick to it.

Two aspects of EMR implementation must be addressed. The first planning step should always emphasize practice issues: goals (increase productivity, remote access to patient data), budget constraints, information needs (HEDIS, provider profiles), employee skills, etc. The second planning step should focus on EMR products, vendors, and potential implementation issues (disruption of office routine, staff training, etc.). Table 13-1 presents an EMR implementation plan outline. The suggested completion times assume a practice at a single site with three to four physicians.

Notice the time allotted for the goal statement, process identification, and process analysis steps. These first steps, which are dedicated to understanding the fine points of how a practice operates, are the most important of the group. It is in these steps that you give substance to the goals that led

Table 13-1   EMR Implementation Plan Outline.

Planning Step	Suggested Time for Completion
Goal statement	1 month
Process identification	1-2 months
Process analysis	2-3 month
Product evaluation	1-2 months
Vendor qualification	1 month
Creation of a Request for Proposal	1 month or less
Contract negotiation	1 month or less
Implementation	1-2 months

to the idea of implementing an EMR system. Each step has a corresponding chapter in this book to help you successfully complete that step. The remainder of this chapter is devoted to the first step, the goal statement.

The Goal Statement

What problems are you trying to solve? Frame your answer in the most concrete terms possible. Are you hoping to increase productivity, reduce FTEs, improve access to patient data, or perform outcomes analyses? These are a few of the reasons most often given for investigating EMR systems. Unfortunately, the next step is frequently a call to an EMR vendor. The more appropriate action would be to look at the problem closely and determine why it exists. A good way to start the problem definition step of your implementation plan is with staff interviews. Have each person create a list of common problems that they regularly encounter, then group them by type. The most common reasons for needing an EMR are discussed below.

"We Want To Increase Productivity"

If increased productivity is the goal, it would be very helpful to know why productivity is less than desired. Productivity is a fairly vague concept in many practice situations. If you wish to increase productivity, you must first define it in terms of what happens on a daily basis in your practice. Let us assume that in your practice productivity is defined as the number of patients seen per day. The obvious next step is to determine why more patients cannot be seen each day.

If a good deal of time is spent looking for charts or if needed information (lab reports etc.) is frequently unavailable, then poor productivity might be related to time spent looking for charts or missing patient data. Assuming that locating charts during patient visits is an issue, it would be helpful to categorize this as a chart access problem.

Once chart access issues are on the table, try to determine if there are other chart access problems. Remote access to patient data, especially while on-call, is a well-recognized access issue. Similarly, concurrent access (multiple users at the same time) may be an issue in large practices where more than one provider may need access to the paper chart at the same time. Finally, the simple, but very common, problem of temporarily misplaced charts is one that many practices deal with daily.

Once you are satisfied that you have a fairly complete problem list, turn your attention to understanding why these problems exist. At this point you are trying to determine which problems may be solved by a change in administrative policy and procedures as opposed to those which can only be solved by an EMR. Consider the example of an office where there is a 30-minute lag-time between patient sign-in and placement in an examining room. If the delay is due to problems locating the patient's chart, then an EMR system may help. However, if the delay is due to poorly trained staff, an EMR system may actually result in a decrease in productivity. Table 13-2 lists common causes of low productivity. No amount of technology will resolve these issues; sound administrative policies are required.

Table 13-2   Common Issues That Affect Productivity.

Poor staff training

Poorly defined staff duties

Lack of formal administrative policy

Ineffective methods of handling telephone calls

Ineffective methods of managing charts

Ineffective methods of incorporating information flow into the practice (labs, x-rays, referrals, etc.)

Poor resource scheduling (e.g., procedure suites)

"We Need To Perform Outcomes Studies"

If you take care of patients covered by managed care plans, chances are that you will want to perform some type of outcomes studies. (Chapters 8 and 9 discussed various types of outcomes studies.) Only a few types are done in most practices. However, they can be quite helpful. Provider profiles, patient satisfaction, and simple performance studies are well within the capabilities of the average practice. Each may be done manually, but an EMR will certainly make things much easier. Of course, proper administrative policies must be in place to assure that data are collected and entered in a systematic manner. A good starting point for profiling is the monitoring of lab tests. Begin by simply looking at the number of each type ordered, then compare ordering patterns for each provider. This is also a good way to implement simple guidelines in a practice. For example, creating a standard set of labs to be ordered for new patients with type 2 diabetes allows staff to more readily monitor variances and determine when labs are missing or late.

HEDIS reports are used to compare HMOs for compliance with generally accepted clinical practices such as the use of beta-blockers in patients who have had a myocardial infarction. Doing these reports manually is very time consuming. If you need this capability, an EMR system is almost a requirement.

Outcomes studies require data that are valid and complete. Review your practice with an eye towards standardizing as many common activities as possible. You may, for example, reduce the number of laboratory services, thereby decreasing the number of lab order forms and the number of names for different combinations of common lab tests (e.g., chem-7 vs. electrolyte panel). Do you have a method for assuring that all diabetic patients receive yearly eye exams? Do you conduct chart reviews to determine if all required documentation is present? How are common regular interventions such as flu shots recorded? Do you have a special form or flow sheet or are these items included only in the providers note? Table 13-3 list suggestions for preparing your practice for outcomes studies.

"We Need To Get a Better Handle on Costs"

Cost control is a major issue for many practices, especially for those with significant numbers of capitated patients. Electronic medical records can help in this area. However, an EMR system alone is not enough; your practice management system is important as well. When dealing with capitation the costs (depending upon the amount of risk taken on by the

Table 13-3   Steps for Preparing for Outcomes Analysis.

Implement standard preventive health measures.

Create a process for doing internal chart review.

Implement standard protocols for accepted clinical practices (ACE inhibitors for CHF, inhaled steroids for asthma, etc.).

Standardize documentation for common procedures and interventions.

Table 13-4   Suggestions for Monitoring Patient Care Costs.

Review disposable supplies for unnecessary use/overuse.

Review practice guidelines for common diseases for suggestions for best use of diagnostic studies and interventions.

Look at antibiotic prescribing habits for overuse.

Look at outside referral patterns for common procedures/diagnoses.

Review emergency room visits, emphasizing patients with the following diagnoses: asthma, chest pain, headache, URI, UTI, abdominal pain.

Review use of patient educational materials/walk-out instructions.

practice) generated from a patient encounter are derived from three main sources: diagnostic interventions (labs, x-rays, procedures), referrals, and therapeutic interventions. Begin your analysis by reviewing use of medications and diagnostic studies by diagnosis. For example, in managing patients with headaches, how often do you order CT scans or refer to neurologists? How often do providers order electrolyte studies for patients taking diuretics?

Many common prescribing habits may confer little real benefit to the patient yet generate costs to the practice. An excellent example is the widespread use of antibiotics for viral upper respiratory infections. Another cost-saving practice that is also good medicine is the use of prophylactic medications for patients who suffer from migraines. Effective prophylaxis may result in less use of expensive pain medications and fewer emergency room visits. Table 13-4 offers suggestions for reviewing practice patient care-related costs.

"We Need To Create Provider Profiles"

Provider profiling is increasingly becoming an issue for practitioners. The need to be well-informed concerning use of labs, procedures, medications, and referrals is present even in markets where managed care is not yet an issue. The mechanics of profiling is relatively straightforward. A good place to begin is one test or test category such as chest x-rays. A paper-based system can easily be set up for a small practice. Keep a log of tests ordered, match with diagnoses, and periodically tally tests ordered per diagnosis. Of course, doing this for a large number of tests or diagnoses will require some type of computerized database. However, the discipline and administrative processes needed to assure data capture and validation may begin using a manual system. Once profiling data become available, the next step is to use the data to understand practice habits.

Provider profiling is but one of a number of types of outcomes studies. Though it covers only provider actions, it can provide a practice with a very powerful method for monitoring and increasing its use of evidenced-based medicine concepts. In addition, profiling aids in understanding how patient care interventions contribute to costs.

Table 13-5 offers profiling initiation suggestions.

"We Need Better Access to Patient Information"

Timely access to information is a cornerstone of good patient care. Large practices and those with multiple sites are most likely to have problems with chart access. Remote access (i.e., access to records while the physician is on call or simply away from the office) should permit easy and rapid access to patient data. This is perhaps one of the clearest benefits of EMR technology. Of course, good data sets are not a function of EMR technology. Like many other things in a practice, quality data collection requires well-defined administrative policies that are adequately enforced. There-

---

Table 13-5   Profiling Initiation Suggestions.

Put in place administrative processes for logging all tests, procedures, and referrals along with diagnoses.

Conduct at least quarterly reviews of usage patterns.

Compare practice patterns with widely accepted guidelines.

Make quality improvement an issue in assessing practice performance.

fore, even though timely information access is a perfect application of EMR technology, the groundwork must be laid via administrative policy and a healthy respect, by all involved, for the importance of properly managing patient information.

Sit down with your medical records staff and review any issues they may have about policies. Ask for suggestions for new policies or changes to current ones. Standardize forms placed on charts, look for redundant forms and practices, and optimize those procedures deemed worth keeping. Obviously, staff training is a major component of sound patient information management activities.

This is also a good time to look at communications with outside consultants or facilities. Can paper-based reports be transmitted in electronic form? Would consultants be willing to send reports via disk, e-mail, or fax? Try polling consultants/groups with whom your practice has frequent interactions to determine if better ways of moving patient information can be agreed upon. Finally, when evaluating EMR systems, look for systems that permit easy import of outside data and allow for remote access with good security protocols.

Parting Advice

You are about to start on a journey that will never really end. New technologies will appear; new reporting requirements will be mandated; your needs will evolve. Therefore, it is very important that you keep your goals firmly in mind. Monitor and evaluate your practice on a regular basis and look for inefficiencies and opportunities to improve. Remember, successful implementation of an EMR system very much depends on your ability to identify and analyze your information needs. Chapters 14 to 20 will guide you through each step. Take your time.

14 / How To Use Consultants Effectively

Erica L. Drazen

Why Use a Consultant?

There are four basic reasons businesses hire information technology consultants:

1. *To access skills that are needed on a one-time or intermittent basis.* Selecting and implementing an electronic medical record (EMR) system is a process that a practice will undertake no more than once every five years. It is impractical to acquire office staff who are skilled in all facets of information systems planning, selection, or implementation for what amounts to episodic needs. Consultants present a reasonable solution, offering ready expertise in a timely and cost-efficient manner.

2. *To supply in-depth knowledge that is not resident in the organization.* Along with their technical expertise, consultants bring an insider's knowledge of key vendors, products, and services. The EMR vendor world changes frequently. Technology is continually evolving, and products may fail to take advantage of significant advances. New vendors enter the market and others close their doors. A vendor's business fundamentals may change through market success, partnerships, mergers, or acquisitions. In the absence of a dominant EMR vendor, market shifts affect all players. Keeping up to date on the status of available products and vendors requires an on-going data collection process. Interpreting changes requires an understanding of the history of the market and the market participants.

3. *To provide an independent viewpoint.* In a market with so many vendors and so little long-term experience, vendors offering "solutions" can deluge physicians and physician office staff. This frequently causes more confusion than clarification. It is also not unusual for different participants in the decision process to have very different priorities and viewpoints. A

physician with a hospital-based practice may be partial to a product offered by the hospital's vendor. Another physician may prefer to purchase a system she has used in a prior institution, and a third may think the system offered by his son's company must be the right one. It is often very helpful to be able to off-load some of the tough political calls to someone whose only interest is doing what is best for the overall practice and who will leave at the end of the project.

4. *To provide supplementary resources for a short period of time.* The final reason to hire a consultant is for an extra set of hands. The consultant who has learned your business by helping you through the planning and selection process is in an ideal position to help you or the vendor implement the selected system.

A Glimpse into the Consulting Business

To select and use a consultant effectively, it is helpful to understand the economics of consulting. Consulting firms hire skilled professionals and make major investments to assure those professionals expand their skills and build their knowledge base. The "product" that the consulting firm sells is time. Since "time" has no shelf life, a successful consulting firm must maximize the time available staff are working on client projects. This results in lower costs for the consulting firm and hence lower rates for consulting services.

One challenge in providing services to the physician market is that the time to sell a project is almost as long and involves a similar effort to selling to a large health plan or IDN, yet the revenue will be smaller. Also, smaller projects offer less flexibility for the consultant to reallocate staff time among tasks if there are delays in scheduling meetings, waiting for decisions, etc. The ideal client understands what he wants from a consulting project, designs an efficient approach to selecting the consultant, recognizes the need to work with the consultant in developing a plan, and commits to minimizing the changes to that plan. An effective collaboration between a consultant and a physician practice needs to recognize the realities of one another's business.

Finding a Consultant

How does one find a consultant? One may look in a consulting directory, wander the trade show at meetings, or ponder the advertising in trade magazines. However, the most common, and perhaps the best, way to select a consultant is through a personal referral. Whom do you know that recently made a similar EMR decision? What consultant did he use? What consultant does the hospital or health plan use for Information Technology planning or selections? Does it have experts in EMR systems?

National consultants who have specialized health care practices include Arthur Andersen, Deloitte & Touche, Ernst and Young, First Consulting Group, and Superior Consulting. Consulting firms who are multi-industry move in and out of health care. A good source of consultants who have a current commitment to clinical systems can be found by checking the Board of Directors of the Computer-Based Patient Record Institute (*www.cpri.com*). The Center for Health Information Management attracts most of the payers in health care, not only those who specialize in clinical systems. Its membership roster also provides contact names and e-mail links (*www.chim.org*).

However, none of the approaches listed above is the right *first* step when selecting a consultant. The first step is to decide 1) why you need a consultant, 2) what you want the consultant to do, and 3) what your selection criteria are. At a minimum, items one and two should be shared with the consulting teams you are considering.

Selecting a Consultant

Four elements are essential to selecting the right consultant: skills, knowledge, fit, and bias. The optimal balance of these elements depends on the role you want the consultant to play. The elements are attributes of both the individual consultants you will be working with and the attributes of the consulting firm. Except when dealing with individual consultants, the firm and the individuals both need to be evaluated to select the ideal consultant.

Skills

Skills in developing information technology plans, working with groups, selecting applications, and implementing the EMR system are mainly attributes of the staff who will work with you. Until you can commit to a start date and an estimated level of effort, it is impossible for any consulting firm to identify the staff that will be working with you on a project (because of the "shelf life" problem associated with consulting firms). However, it is still important for you to meet, evaluate, and interact with the staff that will be assigned to work with you.

If you expect a consulting firm to assist you in planning, selection, and implementation of your EMR system, it is important to evaluate whether a consulting firm selected for an earlier task (e.g., planning) has skills in selection and implementation also.

Knowledge

When you are looking for a consultant to help with an EMR project you want more than generic skills. You want someone who is knowledgeable about your business and the EMR industry. You should be in a good position to judge the knowledge of your business. You can ask, "What are the challenges you have seen in similar projects for similar organizations?" "How have you dealt with them?" "What value should we expect from this project?" "How can it be measured?" If the answers to these questions ring true and the consultants demonstrate operational knowledge in similar settings, you can feel comfortable. Another (useful but dreaded) test is the pop quiz. Twenty-four to forty-eight hours before interviewing the consultant, you present a real-life issue you have faced or are currently facing and ask for advice during the interview.

Presumably you expect an EMR to provide benefits to your organization. To make sure you achieve this goal you need to have realistic expectations, select an EMR system that provides the right support, and be willing to redesign processes to use the system effectively. Any consultant should be able to provide information on what goals have been achieved in other sites and what features and redesign are essential to attain the desired benefits.

At the current pace of change in industry players, products, and technology it is impossible for any one person to have complete knowledge of all industry products. A consultant should be able to cogently review the industry leaders and a few vendors on the "watch" list. However, there is no assurance that any of these vendors is right for you. You certainly do not want to pay for a comprehensive inventory of vendors. Therefore any consultant should have a database of vendors that they can match to your needs. You will want to check:

- Size of the database (number of vendors)
- Topics covered (at a minimum: product features, technology, business metrics, implementation experience)
- Sources of information (not solely from the vendor itself)
- Currency of information and the updating process

Any consultant who does not regularly track more than a dozen EMR vendors probably is not ideally suited to advise on EMR issues.

Fit

Fit is the match between the consultant's style and knowledge and your needs. One aspect of fit is chemistry—whether you feel comfortable with the consultant and whether the consultant's interaction with staff at all levels is appropriate and successful. This can be tested only by face-to-face interaction with the principals who will be working with you. One caution is that sameness is different than fit. In some cases you may want to select a consultant *because* he would not fit your office "culture". If you tend to have difficulty making efficient business decisions, you might want to pick a consultant that does not. If you tend to get mired in detail, you might want a consultant who has a bias toward the strategic level. In general, you want a consultant who will challenge you but who will not make unnecessary waves in your organization and you definitely want someone you can work with for several months. For the reasons discussed earlier, no firm can commit a team to a project until a start date is established; however, you should be able to meet the principals who will work will you. You may also want to reserve the right to interview and approve any member of the team who will be working on site.

Bias

When considering the potential biases a consultant might bring to the relationship, organizations tend to either worry too much or too little about potential conflicts. The real question is "Does this consultant have a reason to alter his advice to us because of other financial interests?" The most obvious bias is involvement with a vendor. Clearly you run a risk if you ask a potential supplier of your EMR to be your consultant—but this does happen! There are other, less visible biases you need to worry about: the consultant has a direct financial interest in an EMR system vendor or has an exclusive implementation agreement with a vendor. There are also potential biases if the consultant has other business relationships with you. Your law firm or accounting firm may be inclined not to "rock the boat" and could shy away from giving advice that it thinks you are not ready to hear. This could lead you to make a costly mistake in your EMR plans.

Some organizations want a consultant that has no relationship with any vendor that might be considered. This can be a mistake. Many consultants have implementation agreements with vendors; they are certified to install the vendor's product and may sell these services either directly or through the vendor. Implementation experience is very valuable in your consultant because such a person must have in-depth knowledge of the product and a better understanding of the total cost of ownership of that product. Rather than excluding any consultant that has implementation agreements with potential vendors, it may be helpful to select a consultant that has nonexclusive agreements with many EMR vendors.

Independent of your willingness to accept bias, the most important thing is that you understand it. The Center for Health Care Information management has accepted a standard of practice for health care consultants that requires that all consultants reveal any vendor or other potential conflicts that might influence their objectivity. Their code of conduct can be found at www.chim.org/membership/infrastructure. The code can be incorporated into the consultant's contract.

A "bottom line" check for bias is to ask which EMR vendor the consultant's last ten clients eventually selected. One would expect that different size and type organizations have selected different vendors if given unbiased advice.

Other Factors

Most steps in selecting a consultant include checking references. However, any consultant certainly can give you three or four great references. Unless you know the references personally, their loyalty to the consultant may be stronger than their relationship to you. On the other hand, it is unrealistic to ask the consultant to give you a list of all their clients and just randomly call whomever you wish. You would not want to be the recipient of a large number of such calls. A good compromise is to ask the consultant for a list of current clients (for the last six months, year, etc.) and review the list to find references you know personally—or that you think are similar to you. Select a few (two or three should be sufficient), then provide the consultant with the opportunity to make a courtesy call to let the reference know you will be calling.

Any consulting firm that specializes in EMRs probably participates in organizations such as CPRI, AHIMA, or AMIA. Colleagues in these organizations should be able to provide a reference for the firm. In fact, if you cannot get firm references through these sources, you probably should think twice about using that consultant.

The Partnership

There is much talk about "partnerships" today. Every vendor and consultant wants to be your "partner". Clearly what they really want is for you to be their customer. In many cases "partnership" is no more than a buzzword. What makes a real partnership work is aligned incentives.

Any established consulting firm that is dedicated to the health care industry has a built-in inventive for a project to be successful. This is a small industry and consultants know that they must maintain a reputation for the quality of the work and for successful outcomes. However, not all consultants depend on a quality reputation and therefore sometimes it is useful to take more explicit steps to see that incentives are aligned.

One technique is putting the fee or part of the fee at risk—to be paid only if a certain level of performance is achieved. The two questions are "Is there a measurable outcome?" and "Is the outcome within the consultant's control?" If the answer to these questions is "yes", then performance guarantees can be effective. For instance, part of an implementation consultant's fee could depend on a successful "go live" by a specified timeframe. It is also reasonable to hold a software developer accountable for on-time delivery of a working code.

It is more difficult to design incentives for planning or selection engagements. Because they have so little control, it is hard to hold consultants accountable for the accuracy of change initiatives. In these cases, other criteria need to be used to test whether you would want the consultant as a partner. At a minimum you might want to check that the consultant has a process in place for quality assurance, routinely surveys client satisfaction, and is willing to share the results of those surveys.

Contract negotiations are the time that really tests the partnership. Is the consultant willing to share information on project costs by task? Can you have a productive discussion of where the approach could be changed to lower costs? Is the consultant willing to name staff who will be assigned? Two questions that are useful to ask are "What activities are likely to provide marginal value?" and "If we had more money, what activities would you suggest we add to the project?"

Although it will be tempting, beware of consultants who are willing to cut the price of an engagement without changing the scope of work. They may have padded the original bid or cut corners, or they may ask for additional money later when you are in no position to say "no". Small discounts or discounts for prompt start or prompt pay are sometimes offered and may be advantageous to both sides.

Custom crafting of contract language is rarely needed and is costly for both sides. Typically, the consultant has a standard contract; if you have one too, you can compare and negotiate differences. You also might want to review your employee agreement and add any items that are relevant including, for instance, provisions to protect confidential patient information. If you get to the point where you have to pull out a contract to reach agreement, the relationship is over anyway.

Obviously, selecting a consultant is only the first step in building a successful relationship. As part of the final selection process you should agree on a schedule for the work, roles and responsibilities, and products that will be delivered. The most important part of the scheduling is arranging for interviews and group meetings, especially any that will require scheduling physician's time.

Most consultants prefer to work with you rather than independently. However, the collaboration can vary from review at specific checkpoints to a complete joint team effort. If there is valuable knowledge that you can gain from the consultant and apply in the future, you will want to have a joint team. An extreme example would be teaming up on the initial implementation of a system that will be installed in multiple clinics. As the implementation progresses, the consultant staff numbers could decrease and your staff complement could increase. However, typically you do not have the staff available to be a full-time part of the consultant's team. Even in that case, it is vital to have a project manager on your side who has the time available to stay in contact with the consulting team, monitor progress, and provide direction. It also makes sense for your staff to take responsibility for tasks that you can do quicker and more efficiently than the consultant. This might include scheduling interviews (your staff knows how each office works), digging out financial data, or creating an inventory of existing systems.

Finally, it is important to keep channels of communication open. If the project seems to be getting off track, raise the issue early, have an open discussion, and agree on the changes to be made. The decision to invest in an EMR system is an important and expensive one. You need to make sure you are getting the best help and advice available.

15 / From Process Analysis to Statement of Requirements

Patricia L. Hale

Computerization in the medical office can increase efficiency and enhance productivity only if an in-depth evaluation of office processes occurs beforehand. This chapter outlines key steps (Table 15-1) to help you evaluate your present practice processes in preparation for implementation of an electronic medical record (EMR) system. This evaluation should begin several months before choosing and implementing EMR to allow you to streamline and enhance areas of difficulty in the office process and to ensure as smooth a transition as possible. This can help decrease some of the initial negative impact of transition to EMR that inevitably occurs.

Identification of Key Office Processes

When physicians evaluate EMR systems, we all have the general tendency to emphasize the areas with which we are most familiar. Specifically, vendors will usually spend as much time as possible showing you the features for physician documentation. Although this is a key area to review when choosing an EMR system, it is equally important to realize that many other office processes actually overshadow this EMR function. Each of these other processes must be reviewed and streamlined to fully take advantage of the improved efficiency an EMR can provide. The processes in most medical offices can be roughly broken down into the areas listed in Table 15-2.

Integration of patient registration, appointment scheduling, and billing between practice management and scheduling software and the EMR results in improved efficiency in multi-specialty group practices. (Chapter 6 provides details on the business processes in a typical medical office.) In ad-

Table 15-1   Major Steps from Process Identification to Statement of Requirements.

Major Steps	Components of Each Step
Identify Key Processes	Classify all office processes into the following groups: • General office management tasks • Patient/Visit-specific tasks • Integration with entities outside the office
Analyze Each Process	Evaluate all office processes and place into the following groups: • Optimized and working well • Present but functioning poorly • Not available but needed
Assign Implementation Plan to All Processes	Assign each process to one of the following groups: • Duplicate successful processes • Modify inefficient processes • Transform old processes and add new ones
Identify Barriers to Implementation	Classify potential barriers into the following groups: • Workflow • Data entry • Integration • Personnel
Prepare Patient Scenarios	Separate key functions to be evaluated into the following groups: • Most common patient • Most complex patient • "Wish list" for ideal future practice

dition, practices that have a large hospital component can also benefit from integration with their management and scheduling systems. In these types of practices, such integration should have a high priority. Although most of these processes occur through the use of practice management and scheduling software, tight integration of the processes with an EMR is needed to preserve or improve office efficiency. Staff time is always one of the highest costs in a practice. Duplication of data entry is one obvious element of the evaluation of this process. Increased efficiency can occur if the nursing staff

Table 15-2   Common Medical Office Processes.

Common Office Processes	Key Components
General Office Management Tasks	• Patient registration/Appointment scheduling • Patient billing • Physician/Provider scheduling • Nursing/Other support staff scheduling

Patient/Visit-Specific Tasks	• Review and filing of test results, letters, and miscellanous forms
	• Recording of phone messages
	• Documentation of advanced directives
	• Patient visit documentation
	   –Nursing/Medical Technicians/Staff
	      Vital signs and other visit-specific documentation
	      Medication review and prescription ordering
	      Test and referral scheduling
	   –Provider/Physician documentation
	   –Wellness issues (review and documentation)

Integration with Entities Outside the Office	• Hospital Information System
	   –Demographics and billing information for inpatient care and procedure services
	   –Reporting for lab, x-ray, and other test results
	   –Hospital dictation
	• Other Physician Offices
	   –Patient demographics and billing information
	   –Consultation notes, office procedures, and test results
	• Integrated Health Care Delivery Systems
	   –Insurers
	   –Home health care agencies
	   –After-hours clinics and regional hospital urgent and emergency care centers

can enter appointments into the scheduling system easily while working within the EMR system. Multi-specialty practices will find this feature especially helpful in providing efficient scheduling of referrals and tests at the time of the initial patient appointment.

Any practice with a large hospital component should also prioritize possible integration with hospital information systems in the evaluation of an EMR system. Patient billing and demographic information should be accessible between information systems, but integration with large hospital systems is often more complex and costly and requires a long planning process and the determination of the possible financial impact.

The small group or individual practice may only require simple integration of demographic information to avoid duplication of data entry and may not find other major integration features either as important or financially feasible. Vendor selection may be significantly affected by the desired emphasis on each of these features.

Physician/provider, nursing, and other support staff scheduling is another feature often emphasized by EMR vendors. Again, these issues are most important for large, multi-specialty and multi-site practices. Small practices can often continue using simple scheduling and billing software if it has worked well in the past. Using key toggle methods to flip between program screens will suffice in the smaller office that is simply duplicating the paper-based schedule book on-line. In larger practices, multiple phone calls and duplicate data entry as well as constant rescheduling issues make the efficiencies gained from more complete scheduling features worth the time required to set the system up and integrate it into the workflow of all of those involved.

Patient and Visit-Specific Tasks

The paper-based medical record has gradually grown to include a number of patient and visit-specific processes resulting from the need to collect, review, and store diverse information from multiple sources. The review and filing tasks often occur between patient visits, but the information must also be readily available to refer to when patients or other providers call and at the time of the next office visit. These tasks are commonly targeted in vendor demonstrations, but to achieve a truly efficient system all of the information must be available electronically. Will this be possible in your office? Will some information need to remain in paper form? If electronic and paper records will coexist following EMR implementation, strong emphasis on process analysis will be required to maintain efficient workflow and information access. (Chapter 7 gives a more detailed discussion of this topic.) A specific list of all types of information and their ability to be transferred to an electronic form should be prepared for each physician before reviewing EMR systems. The easiest way to do this is to prepare a checklist (Fig. 15-1) of patient information and do a survey of each physician's needs. A one-week collection of the results for each physician should be sufficient to give a reasonable sampling of potential needs.

Patient Information	Monday	Tuesday	Wednesday	Thursday	Friday
Total patients seen					
Lab results reviewed (divided into different lab sites if necessary)					
X-ray results reviewed					
Physician referral letters					
Home health care reports/orders					
Other practice-specific test results (e.g., EKG, echo) reviewed					
Insurance information, eligibility and formulary rules					
Health maintenance review					
New/refill prescription orders					
Reviewing PDR and drug interaction information					
Hospital procedure or discharge dictation					
ER sheets					
Protocols and guidelines					
Medical reference material					
MEDLINE search					
Diagnostic support information					
Patient education materials					

Figure 15-1 Survey form for provider access of patient-specific information during an office visit. (Have each provider mark each time the specific type of information listed is accessed.)

Integration with Entities Outside the Office

Many of the most useful features of EMR systems for storage of diverse information require integration of multiple information sources. Issues of integration with outside testing facilities should be investigated long before the vendor selection process. Failure to look at integration issues before vendor evaluation can result in major barriers at the time of implementation.

The most common information needs requiring integration with hospital systems include demographics and billing information for inpatient care and procedural services; test reporting for lab, x-ray, and hospital-based procedures; and dictated provider notes for procedures and tests done in the hospital setting.

Hospital information systems can be a major challenge in this regard because they often involve a combination of complex information systems as well as associated administrative complexities that make integration difficult. It can take months or even years to establish and implement integration with such systems. If integration is required to access a major proportion of needed information, time and resources should be planned to begin this process before EMR vendor analysis begins. Although it seems that using identical systems to those available at the hospital would make integration easier, the difference in design issues for outpatient office patient care and in-hospital care can make these systems inefficient, unwieldy, or difficult to modify for an office practice setting. Vendor selection should still be based on the list of features determined through careful process analysis, not on pressures to use the same vendors as existing hospital systems.

To achieve a truly paper-less office, integration with information systems from other physician offices will also be necessary, but that is often not feasible. The volume and frequency of access to this type of information should also be evaluated before EMR selection. Information accessed from other physician offices usually includes patient demographics and billing information, consultation notes, and office procedures and test results. If the volume is relatively small but access is frequently required, scanning or manual data entry of this information may be worthwhile. If the volume is great or access is infrequent, continuing a paper storage system with hopes for direct electronic integration in the future may be a more workable solution.

Integration with information sources in integrated health care delivery (IDS) systems includes all of these challenges and barriers combined. Ideally, integration between insurers, home health care agencies, after-hours clinics, and hospital emergency care centers may provide increased levels of efficiency throughout the system. Realistically, integration issues provide barriers that may prevent this process from occurring for most medical practices. If sophisticated, integrated information systems are not already available within an IDS, looking at features of an EMR system that emphasize such capabilities should not be a priority. Asking vendors about future plans and system flexibility is probably a reasonable method of assessing this area during the review process.

Individualized Provider and Practice-Specific Processes

When detailed evaluation of office processes occurs, it quickly becomes clear that no two medical practices are the same. There are different types of practices, patient bases, information integration needs, insurer bases, and patient visits. Patient-specific variations that influence the office process are listed in Table 15-3.

Primary care medical practices may be similar in patient visit types (e.g., emphasis on return visits in an internal medicine practice) but differ in insurer base, size of practice, and level of integration between multiple practice sites.

Specialty practices often have a larger population of new patients with a greater emphasis on consultative and procedure services. They may also have a greater dependence on integration with hospital information systems and practice-specific procedures and equipment (e.g., Holter monitor and treadmills in a cardiology practice). A list of these specific needs should be developed before EMR evaluation and the priorities identified and included in vendor review. Patient scenarios can provide a convenient and consistent method of evaluating these needs and are described later in this chapter.

Individual Physician Practice Styles

In addition to practice issues, physician-specific habits are amazingly diverse and must be evaluated before implementation of any EMR system. It is crucial to minimize disruption of ingrained patterns of individual providers during the initial implementation process unless significant gains in efficiency can be made. Provider practice habits will be one of the biggest challenges for implementation of an EMR system in any size group practice and can become a major barrier to success.

It is important to account for physician practice styles when evaluating potential EMR systems. Some practice traits will be incompatible with any

Table 15-3   Practice-Specific Process Variations.

Feature	Types
Practice base	• Hospital-based practice • Enterprise-wide systems • Community-based office practice
Practice type	• Large or small group • Multi-specialty • Primary care

Variations in practice-specific integration issues	Is integration a priority with...?
	• Hospital (e.g., surgical specialty)
	• Other practice sites
	• Multiple urgent care clinics
	   –Integrated delivery systems
	   –Insurers
	   –Home health care agencies
	   –Other

Insurer differences	• Managed care penetration • Capitation
Patient visit type	• Mostly consults • Mostly new patients • Mostly repeat patients • Multiple diagnosis/mostly procedures

EMR system. It is important to identify and target these areas to begin the process of change before implementing an EMR.

Physicians vary dramatically in their interaction style with patients; this is often reflected in the complexity and individualization of the documentation of the patient history, ROS, exam, and so on. Most physicians use specific phrasing and personal notation styles to bring texture to their office notes and to make documentation more patient specific. It is important to realize that many EMRs actually try to move away from this type of documentation to more standardized medical nomenclature. The advantages of standard nomenclature are found in the increased ability to query and evaluate stored information. Drop-down lists, for example, enhance this capability. Dictation and free-form notation allow more freedom in documentation at the cost of loss of some of the information management advantages that an EMR can provide. This important issue should be addressed and discussed by all physicians in the group early on in the process of planning the transition to an EMR.

The use of other types of information during the patient visit may also vary dramatically between individual providers. This information can include access to lab and x-ray results, decision support and reference materials, and patient-teaching materials. Specific provider needs for information should be surveyed as discussed previously and included in the vendor analysis.

The various documentation styles of providers (brief notes, SOAP style versus long narratives and letters, drawings, or other provider-specific notations) must be carefully assessed. It is critical to identify workable compromises as well as those areas that are non-negotiable. Again, evaluation and planning are required before vendor selection.

The willingness and ability of providers to adapt to various data entry methodologies is also a very important issue that should be evaluated long before vendor selection. Physicians often use a variety of data entry methods. Many physicians still depend on the use of handwritten notes. Obviously, new skills will be needed to change to automated information entry. Experimentation with different types of data entry may be helpful before EMR evaluation has begun. Most EMR systems will allow data entry through both keyboard and voice-activated dictation. Technologies for handwriting recognition and other technologies still lag somewhat behind. Drop-down lists are featured in many systems. These lists often include additional notation that was not routinely included in previous data entry methods and often will actually require more provider time for data entry. If routine and repeat visits are a common feature of the medical practice, these methodologies may become tedious and difficult to customize. Stand-alone systems for voice dictation and other methods of data entry can be explored by providers, who then can develop a list of desired features before vendor selection. This process may also take several months.

Analysis of Practice Processes

The goal of process analysis is to evaluate each process area and target it for duplication, modification, or transformation/replacement during implementation of an EMR system. To accomplish this, it will be necessary to evaluate each process first-hand and see how it is presently done. Process analysis will not only provide valuable information but also will allow you to encourage staff involvement that will become indispensable during the future EMR implementation process.

Start by sketching out each process. Think workflow! (See a sample process in Figure 15-2.) Remember, medical software and medical practices are dynamic and require continual evaluation and modification to be successful. Look for what you need now—not what you expect to need in the distant future. Also remember, you can not fix bad information flow with computerization.

If one is interested in improving this process using EMR, then it will be necessary to select systems that support as many of these steps as possible. The ideal EMR system for prescription writing would then include an easily

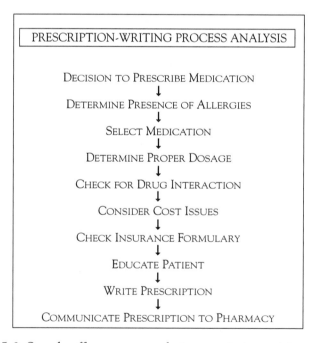

Figure 15-2 Sample office process analysis: prescription writing.

accessible listing of pertinent patient information (name, age, address, tele-phone, insurer with specifics on prescription plan), up-to-date drug infor-mation (on-line versions of current PDR and drug interaction information, drug formularies and costs, and simple patient education materials), and the ability to print to paper or e-mail or fax to participating pharmacies.

Classify each process in specific groups. What works well in your office now? Target these processes for duplication using the EMR system and try not to significantly change them if possible. If your present scheduling and billing software is a success, try to integrate the EMR with it and not re-place it, or only consider replacement with a similar system. What of fu-ture issues? Will your medical practice plan include increased capitation? Will you need the better practice analysis information that a more sophis-ticated practice management system can provide? In these situations, a change to a more complete and integrated practice management system with an EMR may be worth the cost and loss of efficiency during the im-plementation phase. (Ask vendors if a stepped implementation can be done to allow the practice to adapt to the new management system before changing to an EMR.)

Identify processes in need of modification. What doesn't work well now? Can an integrated EMR *improve* them? Areas that often fall into this group include provider scheduling, office communications (possible future use of e-mail and Intranets), HMO eligibility determination and referral processes (possible future electronic versions), prescription ordering and re-newals, and drug-interaction checking. Preventive medicine issues, tickler files, and reminders may be scattered throughout the office in several paper charting systems. EMR systems often provide an excellent method for quick access to this type of information once the initial data entry has been completed. Patient education materials can also be targeted as an area to be modified when the EMR system is implemented. Existing materials should be cataloged and reviewed to develop a list of key types of required patient-teaching materials. An ideal system will provide a large collection of stan-dardized materials (from AFFP or other recognized resources) as well as allow entry of practice-specific materials such as teaching materials and procedural consent forms.

The next step is to identify processes important to the medical practice that are not presently available. The best example of this category of processes is the ability to query patient records for recalls when medication changes are indicated (drug recalls or warnings) and the inclusion of pa-tient-specific protocols, guidelines, and pathways at the time of the patient visit. Another important area that can be targeted for inclusion with the implementation of an EMR system is review of practice compliance with recommended insurer guidelines.

Large or small group practices may also wish to consider including remote access to patient chart information as a new feature to be provided by the EMR system. It is important to list specific features needed in remote access and include them in the vendor evaluation. Table 15-4 lists the major features that should be identified and included in this evaluation.

Finally, do you plan to explore practice-specific profile information that is not presently available to you? Will you be able to implement changes in your medical practice based on this information? Examples of these types of features are

- Practice profiling
- Resource management
- Quality control
- Cost evaluation
- Outcomes research

Table 15-4   Remote Access Feature List.

Access of information from:

- Home

- Hospitals and emergency care centers

- Other urgent care centers

- Other clinic sites

Access of:

- Previous notes

- Problem lists

- Medication and allergy lists

- Test results

- Past medical history and other practice-specific information

---

Many experts recommend fully evaluating query features of any EMR system for the ability to provide this type of practice-specific information. Vendors rarely volunteer to demonstrate query functions, but you should not be dissuaded from including them in your patient scenario preparation because they may become one of the most important ways of improving your practice.

Common Barriers to EMR Implementation

What barriers may prevent successful EMR implementation in your practice?

- Start-up costs
- Implementation-integration into the workflow
- Maintenance issues
- Scalability
- Complexity
- Data entry methodology
- Staff buy-in
- Integration issues with other information systems within and outside the medical practice
- Political issues within and outside the medical practice

Note that the relatively greater amount of information included in an EMR system may actually result in *more* work for office staff and providers. It is usually not realistic to expect a decrease in office staffing when an EMR system is implemented, despite some vendors' claims.

Preparation of Test Scenarios

When the office process identification and analysis is complete, prepare to test office processes with prepared patient scenarios and refine these scenarios when testing potential EMR systems. Start the evaluation at the earliest step of patient contact (scheduling and registration) and continue it all the way to the last step of contact with patient-specific information (referrals, test ordering and scheduling, results review and filing, etc.).

Most medical practices can define three basic patient scenarios (Table 15-5) that cover most of the key components of their practice setting. There

Table 15-5   **Three Test Scenarios.**

Scenario Type	Patient Type	Problem Type	Visit Type	Key Component Examples
Scenario 1 Most common patient	Returning	Routine	Brief	• Access to previous patient information • Data input and ordering • Scheduling
Scenario 2 Most complex patient	New	New	Consultation	• Access to previous patient information • Data input and ordering • Scheduling
Scenario 3 "Wish list" patient	New or returning	New or routine	Any length	• New technology • Decision support • Wireless network and data entry in patient room • Remote access to records • Electronic referrals • Practice profiling and cost evaluation • Resource management and quality control • Outcomes research • "Tickler files" and "To-do lists"

are several advantages to using test scenarios when looking at EMR systems. Often, vendors will emphasize "flashy" features rather than those which support more mundane aspects of everyday medical practice. Using test scenarios will help prevent this. In addition, using these scenarios will often clearly point out one of the common drawbacks of most EMR systems. Many times

EMR systems require clicking through multiple screens to accomplish simple and repetitive office tasks. This problem will become evident when you focus on the step-wise flow using a scenario. Multiple steps for simple tasks can result in severe losses in efficiency. Conversely, it is important to ensure that less common and more complex tasks are still possible without requiring sophisticated computer skills. If you have a significant turnover in office staff, it will be particularly important to include an evaluation of the "learning curve" and software support in one of the practice scenarios.

Let us look at a sample Scenario 1 for a general internal medicine practice (Fig. 15.3). This scenario is the one to which you will want to pay care-

---

Patient: A 73 YO WF with HTN and DM Type 2 comes for a routine office visit

---

Scheduled Visit Length: A 15-min visit is scheduled for both patient contact and data entry

---

Key Components

Access to Previous Patient Information
- Check current problem list (e.g., HTN, DM type 2, menopause)
- Check current medication and allergy/intolerance lists (e.g., blood pressure medication, diabetes medication, sulfa allergy, estrogen intolerance)
- Review last office visit note
- Review recent hospital discharge summary (if appropriate)
- Review lab/x-ray/test results (e.g., chemical profile, HgbA1c, UA)
- Review referral specialist letters and test results (e.g., recent gynecologic exam, Pap smear)
- Check health maintenance issues (e.g., last eye check, foot care, diabetes education, osteoporosis evaluation, immunizations, cancer screening)

Data Input and Ordering
- Entry of vital signs and nursing information
- Entry of provider office note
- Update problem and medication lists
- Prescription writing (with insurance coverage, drug dosing, and drug interaction checks)
- Order tests and referrals (e.g., lab, x-ray, dietician, ophthalmologist)
- Order/provide patient education materials

Scheduling
- Schedule future tests
- Schedule referrals
- Schedule return visits

Figure 15-3 Scenario 1: Simple/common office visit to an internal medicine practice.

ful attention concerning the overall efficiency of patient and information flow. You should choose the most common patient seen in the typical practice in your group, tying in as many general features as possible. When this patient scenario is used to look at the EMR system, do not let irrelevant features distract you; concentrate on the actual speed and efficiency of tasks because any loss of time handling these patients will have the greatest impact on your practice! You may even want to actually time the processes of data entry and access and/or count the number of screens that must be accessed. Unless you plan to have computer stations for each employee, beware of vendor claims that more efficiency is possible by customized screens. Imagine patient and practitioner flow and look for possible conflicts.

Summary

Successful choice and implementation of an EMR system requires a great deal of preparation before the review of vendor products begins. Careful identification and analysis of key office processes are necessary before approaching vendors with a list of required and optional features. This effort can result in the production of very useful patient scenarios that can keep your vendor evaluation on target and limit the amount of time wasted for vendor demonstrations. In addition, this evaluation can also target areas that can benefit from productive change even before the implementation of EMR, resulting in cost savings. Duplicating successful processes and changing only those processes that are not presently optimized will lead to less disruption and lower costs. Office and provider anxiety over the inevitable changes that occur with EMR implementation are also reduced when staff members are included in the processes of analysis and goal setting. Though somewhat tedious, time spent on this segment of preparation for an EMR system is often extremely productive and can prevent many implementation problems.

APPENDIX

The medical office process analysis checklist on pages 331 to 333 can be used to construct patient scenarios and to review the EMR features most important in a particular practice setting. Each area should undergo detailed analysis so that other categories can be added to the checklist.

MEDICAL OFFICE PROCESS ANALYSIS CHECKLIST

Process	Feature	Feature Not Needed	Feature Needed	Duplicate (Working Well Now)	Modify	Transform, Replace, or Add	Comments
General Office Management Tasks							
	Registration						
	Appointments						
	Billing						
	Provider scheduler						
Patient and Visit-Specific Tasks							
	Review of test results, letters, and forms						
	Recording of phone messages						
	Documentation of advanced directives						
	Vital signs and nurse notations						
	Medication review, refill ordering, script writing						
	Test and referral scheduling						
	Provider documentation						
	Review and documentation of health maintenance issues						

MEDICAL OFFICE PROCESS ANALYSIS CHECKLIST *(cont.)*

Process	Feature	Feature Not Needed	Feature Needed	Duplicate (Working Well Now)	Modify	Transform, Replace, or Add	Comments
Remote Access and Integration with Remote Information Systems							
	Remote office or clinic sites						
	Home or mobile office						
	Hospital information system						
	Remote labs						
	Remote x-ray facilities						
	Other test sites						
	Other physician offices						
	Emergency care centers						
	Urgent care centers						
	Pharmacies						
	Insurers						
	Nursing homes or rehabilitation facilities						
	Public health agencies and home health care agencies						
Practice Base							
	Primary care						
	Specialty care						
	Mixed primary and specialty care						
	Hospital-based or enterprise-wide system						

MEDICAL OFFICE PROCESS ANALYSIS CHECKLIST (*cont.*)

Process	Feature	Feature Not Needed	Feature Needed	Duplicate (Working Well Now)	Modify	Transform, Replace, or Add	Comments
Practice Site							
	Single office						
	Multiple clinics						
Practice Type							
	Single or small (3–5) group practice						
	Large single-specialty group practice						
	Multi-specialty group practice						
Insurer Mix							
	Fee for service						
	Managed care						
	Capitation						
Patient Visit Types							
	Mosty new						
	Mostly repeat						
	Mostly consults						
	Mostly multiple or complex diagnosis						
	Mostly procedures						
Data Entry							
	Free-hand notation						
	Dictation/ transcription						
	Voice dictation						
	Keyboard entry						
	Other						

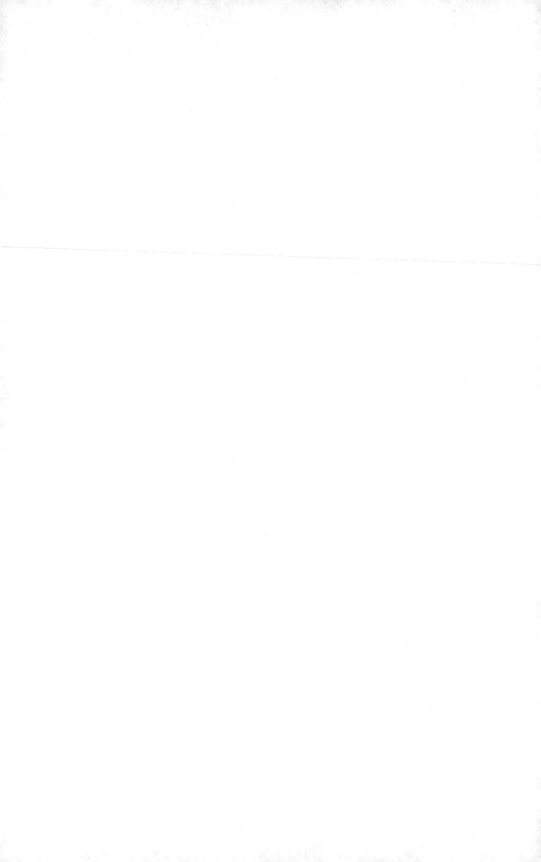

16 / Evaluation of Features

Jerome H. Carter

E valuating the various types and features of electronic medical record (EMR) systems is never easy. A major impediment is the sheer number of available products. At last count, more than 200 companies offered products in this category. Another hindrance is the lack of agreement on which specific features and functions all EMR systems should provide. Unfortunately, no organization or agency has the authority to set requirements and to certify or approve products. Finally, every practice is different; what works well in one might spell disaster in another. Therefore, selecting an EMR product to meet your needs requires a careful, well thought-out strategy. A sound evaluation policy should occur on two levels. The first level involves the analysis of clinical and business processes; the second, analysis of product-specific features and functions. Once the results of these analyses are available, then and only then should attention be given to evaluation of specific products. If you have skipped this vital step, save yourself future headaches; go back and complete it.

The Role of Process Analyses

The lack of a standard definition for EMR and the desire of vendors to differentiate their products has had the practical effect of encouraging significant variation in product functions, features, interfaces, and technical quality. Comparing apples to apples is nearly impossible. What is possible, and very doable, is comparing your process support needs to the features and functions of an EMR product. Chapter 15 offered guidance on performing process analyses and using the results to create a Statement of Requirements. The requirements are a listing of all of the functions that you require an EMR product to provide in order support your practice needs. This information is later combined with very specific questions for EMR vendors concerning their business activities, financial health, etc., to form a document referred to as a Request for Proposal (RFP) (see Chapter 18). The RFP serves two purposes. First, it provides a formal means for telling vendors what you need their product to do for you. Second, it may be used as a resource document for conducting formal product evaluations, demonstrations, and site visits. After all, it contains a statement of what you think is important in a product. This is a key point. Too often organizations spend months creating an RFP and use it only to solicit a response from vendors. Avoid this costly mistake and treat it as an active on-going statement of your needs. Keep a copy handy and refer to it often during the evaluation process.

Getting a Handle on EMR Features

The features and functions incorporated into EMR products are derived from product designers' understanding (or lack thereof) of the features, functions, and uses of paper-based charts. Your ability to effectively select and use an EMR product will also depend upon how well you understand the paper chart and how you use it. For example, there are undoubtedly some activities that you wish to speed up (e.g., determining all medications a patient is currently taking) which would be faster using a computer. With an EMR new capabilities not available with paper charts (e.g., quickly finding all patients taking a specific drug) exist, but they may not be obvious if your desired-features list is formed solely from interactions with paper records.

Uses of the Medical Record

The Institute of Medicine Report on computer-based patient record systems divides medical records usage into two categories: primary and secondary. Looking up an old EKG result, checking a medication list, reading an old progress note, and so on, are primary uses. Primary uses are those that involve direct patient care. Clinicians tend focus too much on primary uses when evaluating products. Secondary uses may be thought of as nonclinical analytical uses (outcomes analysis, cost studies, regulatory reporting, etc.). Secondary users tend to be researchers, educators, and regulatory bodies. However, with the rise of managed care secondary uses (profiling, HEDIS, capitation rate negotiation) have become very important. When using paper records primary and secondary users have specific forms or processes that they use to maximize the value of the chart. Thus, if a doctor wishes to record more preventive health data, a form is added to the chart and a protocol for using the form is created. Administrators attempting to meet regulatory reporting requirements often take a similar approach.

Obviously, the paper chart with all of its failings is quite flexible and useful. Unfortunately, the ease with which one can expand the uses of the paper chart can make it difficult to appreciate its true complexity. It is exactly this failure to appreciate the true complexity of the paper chart that makes selecting and using EMR products so problematic. A good EMR product makes allowances for the needs of both primary and secondary users of the medical record. Since adding new features is not simple, a good deal more forethought is necessary to build a good product. Similarly, selecting a product will be difficult unless *all* potential users have a good understanding of their needs and can articulate those needs sufficiently to vendors, consultants, and information systems professionals. Table 16-1 lists the primary and secondary uses of the medical record that should aid in formulating a good conceptualization of the various uses of an EMR.

Table 16-1   Primary and Secondary Uses of an EMR.

Primary Uses and Required Features

Progress notes

Problem list

Medication list

Drug information and prescription management

Laboratory and test reports

Preventive health support

Referral creation

Guidelines and protocols

Patient education

Secondary Uses

Provider profiling

Patient utilization information

Quality report cards

Performance reviews for practice guidelines, protocols, and pathways

Outcomes analyses

What Features Should EMR Have?

As mentioned earlier, there is no formal standard that sets forth a formal list of EMR required features and functions. However, a workable checklist (see Appendix C) has been derived from an analysis of important primary and secondary uses, the features of available products, and a review of common office and clinical processes that appear amenable to computerization.

For the purposes of this book, three categories will be used to organize EMR features and functions: chart, analysis, and technical. Chart features are those that clinicians use in delivering care. Researchers and administrators will want to look closely at analysis features, and information systems professionals will find the technical feature list helpful.

The evaluation criteria offered in this chapter and Appendix C are intended to act as a guide to understanding which features are generally available and immediately useful, and which are worth "wishing" for but not needed right away. *Product features deemed to be essential are shown in the tables and checklist in roman type; "wish list" items appear in italics.

The proper time to use this set of criteria is after all of the process analyses have been completed. The criteria may then be used to help create an RFP and specific evaluation instruments for hands-on product evaluations, demonstrations, and site visits. Look through the criteria and for each feature area (e.g., medications) determine which are *required* for your needs. It is your personal list of required features that will determine the ideal product for you. It is also very important that the needs of clinicians and administrators be addressed when deciding on required features; be mindful of this during the product evaluation. Whenever possible, make feature requirements determination a committee decision with all parties represented. Each set of criteria is accompanied by a brief discussion of meaning and significance.

Chart Features

Medications

Medication management is an important part of clinical practice. At a minimum, an EMR package should provide the ability to maintain medication and allergy lists, write prescriptions, and automatically alert the practitioner to any drug allergies (Table 16-2). If a prescription writer is present, then automatic drug interaction checking would be a very desirable addi-

---

*The evaluation criteria and checklist are adapted from *Electronic Patient Records for the Office-based Practitioner.* Copyright © 1998 by Jerome H. Carter. All rights reserved.

Table 16-2   Medication Features.

Medication list

   Long-term

   Per episode

   Active/inactive

   Failed after trial

Allergy list

Automatic allergy warning

Prescription writer

   E-mail or fax to pharmacy

   Maintains prescription history

Maintains formulary information by insurance plan

Drug interactions

   Multiple drug-drug

Practitioner-specific medication list

Drug information

   Side effects

   Adverse reactions

   Overdose

   Dosages

   Forms supplied

Reports by

   Patient

   Medication

   Provider

Product features deemed essential are in roman type; "wish list" items appear in italics.

tional feature. Note that, if this feature is available, one must assure that the feature can be enabled and disabled by the user and that the number and types of interactions reported are adjustable. Advanced medication features include formulary tracking by insurance plan, provider-specific medication lists, the ability to e-mail or fax pharmacies, on-line drug information on side effects and adverse reactions, and the ability of the user to add new drugs/prescriptions to the system. Provider-specific medication lists allow each provider to create a list of drugs and dosages that he or she uses most often. This saves time by removing the need to scroll through long lists of medications each time a prescription needs to be written. Minimal report capability should offer the ability to search by patient, drug, and provider. Finally, a link to the *Physicians' Desk Reference* or other on-line drug databases for reference purposes is a desirable feature.

Laboratory/X-ray/Pathology Reports

Perhaps the most useful and yet most difficult feature to obtain in EMR is automatic downloading of laboratories and other types of test reports from

---

Table 16-3   Laboratory/X-ray/Pathology Features.

Maintains test history

    Patient

    Provider

Permits automatic data download from outside facilities

Permits uploading of orders to other facilities (e.g., lab orders)

Maintains profile of available tests/indications

Flags abnormal results

    Permits tracking of abnormal lab followup

Permits creation of panels

    Disease specific

    Patient specific

    Population specific

Alerts for redundant testing

Guideline-aware order entry

Reports by

    Patient

    Test

    Provider

Product features deemed essential are in roman type; "wish list" items appear in italics.

outside facilities. In this regard, providers who work in integrated systems sometimes have an advantage. However, some major independent laboratory companies do offer an automatic download feature. The minimal Lab/X-ray/Pathology features set (Table 16-3) consists of test history by provider and patient, automatic flagging and tracking of abnormal results (panic and delta checks), and the ability to create specific test panels. Advanced features in this setting provide more decision support during the ordering process in the form of alerts for redundant tests, guidelines-based ordering, and the ability to generate reports by patient, provider, and test. Test information profiling that provides information on indications and significance of results is a rare but very useful feature.

Telephone Calls

Telephone call management features are geared to improving documentation. These features are increasingly found in many EMR products (Table 16-4). If present, they can be very useful and aid in reducing potential liability risks. A good call management system may help to reduce unnecessary office visits while helping to monitor patients via tracking functions. For example, during cold and flu season, it might be possible to keep a list of all pa-

---

Table 16-4   Telephone Call Features.

Maintains call history

    Patient

    Site

    Provider

    Number called from automatic dialing

Captures call reason and action taken

Provides alerts and reminders for required followup

Report by

    Patient

    Provider

    Call reason

    Call action

Product features deemed essential are in roman type; "wish list" items appear in italics.

Table 16-5   Diagnosis Features.

Problem list

   Long term

   Per episode

Guideline-based advice

Access to knowledge resources

   Internet

   Practice guidelines

Report by

   Patient

   Provider

   Diagnosis

Product features deemed essential are in roman type; "wish list" items appear in italics.

tients who contacted the practice and were given advice to manage their symptoms. Tracking functions would then allow the provider to find all patients who had called with cold systems and review treatment instructions. Patients who might require follow-up could be easily identified and flagged for a second call or office visit. Capture of "call reason" and "action taken" makes this type of patinet management aid possible and relatively easy.

Diagnosis Features

The problem list is the most important feature in the area of diagnostic features (Table 16-5). The ability to list and view long-term problems separate from those which are acute and limited is a potential time- saver. Guideline-based advice or access to decision support (QMR, Iliad) and other forms of clinical knowledge resources (e.g., electronic textbooks) are advanced features. As information systems evolve this chart feature is likely to garner more attention. Alerts and reminders for diagnostic tests or preventive medicine interventions find their most natural use as part of the diagnosis or ordering processes. In particular, on-line, context-based access to diagnostic decision support information would be a real time-saver for many busy clinicians.

Table 16-6   Referral Features.

Maintains list of referral sites and providers by

Specialty

Reason for referral

Location

Maintains referral history

Patient

Provider

Site

Reason/diagnosis

Maintains list of approved providers/sites by

Insurance plan

Provider preference

Report by

Patient

Provider

Reason/diagnosis

Referral site/provider

Reports by e-mail attachments

Store and forward technology for images

Product features deemed essential are in roman type; "wish list" items appear in italics.

Referrals

Referral management features (Table 16-6) can greatly increase practice productivity. Aside from providing the ability to monitor patients' adherence to referral advice, features that provide insurance plan-specific referral guidance are particularly helpful in managed care environments. All systems should provide a list of referral sites and providers. The ability to adhere to insurance plan referral preferences and provider preferences constitutes advanced capabilities. A key productivity feature, especially within group practices with multiple practice sites, is the ability to send and receive consult requests via encrypted e-mail.

Preventive Medicine

Managed care has made preventive medicine features (Table 16-7) a major reason for buying an EMR system. Patient intervention histories (list of all interventions done for the patient to-date) , provider-defined alerts, and the ability to create user-defined protocols by age, sex, and disease state are essential. Similarly, reporting in this area must be fairly sophisticated and should provide multiple reporting views. Protocol-based reporting (e.g., a listing of all patients undergoing a standardized treatment process or patients being treated with a locally or nationally created practice guideline or protocol), support for SF-36 (a standardized instrument for determining health status such as ability to perform activities of daily life), and other measures of health status should be considered advanced features which few EMRs currently provide.

Table 16-7   Preventive Medicine Features.

Maintains patient intervention history

Permits design of intervention protocols by

   Sex

   Age

   Disease state

   Insurance plan

Permits guideline-based protocols

Provides user-defined alerts

Report by

   Patient population

   Patient

   Provider

   Diagnosis

   Protocol

Health status reports

   SF-36

Product features deemed essential are in roman type; "wish list" items appear in italics.

Clinical Encounter

Capturing the results of the clinical encounter (Table 16-8) is without a doubt the most problematic issue in EMR selection. Two very important needs collide here: creating an accurate description of the encounter in a readable form (primary use) and creating a searchable description of the encounter that can be easily analyzed (secondary). Most EMR systems handle progress notes as plain text, which is not suitable for analysis. Notes may be typed into the system or imported after transcription. Even systems that permit voice or pen-based input usually capture notes as plain text. Templates provide a boost in productivity for those who are comfortable with their use. Ideally, a number of templates for common problems should be provided with the system. Also, creation of templates by providers should be supported as part of the basic product.

Disease-based guidelines/protocols and coded, searchable notes are advanced features found in very few products. Pay close attention to this area; it often will determine whether an EMR system becomes a valued tool as opposed to a continued source of regret. Ask specific questions.

If notes are typed directly into the system, determine if a medical spell checker is included. Are user-defined document templates available? If transcribed documents are downloaded, ask if special software is required

---

Table 16-8   Clinical Encounter Features.

Progress note

  Plain text

  Encoded and searchable

    Vital signs

    Clinical findings

E&M templates

  Defined by end-user

    Specialty specific

Disease-based guidelines/protocols

  Defined by end-user

    Specialty specific

Product features deemed essential are in roman type; "wish list" items appear in italics.

(as opposed any standard word processor). What file formats are supported? Can notes be exported? How is tampering prevented? What type of input devices may be used (voice, pen, keyboard, etc.)? Direct input of clinic notes by providers, when possible, can be one of the most cost-effective features of EMR implementation. Finally, what type of query capability exists?

Patient Education

Patient education materials, especially drug information, can be very useful in a busy practice (Table 16-9). If patient education materials are provided with a system, make sure that they are derived from an authoritative source and are updated frequently. All materials provided should be modifiable by the user. Many systems now provide access to the Internet from within EMR. If this feature is present, the headache of trying maintain an up-to-date patient education materials almost disappears. The Web is a great source of quality patient education materials.

Analysis and Managed Care

The information needs associated with managed care spring from the need to analyze population-based patient data. In order for a system to provide usable data analysis capabilities, it must be designed with certain features (Table 16-10). Foremost among them is a database, preferably relational (not set in stone), which stores discrete coded data items. Note that the presence of a relational database alone is not sufficient to guarantee that a system is able to conduct useful analysis. In addition, the data must be coded using a standard vocabulary and the database must capture the true relationships that exist between items in the database. For example, if one wishes to analyze the cost of antibiotics for the average patient diagnosed

---

Table 16-9   Patient Education Features.

User definable

Preloaded

Updated regularly

Web access to educational materials

Product features deemed essential are in roman type; "wish list" items appear in italics.

with bronchitis, the database must contain links between various combinations of these items. Unfortunately, it is not possible during a demonstration or site visit to determine if the underlying architecture of the system is

Table 16-10   Managed Care Features.
Provider profiles
Medications
Labs
Referrals
Preventive health
Site profiles
Medications
Labs
Referrals
Preventive health
Outcomes by
Guidelines/protocol
Provider
Disease
Site
Predefined reports
HEDIS
JCAHO
Cost analysis
Medications
Labs
Disease
Protocols
Referral
Patient
Provider

Product features deemed essential are in roman type; "wish list" items appear in italics.

able to support a full range of analyses. In order to determine if the system that you are considering is capable of performing useful analyses, it is best to request a demonstration using data from your practice site or to discuss this issue with other practices already using the system. Another approach is to obtain a working copy of the program and use it for a brief period to see if it performs as desired. The features listed below should be considered essential for all but the most basic EMR systems. Perhaps one of the more useful, standard reports that a system might offer is HEDIS (Health Plan Employer Data and Information Set). HEDIS is used to collect data on health plan performance. Although the data elements required are fairly simple, they often require time-consuming chart reviews to obtain an adequate sample. An EMR system with this capability would be very valuable to many practices.

Profiles and other types of reports might be helpful to administrators and medical directors. Ask to see demonstrations of these features with data taken from your practice.

Communications and Infrastructure

The technical issues involved in selecting an EMR system can be somewhat intimidating. However, it is often not as difficult as it may seem because there is only a relatively limited number of acceptable options and knowing what they are and why they are important is not difficult to learn.

Communications

Remote access allows you to access a computer without being physically present (e.g., calling into your office computer from a computer in your den). Remote access is a very desirable feature and along with e-mail, fax, and Internet capability, greatly increases the value of an EMR system.

For practices that desire to conduct in-depth analyses of data, the ability to export data to statistical analysis programs or other systems is an essential feature. Data repositories and warehouses are very large database systems that may have links to EMR systems (see Chapter 4) and help to support patient care and data analysis. Both systems are suited to only the most sophisticated information systems environments. The ability to import data is also very important. This may be especially true during the initial phase of implementation when lack of importation features may result in having to retype old data into the new system.

Decision Support

Decision support may be thought of as occurring on three levels (see Chapter 8). The first level encompasses basic report functions (e.g., find all patients with history of myocardial infarction not currently taking a beta-blocker). Here you are able to group patients, providers, or interventions based upon your parameters. This level of decision support capability relies upon the data stored and the reporting capability of the software package. The next level of decision support is arrived at via the provision of integrated access to reference materials local or via the Internet (drug databases, electronic textbooks, etc.). Ideally, these materials are available within the context of the user's current activity. For example, if a diagnosis of new-onset atrial fibrillation is about to be made, selection of a hypothetical "Reference Button" will bring up the appropriate chapter of an electronic textbook. More advanced decision support capabilities require the availability of sophisticated statistical analysis or pattern recognition functions within the EMR or via seamless interface to stand-alone analytical tools. These functions would seldom be used by clinicians. Rather they are provided for researchers and administrators interested in outcomes, cost, and provider or patient profiling.

Operating Systems

Unix and Novell have been the dominant EMR operating systems, but Windows 95/98 and Windows NT are rapidly gaining ground and most new systems are appearing first on these platforms. Client/server (see Chapter 2) is a mode of computing in which the database and applications reside on a central computer (server) and other computers (clients) make requests to this server to either save or retrieve information. Each type of computing component is referred to as a "tier". Most systems consist of two tiers: the client computer, with which the user interacts directly, and the server, with which client computers interact. Sometimes the efficiency of client/server operations can be improved by adding a second server. In this case, the database resides on one server and the rules for using the database and other applications reside on the second server. This type of set up is referred to as a "three-tiered" client/server environment. Three tiers are best suited to larger practice sites (e.g., hospitals and very large group practices).

Data Types and Storage Formats

Although not essential to EMR functioning, the ability to store sound, video, and graphics may increase the utility of an EMR product for some practices. If these types of data are accepted by an EMR, be sure that they can be searched and indexed as easily as text data. Files are stored on disk using a very specific format. The format is chosen by the product's designer who may or may not make the details of that format public. Your ability to move data between programs is limited by the file format that the program uses. Be sure to clarify with the vendor its policy on letting others know the details of its file format. A vendor may use its file format to prevent you from migrating to another product in the future. Be very careful when asking about this matter.

Standards

A number of attempts have been made to make the sharing of medical information easier. Health Level-7 (HL7) is a standard promoted as a means of permitting easier communications between computer systems. Any EMR system under consideration should support this standard. ICD and CPT codes are standards for billing and recording diagnoses and represent the most widely used coding standards. Common Object Request Broker Architecture (CORBA) is a new standard for handling object use by software programs sharing a common environment. CORBA technology is only now beginning to appear in EMR systems. It is not essential that a system utilize this technology at present, but it should be considered a plus if it is included. MEDCIN and Read codes are vocabularies for recording the information that appears in the progress note. They offer hope to the ideal of creating progress notes that are fully encoded, indexed, and searchable.

Interfaces

Pen-based computers and voice recognition systems may prove to be a boon to those who cannot type with enough skill to use a computer as part of the patient encounter. Pen-based systems no longer attempt to recognize handwriting as their main data input mechanism. Instead, more often they act as pointing devices with the same functionality as a mouse. The most important feature of pen-based systems is portability. Many palm-top systems fall into this category.

Voice recognition systems have improved significantly over the last few years; clinical systems can now accurately recognize continuous speech. Voice recognition, however, despite recent advances, is still very sensitive to accents and other individual speaking traits. The best advice is to try the system out under normal work conditions (background noise, different users) before deciding if it will work for you. Voice recognition systems are relatively inexpensive and worth evaluating. Should you decide to try a pen- or voice-based system, inquire about the availability of medical dictionary or spell-checker add-ons. They will make the job of correcting mistaking less time consuming and frustrating.

Security

Putting data into electronic form always raises the possibility that it may be tampered with or misused. In order to assure proper security for patient information, a practice must implement a combination of office policies and procedures to complement intrinsic EMR security features. Passwords are the most common security feature found in EMR packages. Passwords are only as secure as people permit them to be. They offer an acceptable level of security when properly handled. If your office plans to use passwords, a few precautions may help. Put policies into place making misuse of passwords a serious offense. Insist that your EMR package offers multi-level password access. Multi-level passwords offer additional protection by restricting access to data files based upon the "need to know" (this should be explained). In such a system, each type of file is coded to permit access to certain classes of passwords. The password class for billing clerks would be different than that for doctors, allowing the systems administrator to easily restrict access to lab data to clerks while permitting unencumbered access to physicians. At a minimum, a system should restrict access to files based upon job type.

Audit trails provide an additional security measure. They maintain a record of all file access attempts and permit the systems administrator (the person in charge of maintaining the computer system) to determine if anyone has tried to gain unauthorized access. Authorized users are also logged. Many EMR packages permit the audit trail feature to be disabled; this is a bad idea. Buy a package with automatic audit trail activation that cannot be disabled. Recent gains in computer technology have made user-validation more reliable and may make passwords obsolete. Biometrics, the use of biologically unique markers to provide secure access, has made significant gains recently. Fingerprint, face print, and voice pattern recognition systems are available, relatively inexpensive, and make unauthorized access to data files nearly impossible. Security issues are not limited to unauthorized access. Data validation is equally important. For example, does a system check data input for unlikely values (e.g., temperature of 300°F, blood pres-

Table 16-11   Communications and Infrastructure Features.

Remote access
Fax support or linkage
Word processor support or linkage
Spreadsheet support or linkage
Provides e-mail support or linkage
Internet
   Web-enabled version
Decision support
   Statistical analysis (internal)
   Knowledge resources (access from within EMR)
      MEDLINE
      Internet
Permits data export
   ASCII
   Support for clinical data repository
   Data warehouse
   Statistical analysis packages
Permits data import
   ASCII
   Relational database files
   Application programming interface
Supports varied data formats
   Sound
   Video
   Graphics
File formats supported
   Proprietary
   Commercial standard (Oracle, Sybase, etc.)
   ASCII
Standards supported
   HL-7
   CORBA
   SNOMED
   ICD
   CPT
   MEDCIN
   READ Codes
   LOINC for lab data

Product features deemed essential are in roman type; "wish list" items appear in italics.

Table 16-11   Communications and Infrastructure Features (*continued*).

Interface options
  Pen
  Voice
Keyboard
Graphics
  User modifiable
Security features
Audit trail
  Permits audit trail analysis
    Automatic activation
Passwords
  Text/numeric
  Biometric
    Face
    Voice
    Fingerprint
  Multiple levels by user type
Data validation
Back-up process
Encryption
Operating systems
  Unix
  Macintosh
  Windows 95/98
  Windows NT
  Novell
  Internet based
  Client/server
  Number of tiers
Technology
  Database
    Relational
    Object
    Multi-dimensional
  SQL support

Product features deemed essential are in roman type; "wish list" items appear in italics.

sure of 400/300)? All data stored in an EMR should be subject to some type of validation process. Insist upon it! Since patient information may be shared between sites or other business entities, some form of encryption should be available either within the EMR package or as an add-on option. Automatic encryption of files saved to disk is a valuable form of data protection and systems.

A final security matter is that of file preservation. Here again, office policy comes into play. Back-up, file storage, and disaster-recovery procedures must be set by the systems administrator. This is an area where many businesses fall short with painful results. Select an off-site storage location for all data files. Backups should be done at least once each day; in busy environments, multiple times throughout the day. Look for EMR packages that permit on-line back-ups (i.e., copies of all files stored on the computer's disk drives can be copied for storage while the computer is being used). Other measures such as mirrored backup (using two separate drives to hold identical data) and fault-tolerance are found at the level of the operating system. These measures help to keep your practice running through many types of computer problems. Give serious consideration to making them a part of your EMR setup.

Table 16-11 summarizes the communications and infrastructure features.

17 / Vendor Analysis

Sarah T. Corley

The first step in evaluating vendors is to identify those who make products suitable for your specialty and practice situation. Professional meetings are an excellent opportunity to meet established vendors who have products designed for your specialty. Medical journals often review different software packages. Many Web sites and search engines provide links to electronic medical records (EMR) vendors as well. Web sites that have links to vendors as of publication date include *http://www.computingforclinicians.com/product_information2.htm, http://dir. yahoo.com/Business and Economy/Business to Business/Health Care Management/ Practice and Information Management/Medical Record Systems/,* and *http:// www.aafp.org/fpm/20010100/45elec.html.*

A number of magazines provide reviews or lists of software. *Health Data Management* publishes a resource guide that is available on the Web at *http://hdm.fgray.com/html/buyers/list6.htm.* MD *Computing* publishes annually a medical hardware and software buyers' guide. *Healthcare Informatics* has an annual resource guide in its December issue; this is not available on-line but may be ordered from its Web site at *www.healthcare-informatics.com.*

Vendor Evaluation

Vendors should be evaluated in a systematic fashion using similar criteria. Figure 17-1 is a worksheet that may be used as a template when evaluating potential EMR vendors.

Company
URL
Contact Name
Phone Number
E-mail
Fax Number
Years in Business
Operating Systems (DOS, Windows, Unix)
Number of Installed Sites
Number of Users
Medical Record
Appointments
Billing
Decision Support
Web Browser Interface
SNOMED for Structured Data Entry
Drug Interaction Checking
Lab Interfaces
Cost of Interfaces
Hardware Required
Local Support
System Cost (Per User, Per Workstation)
Cost of Upgrades/Year
Cost of Support/Year
Cost of Training/Year
Frequency of Upgrades
User Groups
Data Entry Modes (Keyboard, Mouse, Light Pen, Voice, Dictation)
E-mail and Messaging
Handheld Interface
ASP
Comments

Figure 17-1 Vendor Worksheet.

Length of Time in Business

It is useful to know how long a company has been in business. Some vendors may have long-established businesses selling other products but are just starting in the EMR business. Although a vendor who has been selling EMR systems for many years may not necessarily be more stable than a newly established company, there will be a better opportunity to evaluate how well the company responds to the changing needs of users.

Next determine how long the vendor's EMR product has been on the market. For each EMR product it is important to determine the number of actual copies sold and the number of users at each site where the software is installed. These are important distinctions. It is possible for a vendor to have sold only one copy of an EMR package to a very large practice and truthfully state that they have more than 500 users, which is, of course, quite different from having sold 500 copies of the software. In the former example, local users of a single product copy may be referred to as "seats" or "licensees".

Customer Profiles

Request a list of clients with practices of a similar size and composition to yours and request three references. Find out the total number of software licenses *sold* each year over the last three years and the total number of software licenses *installed* each year over the last three years. Some software that is sold is never installed, so these lists may be different. If there is a significant discrepancy between the number of systems sold and the number installed, this can be a red flag that the company has a problem with its support and training divisions. Also find out if the vendor's annual sales are increasing, decreasing, or flat. Mature products may have flat sales but should have a large market share. If a product is new, then increasing sales may be the only means available for estimating market share or customer base.

Obtain the name, address, and telephone number of clients representing the ten most recent sales and the ten most recent installations. Often they can provide information about how smoothly the current sales and training force is working. Ask for a complete list of all clients using the product with name, address, telephone number, date purchased, and the date of first productive use. These users can provide background information about how the company has met their needs over the years. If you personally know any users of the system, call them in addition to the three recent references for similar products already given. Determine if there is a users group and whether they attend meetings. If so, ask for an appraisal of their usefulness. Well-developed user group meetings can be an excellent source of helpful advice in optimal use of EMRs.

Medical software is very complex, and software developers write manuals whereas full-time medical practitioners do not. Experienced physician users can help a new user use the software more efficiently. Beta-testers can offer insight into the latest releases. Some physicians may have written programs that are compatible with the product and may offer it as shareware. Find out if there is a regular newsletter published with useful tips and if there is a Web site or Listserve.

Public or Private Corporation

Request audited financial statements for the last three years and a banking reference. If you are making a large monetary investment in a software package, you want to be sure that the company will be in business for years to come and will be able to provide upgrades and technical support. For publicly owned companies, you should search the records for details on finances, funding, and profit-and-loss statements. Security and Exchange Commission reports are available on-line at www.sec.gov. For privately held companies, bank references must be requested and checked.

Upgrades

Compare the major releases planned for each of the software packages and the release and implementation time frames. Check with users to confirm that information the vendors have provided about the frequency of past upgrades is accurate. A major upgrade at least once a year is desirable in an EMR product to keep up with changes in technology and medical practice. References should also be asked whether the upgrades provide valuable features or just cosmetic changes.

Mergers

Ask about mergers, especially if the company has purchased or merged with another company or other companies within the last two years. If so, try to determine if all software products have been supported during this period and whether current users were offered upgraded products. The EMR market is rapidly evolving, and as companies purchase complementary products to speed the development/product releases process, they have left users of orphaned systems without any support or upgrades. *Caveat emptor!*

Litigation

Ask for details of any current or pending litigation. Does this litigation involve users, corporate partners, or the government? Litigation can take away money and time that would otherwise be spent improving the product. Do not buy products from companies that are having legal difficulties with customers. This is never a good sign. Other types of litigation must be judged on a case-by-case basis.

Corporate Partners

Obtain a listing of all the vendor's technology and/or distribution partnerships and alliances. Obtain the names of all partners, along with name, address, telephone number, and a brief description of the nature of the relationship. If partnerships involve software packages that are intended to work together, ascertain the level of integration (user groups and clients are helpful here). These partnerships can be detrimental if they restrict the types of operating systems or peripherals supported. For example, if you already have a UNIX or LINUX operating system and your vendor institutes a partnership with Microsoft, your operating system may not be supported in future releases. Other examples could be limited interfaces with EKG machines, blood glucose monitors, or electronic claims warehouses. Problems can also arise if the second company becomes financially unstable or starts requiring concessions from the vendor you have selected.

Development and Technical Support

Determine the total number of employees within the organization that are directly and exclusively associated with the EMR product. Break this down by department and quantify the average tenure of employees in Marketing and Sales, R&D, Maintenance, Quality Control/Quality Assurance, Technical Support, Client Services/ Installation, Field Service, and End-User Support.

Tenure in the sales and marketing department is much less important than in support and training. Try to ascertain whether the company has adequate resources to train new users. Are there well-written user manuals? Have the trainers had experience with sites similar to yours? A longer tenure will have given them more opportunity to work with disparate practices and improve training material. Computer software support in general has a high turnover rate, but, again, the longer the average length of em-

ployment, the more likely the company is to have encountered your particular problem and to have a rapid solution for you.

Product Viability

A product, even a great one, is only as good as the latest version. Research
and development (R&D) spending is very important to the continued viability of a product. Look at the budget dollars set aside for R&D as well as
the number of personnel. Often when companies are strapped for cash,
R&D spending is one of the first areas to be cut. Insufficient spending for
R&D translates into a product that will not be kept up to date. Avoid products with poor R&D support. You should look for at least as many employees involved in support and R&D as there are in sales. An average tenure of
at least one year in support and two years in R&D should ensure that the
employees are familiar with the product. The longer the length of employment, the more likely it is that the company can devote energy to improving the product rather than training replacement staff.

Ask about annual R&D plans in the area of EMR systems for the next
three years and current and projected expenditures for R&D activity in
both absolute terms and as a percent of gross revenues. Investment in R&D
will ensure that the product will continue to keep pace with changes in the
field and with the needs of the users.

Compare various data entry modes and determine whether they are
currently functional, in development, or planned for the future. These may
include speech (voice) recognition, graphics- or icon-based interfaces,
touch screens, light pens, decision support, Internet integration, or wireless
transmission. If you have a large practice, you may want to have many different options of data entry. If the practitioners have always dictated, the
ability to use voice recognition in the program can keep dictation costs
down and allow direct data entry without physician revolt. Practices with
residents or medical students may be more interested in the decision support features and Internet integration.

Interfaces

Is the company's software HL-7 compliant? What data interchange standards does the vendor adhere to? Which lab companies have functional interfaces with the software? To save time on data entry, a complete EMR
should be able to download lab results directly from the lab into the individual patient's chart. If the EMR does not employ a standard such as HL-7,

it may be impossible or very expensive to download labs or exchange information with others. Which medical management packages have successful interfaces with the software? If a practice plans on keeping its current medical management software, an interface can eliminate the need to enter demographic data twice. You need to know the cost of the interface with your practice management system, because this is usually an additional charge. Find out if this is a total turnkey price or if it is an hourly charge. Expenses can increase rapidly when custom interfaces must be written.

Cost Comparisons

When analyzing costs, be sure that you are comparing comparable proposals. It is helpful to separate the costs of hardware, software, installation, training, technical support, and upgrades. That way you can estimate the total costs of each system.

If a vendor requires that you purchase hardware from it, list the exact specifications of what will be provided and the total cost. Compare that cost with the cost of commercially available hardware. Hardware costs are dropping rapidly and bargains are easily available. If hardware is provided, what is the length of the contract? Is it leased or purchased? Most equipment is adequate for about three years, but improvements to both hardware and software can render the hardware obsolete after that. It is very important to have service costs included. A practice that is "paperless" must have guaranteed immediate service on the server and at least next-day service on the workstations.

When evaluating the costs of the software itself, you should list the total cost per user. That way, if the practice grows, you will already have the dollar amount needed to increase the number of licenses. Most vendors will have a lower cost if more licenses are purchased so you may wish to group the prices (e.g., 1 to 10 licenses, $3000 per user; 11 to 25 licenses, $2500 per user; etc.). Compare the costs for regular updates for the drug interaction package and software updates. If this is a flat rate, note whether the rate is guaranteed for any period of time. If you are considering separate components in addition to basic EMR, such as a billing and scheduling package, those prices should be itemized separately.

Training Services

Training costs can be very expensive. You should itemize training costs by the number of hours and number of users to be trained. You should list the number of hours of training the vendor suggests and whether any training is included in the cost of the software. You should also note if the training is on or off site. If it is to be off site, you must factor in travel costs for those attending the training; if it is to be on site, you need to include the costs of the trainers' expenses if they are to paid by your practice. You should check references on the assigned trainer before paying for the training. The quality may vary widely between trainers from the same company.

18 / Creating a Request for Proposal and Negotiating a Contract

Sarah T. Corley

Defining a Request for Proposal

A Request for Proposal (RFP) is a document used for comparing different products. It must include detailed information about the needs of the practice so the proposal can be tailored appropriately. The process of designing an RFP will help in assessing and setting priorities for product features. Responding to an RFP requires a significant time investment by the vendor, so the practice should strive to present a concise document to a few select vendors.

Determining the Need for a Request for Proposal

The intent of the RFP is to specify *exactly* what the practice is looking for in a product, including hardware, software, maintenance, and training. The vendor's response will indicate whether the desired features are available in their current product and, if not, whether the desired features are in development. The reply should also provide detailed cost information. Because responding to an RFP may be very labor intensive for a vendor, it may be unwilling to complete one if they do not think the buyer is serious. To make sure the practice appears serious, it should complete a rigorous self-evaluation before designing the RFP (see Chapters 13, 15, and 16). Send your RFP to only two or four companies. Appendix D is a sample RFP that may be used as a template when designing your own.

Gathering Background
Information About Your Practice

Before you select an electronic medical records (EMR) system to speed or fix the problems identified in your practice, you must know how the current system is working. Start by collecting information about how well your practice functions. The information needs to be detailed and should involve several months of self-examination and study (see Chapters 13 and 15). This information, along with desired product features, should be provided to the vendor as part of your RFP.

Number of Users

How many staff will be using the system? Most software packages are sold by the number of licenses. You should know the maximum number of users who will require access to both software and hardware at any given time. Do not make the mistake of underestimating future needs; plan for all potential users, not just those who are present initially.

Number of Workstations

Remember that a paperless office usually needs more than one workstation per user. Physicians will need terminals in the exam rooms and in their offices. The staff will need access to workstations throughout the office. As with the software, do not underestimate the total number of workstations required.

Computer Experience of Users

To accurately estimate training costs, the computer literacy of all staff must be taken into account. Training costs are often based on an hourly rate, and you do not want to unnecessarily spend expensive training time going over the basics of learning how to log on/off, using a mouse, and other basic computing skills. If few staff have even minimal computer skills, it may be cost-effective to pay for those staff members to attend basic computer classes at a local community college (if the practice is large, on-site training is a reasonable alternative). This approach will ensure that money spent for on-site EMR training will not be wasted.

Computerization of Tasks

Consideration of how the EMR system will be used should be an early part of the selection process. Will the practice be paperless? If so, then each staff person must have his or her own terminal and user license. It will also require workstations in the exam rooms, labs, and other areas where the staff must have access to the information. A paperless office requires other changes in the office work flow as well. Instead of simply filing documents from outside sources, they will have to be scanned into the EMR system. Labs will require an electronic interface so that results can be downloaded automatically into your EMR system. If computerized EKGs will be used, the computer station in the exam rooms must be close enough that the lead from the EKG machine can be attached to the computer adapter. Will scheduling be included with the EMR system? Will phone messages be handled through internal e-mail? Will nurses be entering their own notes for procedures such as immunizations, allergy shots, and ear washes? A paperless office greatly increases data entry requirements, so plan accordingly.

Existing Software

Integrating current software with newly arrived EMR can be a difficult and time-consuming process. In many offices a practice management system (PMS) will already be in place. You may be able to avoid duplicate entry of demographic data if it is possible to interface your EMR to the PMS. Interfaces exist for many popular PMS systems. Be sure to ask EMR vendors which practice management systems they provide interfaces for. If there other programs you wish to keep, you must be sure that the platforms are compatible. Incompatibilities may arise because of operating system (e.g., Unix versus Windows) or hardware (e.g., Intel-based systems versus RISC) differences. If you plan to change operating systems, you will need to know which current programs will be compatible with the new operating system. Also, be sure there are programs available for the new operating system that meet all your needs. Even when new software is found, problems may occur because of differences in how files are handled. For example, if you are changing your word processing program, you may need to plan for time and money spent reformatting documents.

Existing Hardware

If you plan on keeping existing computers, they will need to be itemized by processor speed, hard-drive size, and amount of RAM. All software programs will have minimal hardware requirements and optimal hardware requirements. It will aid in a smooth transition if your new hardware meets the optimal requirements of the EMR system, because minimal requirements often result in frustratingly slow response times.

The Budget

EMR software varies widely in cost, and the practice budget should be used to narrow down the choice. Be realistic about budget issues: It is much too easy to take on an unmanageable debt load. Keep in mind that new systems tend to make offices less productive for a period of time after installation, so do not assume that income will immediately increase; it is more likely to decline slightly or stay flat. Try to avoid being seduced by features for which you may have little need. Twenty-five features that you use often are better than 100 features that serve only occasional needs. Do you wish to be paperless? This is more expensive initially than leaving some items in paper form, although cost savings occur over time. The vendor should know your budget range so that realistic proposals can be made.

Choosing Who Will Determine Needed Components and Select the System

The practice needs to decide who will make the final decision. Will it be an individual or committee decision? Some techniques for arriving at a consensus are detailed in an article by Chocholik et al (1). Ideally, the RFP should reflect what has been learned from the analysis of your practice and the goals that you have set (see Chapter 13). The decision-making mechanism should have been created and tested during the problem definition and process analysis. If this is the case, the decision as to which system to buy and what features are essential will be a natural outgrowth of the completed analysis. If you have not created a formal process for analyzing your practice and arriving at product-related decisions, then go back and do so. Otherwise, it is likely that you will pay a stiff price in dollars and disruption.

Typical Components of a Request for Proposal

An RFP should have four basic sections: practice information, vendor information, product features required, and support and services. Provide the vendor with detailed information that reflects the size, scope, and future plans for your practice. The vendor will use this information to determine if you are really a potential customer. For example, if your budget is too low or your practice is smaller than what the vendor is accustomed to working with, then early on the vendor can withdraw from consideration and save everyone time and frustration.

Just as the vendor may use practice information to determine that you are not a good prospect, you will use the information provided by the vendor to make the same determination (see Chapter 17). Length of time in business, financial stability, percentage of dollars spent on research and development, and support available are helpful factors in determining the viability of the vendor.

Assuming that the vendor appears to be profitable and stable, you may turn your attention to reviewing product features. Be detailed and specific when identifying desired product features. Use the feature list provided in Appendix C to create a list specific to your practice.

A smooth installation requires attention to support and services. Use the RFP process to identify vendors who will provide the level of support that you require. Typical issues are training, technical support, provision of interfaces, and updates. Each of these should be spelled out in detail and, once agreed upon, should be written into the contract (see Chapter 20).

Negotiating a Contract

The contract often becomes a source of misery for many practices. Too often a practice will trustingly sign a standard contract, which is usually written to favor the vendor, without carefully reading its content. This is a serious mistake. Always read the contract carefully, then have your attorney look at it. Do not accept *any* terms that are not favorable to you.

When negotiating a contract, consider your areas of strength as well as the vendor's weaknesses. If you have a large, high-profile practice, you should be able to negotiate a discounted rate based upon the visibility and marketing advantages that accrue to the vendor if the implementation is successful. If the vendor is just starting out and has no existing installations, you should *never* pay full price (your practice will be a beta test site whether or not it is labeled as such). If the vendor has a product with functional installed sites but is moving into a new geographic market, you may be able to negotiate a discount based on the uncertainties of local support and the benefits to the vendor of your practice being a local reference for other interested buyers. If you are buying a large number of user licenses either for your practice or as part of a local consortium of physician buyers, you should ask for a volume discount because installation and training costs can be shared.

Everything that is being purchased should be listed in detail in the contract. If you are purchasing hardware from the vendor, you must detail, exactly, the manufacturer, model, year, hard-drive size, memory, network card speed, modem type and speed, size of monitors, and types of keyboards. Nothing should be assumed. Hardware service contracts should also be spelled out in detail, including the timeframe for service on both the server and workstations as well as whether this is on or off site. The contract should specify hardware and service costs and whether installation/setup costs are included.

The contract for your network should include the type of cable to be laid, the speed of the network cards, the type of hub and any routers, and the type of network software. It should specify the maximum number of network users and the costs of increasing network connections. If network maintenance is included, the contract should detail the costs and timeframe of support as well as the contacts for service on weekends and holidays. The contract should specify any pre-implementation services to be provided along with the timeframe for such assistance and any costs for those services. All software should be itemized in the contract by the modules included, number of concurrent users, cost per user, and total system cost. It should identify the maximum number of users and the incremental cost of adding users. If the company makes other modules, which the practice is not currently purchasing, the costs of acquiring them later should be set at the time the contract is signed. The costs and frequency of upgrades should be listed in the contract as well as the length of time that upgrades will be available at that price. Try to negotiate a set price for the next three to five years if possible, so that you may budget appropriately.

Training costs should detail the number of trainers to be provided, the number of trainees allowed, and the number of hours of training included at the agreed upon price. The contract should specify the cost of additional training at a daily or hourly rate. Make sure this price is valid for the next year or two because employees often require additional training. Additional training after 3 to 6 months will often improve their efficiency once they are familiar with the system. If the trainer is traveling from a distant site, the contract should specify the maximum amount that will be paid for living and travel expenses.

If the software requires customization, the fees should be listed along with the services to be provided. A practice should always try to negotiate a flat-fee for the customization of office forms, billing, and demographics information. You should also try to negotiate a flat rate for lab interfaces, and the contract should specify that final payment will not be made until the interface is completed and functional. If progress note templates cannot be created or amended by practice staff, have the cost for this service clearly stated in the contract.

Technical support is crucial to successful EMR implementation. The contract must identify who will be providing these services, at what hours (9–5 or 24/7), and at what cost. If the vendor provides support outside of regular business hours, determine whether these services are charged at a higher rate than those rendered during business hours. Be sure that you have phone numbers, e-mail addresses, fax numbers, and pager numbers so that you can contact technical support at any time.

Remember, if an agreement is not in the contract, it is not binding. Read all contracts carefully and do not be afraid to negotiate the best deal possible.

REFERENCE

1. **Chocholik JK, Bouchard SE, Tan JK, Ostrow DN.** The determination of relevant goals and criteria used to select an automated patient care information system: a delphi approach. JAMA. 1999;6:219-33.

19 / Gathering Information: Site Visits and Demonstrations

Bruce Slater

S ite visits and product demonstrations are some of the most enjoyable parts of working with a vendor. They are vitally important to the evaluation of a product, and offer a welcome change of pace for the EMR selection team. The excitement of a road trip or welcoming a visitor can liven up even the dullest vendor/product evaluation process.

Site Visits

Why Make a Site Visit?

The purpose of a site visit is to see the vendor's product in use in an environment very similar to yours. The two operative features are making sure that 1) what you are seeing is very similar to what you are buying and 2) the group you are visiting is very similar to your group.

Who Should Visit the Site?

The team leader should be the person with overall responsibility for vendor selection at your institution. The team size should be small; three to five people are reasonable unless your site is very large. If your team size is larger and there are no "nonessential" members, consider making two visits or visit two sites rather than imposing a large group on the host site. It is quite possible to overwhelm the visiting site and create problems for the vendor who has asked the indulgence of the host for this visit. In choosing your site visitors it is important to keep compatible personalities in mind. It may be better to send a fairly knowledgeable yet socially competent person rather than an expert who does not get along well with others. The team should involve a physician leader, administrator or managerial person, and a user of the system. If you are vetting a physician system that nurses also use, then inviting a nurse is wise. If the system involves administrative systems such as scheduling, then having a front-line person who deals with patients and schedules visits is appropriate. Similarly, if there is a telephone interface with the product, then a receptionist should be part of the team. If the product has a patient interface, then you should consider bringing along a favorite patient who has some computer experience and can give you the best evaluation.

In fact, all team members should be comfortable with computers. Team members should have a history with your organization so that they know the people who will be using the system and can represent their views. In addition, members of the site visit team should be very comfortable working with each other.

Each person chosen for the team should have knowledge or expertise that can be brought to bear when evaluating a product. The member should have a full set of questions and issues from the sector he represents. Because team size is limited, it is rare that you can bring two people doing the same job to a site. Thus, even though physicians have a lot of clout, it would be a bad idea to take two doctors on a site visit. The same reasoning applies to administrative personnel. If a sector is not represented because of team size limitations, then another member should be given its questions and issues beforehand to ask the vendor and site personnel.

The team has a specific function and when selecting it you should be very careful about your choices. Once members are selected, team composition should be reviewed by relevant decision-makers. To make sure there are no surprises when the team is announced, you should confirm availability before finalizing membership.

Team members should be fair and not go into the evaluation with a preconceived notion about the outcome. It is possible to have "leanings" without prejudicing the evaluation. Team members should be made to understand that they are not being sent to render opinions but rather to objectively gather information. Be careful that an outspoken member does not insult the host organization by "explaining" the faults of the system to the host in the middle of the visit. There will be opportunity for a later, comprehensive review in which any member may voice subjective assessments of all visit-related findings.

It goes without saying that none of the team or their family members should have any financial arrangement with the vendor. Likewise, team members should not receive any direct support or gifts from the vendor. The team should be able to leave its current work for a day or two without untoward results. Support from the institution should be given to the team in the form of time for preparing for the site visit and subsequent writeup. Be careful to select members whose workload permits adequate preparation for site-visit related duties and activities. Site-visiting expertise is a rare but valuable skill. Potential team members who have conducted site visits in the past may be able to provide useful insights even though their present job functions are not directly applicable to the product investigated. Site visiting is an anthropologic skill. Being a professional stranger is a valuable ability.

Whom Do You Interview?

Choosing people to interview at the site is more problematic. Always include line-users to aid in assessing user interface and workflow issues. Managers and administrators may help with understanding the effects of system implementation on job performance, job functions, cost-savings, etc. Request a list of people with whom you will be allowed to visit. This is to assure that you are not being given personnel who cannot answer your operational questions or those who do not understand the higher administrative aspects of the installation. It is important to have the correct balance between users, managers, and administrative personnel. You want everyone to be comfortable with the kinds of people they will meet and the questions they need to ask.

When Do You Make a Site Visit?

The site visit should neither come at the beginning of the selection process nor at the very end. The site visit allows the team to evaluate how a specific product works in a production environment. Therefore, it is essential that the EMR selection process be far enough along to have resulted in a narrowing of the field to a few very desirable products. Do not wait until after you have settled on a single product. Site visits conducted at this point serve simply as rubber stamps and it is too easy to gloss over deficiencies because team members would not be inclined to "disagree" with what amounts to a foregone conclusion. Except for the most complicated multi-function systems, one day should be adequate for a site visit. If travel issues are a consideration, arriving mid-day and leaving the following mid-day can accommodate a complete visit.

Which Sites Do You Visit?

Always select sites that will allow you to answer questions pertinent to your evaluation process. If system response time is an issue, try to visit a site that has a high patient volume or a large number of workstations. Vendor support quality issues are also good site visit topics. However, the best rule is to visit sites that are most like your own in terms of patient volume, revenue, technical expertise, etc. If money is no object, then the sites most like your own with the products most like the one you are considering, regardless of location, are the places to visit. Usually a compromise will have to be made. By limiting the scope and cost of your visit, you limit the number of potential sites. Usually a reasonable compromise can be made in the number of visitors and number of sites so that a good representative visit can be arranged.

A Sample Site Visit: Questions and Logistics

Questions

Divide the functionality of prospective systems into logical groups. For each group develop a set of questions that addresses process and ease-of-use for each aspect of the system. What follows is a sample list of functional groups and possible questions. Study and modify them according to your needs. Review them before your visit. If these questions generate others about your own institution, these must be answered before the site visit. For example, if you have a robust, secure e-mail system at your institution but you had not thought about using e-mail in your clinical system, perhaps this should be addressed in the project design.

Front End
The front end includes patient contacts (in person, over the phone, or via a messaging system), check-in processing for visits, financial verification, insurance confirmation, managed care processing (verifying correct network, co-pays, deductibles, referral verification, and other managed care issues), check-out processing, taking payments, and making follow-up or referral appointments.

1. Is patient look-up easy? Are you prompted with a list of prescheduled patients to chose from?
2. How are patients identified? Is a Soundex feature available?

3. How are potential mismatches dealt with? How do you resolve incorrect matches?
4. Does the system prompt you with financial details for each patient?
5. Does the system integrate with your phone system by using caller ID to bring up the patient's record?
6. Does the system follow your workflow? Can it be made to?
7. How much managed care information does it supply? Is it accurate? Up to date?
8. Is simple cash collection quick and intuitive?
9. Is the scheduling system easy to use?

Clinical Preprocessing

Clinical staff take over and escort the patient to the examination room, take the initial history, vital signs, check medications and allergies, and prepare for the provider. In some systems clinical personnel assist patients in using data collection and education software in the waiting or exam room.

1. Is patient look-up easy? Are you prompted with a list of prescheduled patients to chose from?
2. Are templates provided to enter data? Are they easy to use?
3. Is the system used in the exam room? Can patients "peek" into their record?
4. How easy is it to enter medications or allergies?
5. What are the provisions for security? How long does it take to log-in? How often do you have to log-in?
6. Are there any features that patients can use? Are they easy to use? Do patients like them?
7. Is it easy to check immunizations?
8. Can you easily look up lab and imaging results?

Clinical Visit

During the clinical visit the provider takes a history, reviews past records, examines the patient, plans treatment or further evaluations, documents the visit, creates a superbill, and plans follow-up.

1. Is the system used in the exam room? Is the patient preselected by an aide before you enter the exam room?
2. Is there expert advice built into the system? Is it easy to use?

3. Does the system help with documentation? How much time does it take?
4. Does the system fit into your workflow? What changes do you have to make?
5. Does the system enable you to order labs, images, or referrals?
6. If available, are templates easy to create or change?
7. Can you schedule the patient for a return visit or to see a specialist in your organization?
8. Are clinical guidelines or informal local information available through the system?
9. Does the system enable electronic communication? With patients? With staff? With other providers?
10. What do you like best about the system? What part of the system do you interact with most? Least?
11. Does the system perform as expected? Does it respond fast enough?

Clinical Postprocessing

During clinical postprocessing, staff may give immunizations and certain treatments, collect specimens, and help facilitate referrals or lab tests by filling out forms or getting approval from managed care organizations.

1. Does the system help with immunizations?
2. How does the system fit into your workflow?
3. Does the system save time?
4. Is the system connected to managed care information to make referrals easier?
5. Is there patient education material available?
6. Does the system make it easier to order labs or images?
7. Does the system offer an appointment option/feature?
8. Does the system provide for electronic communication?

Previsit Triage

Clinical personnel, usually nurses, may get messages from patients, usually on the phone but increasingly via e-mail or Web interfaces. They give advice and/or reassurance and pass the message to a physician to approve before or after the fact or for the physician to contact the patient directly.

1. Does the system "pop up" the patient's clinical information when a call comes in?

2. Can you record telephone consultations directly into the system?
3. What decision support tools are available while you are on the phone with a patient?
4. Does the system enable you to message to physicians for assistance? During a call?
5. Can you make appointments for the patient while on the phone?
6. Can you order labs or images through the system?
7. Does the system help you with prescription refills?
8. Can you make a managed care referral for a patient while on the phone?

Back Office

Billing, collections, finance, accounting, and other administrative and management functions constitute the back-office activities that do not directly deal with the patient.

1. Can you view bills easily to answer questions for payers or patients?
2. Does the proposed system make it easier to perform the usual functions of your previous accounting system? Harder?
3. Is the accounts-receivable module easy to use and intuitive?
4. Does the accounts-receivable module fit into your workflow? How much do you have to change it to fit into the new system?
5. What features exist to edit claims before they are sent to the insurance company?
6. Can you access clinical records to correctly code visits?
7. How are the managed care functions interfaced with the managed care companies?
8. What other administrative features does this system have that make it easier to use than other systems?

General System Questions

There are some questions that either do not apply to a specific subsystem or apply equally to all parts of a system. In Question 6 below, the functional model refers to how the system represents concepts. That is, Do you select the data first, then indicate what you want to do with it? or Do you decide first what you are going to do before you select data? In Question 7, the information model refers to how the system represents data or information. For example, is the name represented the same way in all places (Firstname

Lastname or Lastname, Firstname)?

1. Does the system force the use of redundant data entry procedures (enter the same information twice or in two different
places)?
2. Does users find themselves "going in, then backing out" of
menu systems to get where they need to go, or is navigation
simple and straightforward?
3. Does the system make you write down information on paper to
transfer it or use it in another section?
4. Does the system offer a consistent look and feel? Do all dialog
boxes operate the same way? Printing procedures?
5. Do the keys do the same thing in all places in the program? Are
they standard for the platform or idiosyncratic? Does the system
require a template for the keyboard?
6. Does the system operate with the same functional model in all
places?
7. Does the system operate with the same information model in
all places?
8. Is the vendor responsive to problems and inquiries?
9. Are you generally pleased with the functionality and value
from the system? What do you not like about the contract with
the vendor?
10. Would you go with the same system and installation consultant
again?

Training and Installation Issues

Some issues can be brought up in all interviews regarding training. The
"train-a-trainer" system is a good idea. (The vendor trains a cadre of trainers who then train end-users to be peer trainers.) It can be a cost-effective
training method.

1. Did you receive adequate training? Was it from the company or a
"train-a-trainer" system?
2. Was the training done logically? Did it fit your workflow model?
3. In situations where the system did not fit your workflow model,
did you get an adequate explanation of the model it uses and why?
4. Were people present to help you when you went live? How is
phone support?
5. How long did productivity decrease after installation before getting back to normal?

6. What is your local support model? Do you have/need a help desk?
7. Is there on-line training and help functionality?
8. Are there "wizards" to help with complex functions?
9. What was/were the worse mistake(s) you made during installation?

Technical Issues

Technical issues may not be addressed sufficiently if all members of the team are users and administrators. If the team leader has access to technical personnel on-site, then the leader should ask these questions. If the answers are not understood by the team, arrange for a follow-up contact from a more knowledgeable person at your home site.

1. Were the hardware and utility functions adequate for your purposes?
2. Were the sizing calculations by the vendor realistic?
3. How often does the system go down? What is up-time percentage?
4. Is the vendor responsive to problem inquiries?
5. Did the vendor stay on schedule for installation and training?
6. How hard is it to interface with new systems?
7. Has the vendor ever deceived you?
8. Were there hidden or unexpected costs?

Logistics

Ideally, each team member should talk to several people at the site. The team may have to divide so that physicians interview physicians, nurses, and other direct users while administrators talk to managerial and other administrative front-line users. The visit matrix should be worked out well before the visit. Confirm in advance which personnel you will be given access to and that they will have time set aside to answer your questions. Keep in mind that quiet observation of site personnel going about their usual activities can be quite helpful. If possible, try to arrange for actual use of the system by team members (register a patient, log a phone call, make a referral, etc.).

The objectivity of host personnel is very important. It is acceptable to ask what, if anything, was given as a *quid pro quo* (by the vendor to the visit site) for granting the visit. While it is not ethical to specifically snoop around and ask questions of people to whom you have not been given access, there are ways to get confirmation of your host's opinion. While in your host's presence, it is considered fair game to strike up a conversation with a hosting co-worker by asking the co-worker to confirm your host's recently voiced opinions of the system. You may not get a full answer, but if there are hidden issues that your host has overlooked, a few passing comments may suggest further direct questions to your host about aspects he or she is less pleased with.

Extensive planning before the visit is required in order to assure a fruitful visit. Try to anticipate activities that might make team members unavailable (vacations, project deadlines, etc.) and plan accordingly. Keeping everyone on schedule, while being able to change the schedule to accommodate unanticipated opportunities, is a balancing act that only experience can finely attain.

Product Demonstrations

Why?

During the early stages of selecting an EMR system you may want to show your constituents a few of the leading products in the field so the project becomes more real to them. Later, a definitive demonstration occurs as part of a systematic evaluation of several products (finalists); this demonstration should be scripted so you can see how the products perform the features you require.

The initial free-form demonstration may be open-ended and run completely by the vendor sales team. It may include information about the company, how the product fits into the "bigger picture", and why the product is better than the competition's. It should take an hour or more and end with a session that permits hands-on access to the product.

The later, scripted demonstration may be a multi-day affair. There may be several scripts, lengthy interactions, multiple users, and de-briefing sessions. The scripts must be finished before considering which vendors to invite to participate. The scripts must entail tasks that are commonly done and those that are critical. Physician data entry is the heart of an EMR system and must be addressed during any demonstration.

Who?

Vendor Personnel
The vendor usually determines the make-up of the initial free-form demonstration. Typically a number of sales staff are included in the initial group.

Generally, the more senior the vendor personnel who attend, the more you as a customer will get out of the demonstration because sales personnel can only offer so much insight into the past and future development of the product.

The vendor should bring a substantial team to the short-list scripted demonstration. You should meet with senior-level personnel who have the authority to negotiate. Insist on having a physician from the vendor's staff, usually a Vice President, attend the demonstration. If there is no such person available, an early physician-user can suffice if accompanied by a vendor VP level representative. The other vendor personnel should be experienced users of each module featured in the product.

Office Personnel
On the customer side, who attends will depend on the purpose of the demonstration. In the early stages of EMR promotion, a series of sales presentations can be opened to the general audience of all potential users. Open presentations of this type can help generate enthusiasm and momentum for the project. The clinical and administrative opinion leaders should be invited as well as the decision-makers. For a scripted short-list demonstration, a much smaller team should be involved. The lead physician and key administrative personnel should be present, and one of them should sponsor the demonstration. A few persons on the project steering committee should be invited so that three to five might attend the demonstrations of each module. In addition, there should be a team of attendees who will be required to use the module in your institution. You should aim for at least three users in order to have enough for a balanced opinion (but not too many to bog down the proceedings). The criteria for selecting persons to participate in a demonstration are similar to the site visit criteria. Level-headed individuals who have a history with your institution are better than very computer savvy, but socially dissonant, individuals.

When?

The pep-rally type of demonstration should take place early in the process. As soon as administrative approval is given and a team assembled, demonstrations may be given of several products to provide a stimulating beginning to your selection process. The scripted demonstration should occur after the field is limited to about three finalists. The sequence of office demonstration and site visit is not critical and may depend on local factors such as availability of the vendors and the site visit team. If you have a formal set of questions and tasks for the site visit and a script and variations for the short-list demonstration, you could intersperse these as schedules permit.

Where?

The early sales demonstration is best done in an auditorium or small conference room depending on the size of the audience. You will need power outlets, video monitor projection, and network or phone connections as well as the typical audio projection depending on the needs of your presenter. For political reasons you should consider the impact of a sparsely attended demonstration in a large auditorium versus the standing-room-only effect of a medium-size room. The setting of a scripted demonstration is ideally a clinical area. However, you will not usually be able to secure a real clinical or patient area unless you do so during nonpatient hours. Since workflow can be critical to the success or failure of a system, it is definitely worth the trouble of creating a mock-up that represents the physical realities of your clinical area. For example, the mock-up reception area, waiting area, clinical area, and checkout areas should represent the physical realities of your situation. You should supply mock patients to move through the system and interact with vendor personnel using the product.

Basics

The sales-type demonstration requires only a brief introduction of the vendor personnel conducting the show. The audience will usually not be interested in the history of the company, although the company will frequently want to tell you how many years they have been selling this product and why their company is better than the competition. While there may be some merit to a limited review of company makeup, philosophy, and history, this should not take more than a few minutes. An overview of how the product fits into the overall information and patient care system is appropriate. What the audience really wants to see is how the product works, what the screens look like, how data entry is accomplished, how easy it is to navigate through the screens, and how the product is going to improve their daily lives or increase the quality of the care that they give to patients.

The success of the scripted demonstration depends heavily on the script. The script should take at least one patient from initial problem discovery through contacting the provider, getting care, and followup. Other patients can focus on smaller areas of the spectrum of care. Separate patient scripts could involve extensive telephone dialog, changing insurance or demographic information, a nurse protocol, a single-problem primary care visit, a single-problem specialty visit, a multi-problem primary care visit, a surgical procedure, and various administrative tasks and reports. The vendor should bring a system mocked up with adequate clinical data to make these realistic. Be wary of data that has already been entered to "speed-up" the demo.

Addressing Important Issues

The vendor primarily drives the sales demonstration because it is usually given in response to a request for general information. The prospective client should provide guidance on any particular features it wishes to be shown. Failure to properly target a sales demonstration then should reflect poorly on the company or at least on the sales force.

Scripted demonstrations are much more formal and more is at stake. A Request for Proposal is often sent to the vendor. Preparation of a scripted demonstration involves several steps:

1. Determine what problems the EMR system is to address/solve.
2. Talk to your users to understand their needs and workflow issues.
3. Get a specific list of tasks a system must do to provide the required functionality.
4. Get users to suggest scenarios that address the full range of functionality issues.
5. Write detailed scripts for each scenario; include patient dialogue.
6. Make this list available to the companies that you invite to conduct scripted demonstrations.
7. Discuss misunderstandings ahead of time to make sure the vendor addresses the areas correctly.
8. Modify the scripts if necessary and deliver the final version to each company.
9. Schedule demonstrations.
10. During the demonstration have your people play the part of the patient or other outside person.
11. Be prepared to change details slightly to make sure the demonstration has not been "hard-wired" into the program beforehand to make data entry appear easier than it really is.
12. Create and use a weighted grading tool for the demonstration.

Evaluating Site Visits and Product Demonstrations

For each site visit and each scripted demonstration of a system, it is important to objectively quantify your appraisal of the system's performance and how well it meets your needs. This information combined with the cost of the system will significantly enhance one's ability to calculate the value that the system could bring to your enterprise. To organize the evaluation, a formal document should be developed with questions grouped into categories based upon the results of a needs assessments and wish list. Where possible, study documents used by other organizations making similar decisions. When perusing other organization's list of survey documents, consider how closely the other organization's situation resembles your own. As much as is practicable avoid open-ended questions (i.e., create yes/no or multiple-choice questions).

It is important that a means of scoring responses be created. Scoring may be on a 0 to 1 scale or a more conceptual essential/nonessential feature format. For example, if you are in a predominately but not exclusively Novell network environment, you might make a question concerning network platforms have a value of .8 for a Novell-friendly system and .2 for a system that is not designed specifically to take advantage of Novell's features. Alternatively, you may choose to make Novell a requirement, in which case you would include a question indicating a Novell compatibility value of 1.0 and a noncompatability value of 0.0.

To record this quantification, a spreadsheet is a good idea. The spreadsheet follows the outline of the survey. On the spreadsheet record the importance of each question in a category to the overall category assessment. For each category, in a similar way assign a weight or importance factor for the category to the overall decision. Now when you fill in answers for each question you can transfer a numeric value to the spreadsheet and a score will emerge representing an objective measure of the value of a particular system. To facilitate multiple users contributing input to these decisions, you should develop a survey guidebook explaining the importance of each question and the significance of each answer choice.

Summary

Listed below are ten important "Do's" when conducting a site visit or hosting a product demonstration:

1. Do your political homework first to be sure you have support.
2. Make sure the system fits in the enterprise strategic plan.
3. Make sure you get a feeling of start-to-finish function.
4. Be prepared with a questionnaire from each area.
5. Look for common real-life uses.
6. Search for time savers and time wasters.
7. Think about installation, training, and back-office issues.
8. Keep tone even-handed.
9. Evaluate all important features quantitatively.
10. Ask about a work-around plan if a feature is not present.

Listed below are ten important "Don't's" when conducting a site visit or hosting a product demonstration:

1. Don't get caught up in details.
2. Don't get drawn in by hard-sell tactics.
3. Don't let logistic mistakes detract from the evaluation.
4. Don't keep your script exactly as advertised; change details.
5. Don't put problem personalities on your evaluation team.
6. Don't pass judgment during the evaluation.
7. Don't let overly solicitous salespersons sway you.
8. Don't accept vendor comments on relative merits of features.
9. Don't accept unproved bromides like "Everyone Loves It".
10. Don't let presentation gloss over critical dysfunction.

20 / Implementation: Preparation and Training

Sarah T. Corley

Physical Logistics

If you are adding computers to a space that has already been built, you will need to consider the wiring layout for your network. Be sure that you are using a reputable, experienced vendor for network installation. Cables can be damaged during installation, and this will slow the network down or make it difficult to locate problems. If it is a standard cable-based Ethernet network, then Cat 5 cable will have to be run through the walls into the offices and exam rooms and into a central room where the server will reside. If you are using a radio transmitter network, the transmitters will have to be installed and tested. This may take as little as a day if you have a small space and pop-up ceiling tiles, or it may take much longer if you are in an older, plaster-walled building.

Generally, wiring should be completed in two days for a small office and in less than a week for a larger office. (All cables should be tested, found to be functional, and warranted in writing before final payment is made.) It will, of course, take time for this to be scheduled, so allow four weeks from when you contact the cabling vendor to completion of the job. During this time of disruption, you should also consider whether the exam rooms will be conducive to the use of a computer and, if not, they should be reconfigured as well. This may involve building small computer stands with pull-out keyboards and will very likely increase the time required for design and installation. If cables must be run through the walls, you should strongly consider running telephone wires at the same time if you will be using modems. A DSL or T-1 line will provide connectivity via the server and does not require additional phone lines besides the one to the server.

Computers

In most offices, server and workstations are best custom ordered. This allows selection of server features tailored to your specific needs. If you are leasing your equipment, you should allow at least a month for completion of the lease paperwork, credit approval, and shipping of the computers. If you have an existing lease agreement already, this time period will usually require no more than two weeks between order and receipt. Once the computers have been received from the hardware vendor, they will have to be configured.

Many software vendors will have the server shipped to an installation specialist to configure it before sending it to the office. This can cut down on office disruption. The server will need to be configured for the network first, then for your specific application software. This process will usually take two to three days if all goes smoothly. If there are incompatibilities between the software, network operating system, or server, this can take longer. Each workstation will also need to be configured for the network, and printers will have to be added and configured for users. This usually takes about 30 to 45 minutes per machine. If in addition to an electronic medical records (EMR) system you are adding other software applications (e-mail, faxing capabilities, coding software, etc.), installation and configuration will require more time.

Table 20-1 lists requirements for installing your computer system.

Software Installation/Customization

It will usually take at least one day to install the various software programs, add users, configure printers, configure scanners, and set up computer shares. The practice should request that data back-up tasks and related utilities be configured to run automatically as a night-time batch file. Remote access will need to be set up in the office and at home sites if physicians will be dialing into the system outside of business hours.

Many vendors will supply diagnosis and procedure codes with the software, but there is still a lot of customization that must be done. Lab normal values will have to be added; user names, security levels, and passwords must be created. If prescriptions will be printed, the template and fonts will need to be configured to fit on a quarter-page piece of paper. Customization will realistically take about two days if worked on without interruption.

If lab interfaces are to be used, you should plan on at least three months

Table 20-1   Requirements for Computer Installation.

- Written implementation plan
- Wiring diagram with proposed server and workstation locations
- Server specifications for memory, disk drives, communications lines, etc.
- List of workstations and proposed configuration of each
- List of software applications and intended users
- Contract with detailed listing of specific vendor responsibilities for setup, testing, training, etc.
- Communications plan (e.g., Internet connection, fax, e-mail)

from purchase of the interface to the first test download. This is because a functioning interface depends upon cooperation and coordination with the software vendor, the lab, and the practice. The lab must have the capacity to download test results, to design a program for capturing data and sending that data to the office, and to provide data dictionaries so that the data will end up in the appropriate section of the chart. New lab requisitions may need to be designed and printed so that patient medical record numbers and provider ID numbers are captured by the lab and reported with the results. (You may think this is a simple thing to do—trust me, it is not.) Your vendor will probably need to write an interface to allow the downloaded lab files to be uploaded into patient records. There is usually a flat fee for this. The vendor will usually serve as the liaison with the lab and arrange all the preliminary testing. The practice may be responsible for creating a bridging data dictionary so that the lab names used in the practice's records can be matched to the test code numbers used by the laboratory. The matching of practice test names with formal lab test codes is a task best done by someone with extensive experience (in most instances, this will be a physician) with lab names used by the practice. Daunting as this may seem it will only take about four hours if done by a computer-savvy physician or nurse.

Templates, which can greatly speed the entry of progress notes and other clinical data, should be customized for the site. Templates may also help with quality assurance activities by providing for capture of standard data sets for certain diagnoses. Templates for common problems such as "New Diabetic" and "New Hypertensive" may speed data entry while ensuring that the same information is gathered for all patients with that diagnosis, making outcomes analysis much easier. Stock templates provided by the vendor should be reviewed and changes made to reflect the practice style of each physician who will use them. If the user can customize the templates (a very useful feature), then the templates can be further refined as the need arises.

Table 20-2 lists tips for software installation and customization.

Training

Training is the most important aspect of implementation. If the users are not well trained, the system is doomed to fail. If at all possible, negotiate a flat rate for the training package and be sure that expectations and commitments are clearly stated in your contract. The trainer should be an expert in all of the features of the program as well as a good teacher. The staff needs to have basic computer skills to focus on the training. All hardware should be tested and known to be functional before the training session.

Preliminary training for staff members who are not computer literate should be done in advance of the actual implementation phase. This includes users who have only been working in a DOS or pre-Windows 95 environment. It will be difficult for them to focus on software-specific training when they have not mastered the basics of operating systems that offer a graphical user interface. Depending upon the size of the practice, training may be done at a local adult education center or on site (off site may offer a more distraction-free learning environment). If at all possible, employees who have similar work roles should be trained together. This allows the training to be focused on the way that group will be interacting with the

---

Table 20-2   Tips for Software Installation and Customization.

- Create a policy for assignment of passwords and other security issues
- List interface required (lab, hospital, practice management system)
- Install required coding systems (CPT, ICD, SNOMED, etc.)
- Make a detailed list of remote access requirements
- List common problems for which templates are desired
- Review common office forms to determine which may be computerized or eliminated

software. Receptionists/appointment schedulers will use the system differently than will nurses and physicians.

Allow adequate time for breaks so that the staff can have enough time to absorb what is being taught. One full day of training with each group would be the minimum and preferably a second day could be spent with the trainer to help as the staff become acquainted with the system. I recommend setting up another day of training after the system has been in place for three months so that staff members can optimize the way they use the system and also learn more obscure or undocumented features that improve the day-to-day use of the software.

Table 20-3 lists tips for training staff.

Staff Expectations

Staff should be involved from the beginning of the process and kept informed of what changes will occur that can affect their jobs. People in general are very resistant to change, and it is very important that you consider the needs of the staff and also be aware of their fears. Take time to sit down with each member of the staff and discuss your plans for changes in job duties and employment levels. If you anticipate that fewer staff will be required, make the decisions as early as possible. Staff who will be let go should be given appropriate notice, letters of reference (if appropriate), and help in finding new positions (again if appropriate). Above all, do not let fear of job security plague your staff for long periods of time. It may result in unexpected resignations or even malicious acts. If paper records will no longer be kept, the medical records staff may need to be retrained for other functions. While charts will no longer have to be pulled and filed, there will be new tasks. In particular, data entry will become an issue. Outside reports will need to be entered into the EMR system through file

---

Table 20-3   Tips for Training Staff.

- Negotiate a flat-fee for all training

- Have vendor responsibilities clearly stated in the contract

- Note that off-site training may be less distracting and more effective

- Begin training of computer illiterate staff well in advance of implementation

- Set aside time for additional training a few months after installation

---

downloads, scanning, or manual addition. Lab results will need to be entered manually until the lab interface has been successfully implemented. If optimal use is made of the new data, there will be work involved in running reports and contacting patients who may be overdue for health maintenance procedures.

The nursing staff will still have the same duties as before but will need to enter and retrieve data from the computer rather than from a paper chart. You must be vigilant early on to be sure that *all* data are entered in the computer rather than scribbled as notes on the bottom of a consultant's report or a lab sheet. To improve staff buy-in, there should be regular training sessions in the office by "super users" to show other staff members ways to save time and effort using the newly available resources. Physicians should be aware that initially *more* effort will be required to accomplish the same tasks. However, as familiarity with the new system improves, productivity will increase and patient care quality will be enhanced.

Caveats and Advice

Try to negotiate a flat fee with your vendor for items that have the potential to be very time consuming. This would include all types of interfaces, billing, scheduling, and lab. All interfaces, even if designed for the same versions of the same programs, will require individual changes, and unexpected events will always occur. Lab interfaces will always take much longer than you think. Plan for how the data will be entered meanwhile. Do not try to use already busy staff to do this in their free time! It is often most economical to hire a data entry contractor to come in for a few hours on the weekend to enter the labs. If you are not able to change templates or chart format or other items without programming assistance from the vendor, you should try to negotiate a flat fee for a certain number of templates.

Cable wires frequently have flaws, so buy top-quality cable, have it installed professionally, and have it tested and warranted. Get same-day, four-hour service for your server. Get next-day, in-office service for your workstations. The peace of mind is well worth the cost.

Try to get your clinical consultants to send you reports on a floppy disk or through encrypted e-mail as an ASCII file to reduce the need for scanning. If this is not possible, try to have them send reports with a large clear font on plain paper, not letterhead. Plain paper will improve the quality of scanned documents using an Optical Character Recognition system. If documents are handwritten, they can be scanned as an image but it will take up more disk space and will prevent the text from being searched in a query.

Take the time to plan the exam room layouts so that you can maintain eye contact with patients while using the computer. Ask your vendor for suggestions or, better yet, for photos of different practice designs. Plan for the layout of your desk. A traditional desk makes an uncomfortable workstation, so often the best solution is new desks and chairs. Pay attention to the ergonomics of everyone's workstation to avoid lost time.

Table 20-4   Implementation Timeline.

Time to Implementation	Suggested Actions
6 weeks	Finalize EMR contract, work out details of implementation plan
4 weeks	Order computers, servers. Decide on workstation and server configurations and non-EMR software
	Order cabling and set installation date
	Decide on communications options (ADSL, T1, POTS)
	Request interfaces required (lab, hospital, practice management system)
3 weeks	Set policy for assignment of passwords and other security issues
	Begin training non-computer literate staff
	Determine coding systems
	Review vendor templates and begin customization
	Review common office forms to determine which may be computerized
2 weeks	Finalize installation plans with vendors, consultants, and outside facilities
	Adjust patient/procedure schedules for installation
1 week	Begin application-specific training
	Check final system configurations and specifications
	In large practices, create an "implementation problem" team to review problems occurring after the "go live" date
	Review last-minute details with staff

Spend the money for the fastest, biggest processors and computers available. Once you have a computer in place, you will want to add other software: textbooks, the Gail model breast cancer tool, atlases, patient education material, electronic code books, electronic address books, on-line access, and others. Get an uninterrupted power supply for the server and as many of the workstations as you can afford. There is nothing worse than losing a note or an appointment because of a sudden interruption of power in a thunderstorm. It also prevents the data corruption that can occur with a disorderly shutdown.

If a DSL line is available to your office, get one. You can save a lot of money in phone calls by e-mailing lab results and having patients e-mail prescription, appointment, and referral requests to the office and receive electronic replies. Fewer ringing phones also makes the office more peaceful. If you have constant access to the Internet, insurance company sites can be visited and claim status checked. Many HMOs allow you to complete referral requests on-line.

Consider having a professional design a Web page for you. This can include all the material in your practice brochure as a marketing tool. You can include all of your registration materials so they can be completed ahead of time and either printed or electronically sent to the office. This saves a great deal of time for new appointments without the postage and paper costs of mailing forms. You can include links for e-mailing appointment, prescription, and referral requests as well.

Do not print out a copy of your notes. This will double costs because you will have the computer expense plus chart expenses. Staff will always be tempted to pull charts and put handwritten notes in them if they are available, leaving the electronic record incomplete.

Table 20-4 is an implementation timeline that can be used a guide for your own practice

Appendix A
Glossary of Selected Terms

Steven Spadt, Linda Sundberg, and Jerome H. Carter

ADSL	Asymmetrical Digital Subscriber Line, a newly available means for providing high-speed Internet access. A special modem is required. However, regular telephone lines may be used. Download speeds of 1.5 megabits/second are attainable.
ASCII	American Standard Code for Information Interchange, a computer code of characters that consists of 7 or 8 binary values. A total of 256 characters comprise this set. ASCII is a standard for recording text files and serves as a standard format for exchanging files between application programs.
ATM	Asynchronous Transfer Mode, a method of transmitting and receiving data at speeds of up to 622 megabits/second.
Audit Trail	A historical record of access to a file or computer system. Audit trails are useful as an adjunct to other security methods.
Authentication	The process of verifying a user identity. Passwords are the most common type of authentication process.
Biometrics	A method of user verification based upon biologic markers such as fingerprints or iris patterns. Biometric authentication is becoming more popular due to its better resistance to tampering and low failure rates.
Browser	An application that permits downloading and viewing of Web pages. Internet Explorer and NetScape Navigator are the most popular Web browsers.
C++	One of the most popular programming languages, C++ was the first widely accepted object-oriented language. It began the trend towards object-oriented programming techniques, continued today by Java. It is still one of the most utilized languages for developing enterprise-level application software.

APPENDIX A   Glossary of Selected Terms (*continued*)

Cable Modem	A new type of modem that promises speeds of up to six times faster than a dedicated T1 line (the type of connection used by most large organizations). Because cable modems communicate with the Internet over cable TV lines, they are much faster than modems that use phone lines. Costs may be prohibitive, though, because modems are about three times more expensive than a traditional phone modem and monthly fees from cable companies currently average around $50 per month.
CD-Recordable	Compact Disk Recordable (CD-R) is a CD-ROM format that enables one to read and write compact disks. CDs recorded using this technology cannot be erased.
Client/Server	A means for accessing information that resides on a central computer (server) by any number of connected computers (clients). Client/server computing differs from traditional mainframe computing (with dumb terminals) by allowing clients to process retrieved information (smart). This is the major computing style seen in most small- and medium-sized businesses.
Controlled Vocabulary	A list of preferred terms for describing actions, concepts, and findings within a particular domain. In health care a controlled vocabulary might be used to suggest acceptable terms for encoding the progress note.
CORBA	Common Object Request Broker Architecture, a standard for building applications that uses objects as a mechanism to exchange data and services. CORBA applications permit a three-tiered client/server architecture in which the data reside on the server, the requesting application on the client, and the rules for accessing the data within CORBA objects.
CPT	Current Procedural Terminology, a coding scheme used for billing and reimbursement. It provides codes for diagnostic and therapeutic procedures.
CPU	In personal computers, the microprocessor that performs all processing functions. CPUs are predominantly 32 bits (i.e., each can handle 4 units of information at once). Processors that can manipulate 64 bits (8 units) are becoming more widely available.
Data Dictionary	A file in a database system that contains information regarding the records and fields (type, length, access permission) within the database.
Data Mart	A limited aggregate data set used for decision support often containing data from one area or activity (i.e., sales only).

APPENDIX A   Glossary of Selected Terms (*continued*)

Data Mining	The process of extracting information from a database using statistical or artificial intelligence analytical tools.
Data Warehouse	An aggregate data collection containing summarized information that is used for decision support. Data warehouses are usually found in large organizations and contain a wide range of data (sales, costs, revenue, etc.).
DBMS	An application program that manages the creation, storage, and retrieval of data. The most common type of DBMS uses relational architectures.
Encryption	The process of scrambling data by encoding it using a standard scheme (key) that allows only those who have access to the key to unscramble and read the data.
Firewall	Hardware or software that limits access to a computer from a network or an external source. Firewalls often form the first line of security for protecting Web sites.
HEDIS	Health Plan Employer Data and Information Set, a set of performance measures created to assist purchasers of health care services in evaluating the care offered by health plans; often used as a measure of care quality.
HIPAA	The Health Insurance Portability and Accountability Act of 1996.
HL-7	Health Level 7, a standard for encoding health care information that is passed between computer systems.
HTML	Hypertext Markup Language, the formatting code that designs Web pages. HTML defines codes that control the layout and appearance of Web pages.
ICD	International Classification of Diseases, a standard scheme for encoding diagnoses.
Intranet	A network site that functions like the Web except it has restricted use, usually within a company or organization.
Internet 2	The Internet 2 is a project being led by universities, government, and corporations to "facilitate and coordinate the development, deployment, operation and technology transfer of advanced, network-based applications and network services to further U.S. leadership in research and higher education and accelerate the availability of new services and applications on the Internet." This mission of the Internet 2 project is largely in response to the commercialization of the current manifestation of the Internet that has impeded its use for research and educational purposes.

APPENDIX A   Glossary of Selected Terms (*continued*)

Java	An object-oriented programming language designed by Sun Microsystems. A major feature of this language is platform independence (i.e., it is not tied to a particular operating system). It is being used increasingly in the design of Web sites and for the creation of Web-based applications.
Local Area Network	A network that connects computers within a limited geographic area.
Master Patient Index	An application used within health care organizations to assure that medical record numbers are unique.
N-Tier	A design architecture for building database applications, N-tier allows the location of application and database portions (called components) of a system anywhere within a network. This technique is very popular for building systems intended to be made accessible via the Internet, because the client portion of the application can be the Web browser and other portions of the system can be spread amongst one or more machines networked together via the Internet.
Object Database	Unlike the more popular relational database, object databases store data in an object hierarchy rather than in linear records in tables. The database manages the hierarchy of objects. This technique for storage is often more appropriate for systems built with object-oriented methods, because the data need not be mapped between linear records and objects each time the data are stored or retrieved from the database.
PACS	Picture Archiving and Communication System, a system dedicated to the storage and retrieval of radiologic images.
Provider Profiling	A process whereby provider patterns of usage of medications, diagnostic tests, and other interventions are recorded and analyzed.
Query	Usually just a text string, the query is a message passed from some application (or even directly from a user) to a database. The message requests some subset of the data contained in the database. Often times, this term is also used to identify the returned data as well as the request.
Read Codes	A coding system created in the United Kingdom that is designed to permit encoding of the patient record.
Relational Database	A database architecture where data reside in tables made of records that consist of identical fields. Data are accessed using a standard query language (SQL).

APPENDIX A   Glossary of Selected Terms (*continued*)

RFP
Request for Proposal, a document sent to various companies requesting that they submit an application detailing how they will provide the application or service requested.

Server
A powerful, central computer which holds key applications and data that are shared with other computers which communicate with it via a network.

SNOMED
Systematized Nomenclature of Human and Veterinary Medicine, a standard nomenclature for encoding diagnostic information.

SQL
Structured Query Language, a standardized language used to write queries of databases. SQL is most often expressed as an ASCII text string, which is passed to a database as a query. The syntax is mostly human-readable, e.g., "SELECT [Last Name] FROM [Employees] WHERE [Job Title] = 'Manager'" would return all the last names of the employees whose job title is 'Manager'.

T1
A digital carrier that transfers data at the rate of 1.544 megabits/second.

TCP/IP
Transfer Control Protocol/Internet Protocol.

Thin Client
One component of the N-tier architecture, the thin client is the portion of the application that is responsible for presenting the user interface. Thin clients are given this name due to their lack of complex business logic, data, or other functionality, which are all aspects of the system handled by other components. In Internet-accessible applications, the thin client is usually a standard Web browser.

Unix
A multi-user, multi-tasking operating system created in the 1970s that is still used in many computer installations. Much of the current internet was built upon Unix-based systems.

User Interface
The portion of a software application that makes it accessible to a user, the user interface often contains push buttons, text areas in which the user can type information, windows containing information, etc. User interfaces that contain functionality that is accessible by pointing and clicking with a mouse are called Graphical User Interfaces (GUIs).

Voice Recognition
A type of computer input that is based upon speech. Voice recognition may be discrete (pauses between words) or continuous. A number of inexpensive models are available.

Wide Area Network
WAN, a network spread over a large geographic region consisting of connected local networks.

APPENDIX A	Glossary of Selected Terms (*continued*)
Windows NT	An operating system from Microsoft that is designed primarily for corporate PC use, Windows NT is based on a 32-bit architecture like that of its Windows siblings but has features that expand functionality, improve performance, and increase security levels. For running a network, there is a Server version available.
Windows 2000	The newest operating system offering from Microsoft, Windows 2000 is really a family of offerings. Each option represents only minor changes in functionality from the older Windows operating systems (NT, 95, and 98) but is significant in its merger of Windows NT and the 95/98 family. Now, rather than choosing between Windows NT and Windows 98, a user must select from the Windows 2000 line of operating systems.
WORM	Write Once, Read Many is a type of optical disk. Data are permanent once placed on the disk.
XML	Extensible Markup Language.

Appendix B
Electronic Medical Record Resources

Vendors

N.B. This EMR vendor listing is provided only as a guide for the reader. It does not pretend to inconclusiveness. No endorsement of any or all of these vendors is implied or given by the editor or the American College of Physicians–American Society for Internal Medicine.

A⁴ Health Systems
5501 Dillard Drive
Cary, NC 27511
888-672-3282
www.a4healthsystems.com

Accumedic Computer Systems, Inc.
11 Grace Avenue, Suite 401
Great Neck, NY 11021
800-765-9300
www.accumedic.com

Advanced Health Technologies
200 West Adams Street, Suite 1000
Chicago, IL 60606
312-443-5800
www.advhealth.com

Affinity Software Corporation
1600 Providence Highway
Walpole, MA 02081
800-437-4307
www.affinitysoft.com

American Management Systems
12601 Fair Lakes Circle
Fairfax, VA 22033
800-682-0028
www.amsinc.com

American Medical Software
7 GE Professional Park
PO Box 236
Edwardsville, IL 62025
800-736-8456
www.americanmedical.com

Araxsys, Inc.
200 Penobscot Drive
Redwood City, CA 94063
800-932-2729
www.araxsys.com

Axolotl Corporation
800 El Camino Real West, #150
Mountain View, CA 94040
888-296-5685
www.axolotl.com

Azron, Inc.
5950 La Place Court, Suite 250
Carlsbad, CA 92008
760-804-8800
www.azron.com

Berdy Medical Systems
155 Cedar Lane
Teaneck, NJ 07666
800-662-3739
www.uhcd.com/berdy

Brickell Research, Inc.
2490 Coral Way, Suite 401
Miami, FL 33145
305-858-6984
www.brickellresearch.com

Care Data Systems
5455 North Sheridan, Suite 1401
Chicago, IL 60640
888-340-DATA
www.caredatasystems.com

Care Informatiuon Systems
2815 Old Jacksonville Road,
    Suite 201
Springfield, IL 62704
800-590-4100
www.careinfo.com

CareMed Corporation
5565 Grossmont Center, Building 2,
    Suite 2
La Mesa, CA 91942
800-392-6379
www.caremed.com

Cerner Corporation
2800 Rockcreek Parkway
Kansas City, MO 64117
816-221-1024
www.cerner.com

Chartcare, Inc.
1400 Peoples Plaza, Suite 220
Newark, DE 19702
800-438-1277
www.chartcare.com

Chartware, Inc.
101 Golf Course Drive, Suite A220
Rohnert Park, CA 94928
800-642-4278
www.chartware.com

CliniComp International
9655 Towne Center Drive
San Diego, CA 92121
800-350-8202
www.clinicomp.com

Clinical Information Solutions
30 Willow Street
North Andover, MA 01845
800-421-7432
www.aimcare.com

Clinical NetwoRx, Inc.
9400 North MacArthur Boulevard,
    Suite 333
Irving, TX 75063
972-871-7100
www.cnrx.com

Datamedic Corporation
20 Oser Avenue
Hauppauge, NY 11788
800-645-7100
www.datamedic.com

Docs, Inc.
1443 West Sunset Avenue
Springdale, AZ 72764
800-455-7627
www.docs.com

Echo Management Group
1620 Main Street
Center Conway, NH 03813
800-635-8209
www.echoman.com

Eclipsys Corporation
777 East Atlantic Avenue, Suite 200
Delray Beach, FL 33483
561-243-1440
www.eclipsys.com

Electronic Healthcare Systems, Inc.
100 Brookwood Place, Suite 410
Birmingham, AL 35209
888-879-7302
www.ehsmed.com

Enterprise Healthcare Systems, Inc.
11409 St. Andrew's Way
Scottsdale, AZ 85254
602-998-5452
www.ehsiplus.com

Epic Systems Corporation
5301 Tokay Boulevard
Madison, WI 53711
608-271-9000
www.epicsys.com

Epsilon Systems, Inc.
929 Fifth Avenue NW, Suite300
St. Paul, MN 55112
612-636-3890
www.carefacts.com

Experior Corporation
5710 Coventry Lane
Fort Wayne, IN 46804
800-595-2020
www.experior.com

HBO&C
301 Perimeter Center North
Atlanta, GA 30346
800-981-8601
www.hboc.com

HCS
PO Box 2430
Farmingdale, NJ 07727
800-524-1038
www.hcsinteractant.com

Healthcare Data Inc.
5311 Mount Pleasant North Drive
Greenwood, IN 46142
317-884-4812
www.healthprobe.com

Health Care Data Systems
5703 Enterprise Parkway, Box 608
DeWitt, NY 13214
800-950-7111
www.hcds.com

Health Information Systems
2 North Plains Industrial Road
Wallingford, CT 06492
800-562-7069
www.healthis.com

HealthMagic Inc.
1444 Wazee Street, Suite 210
Denver, CO 80202
303-592-1580
www.haelthmagic.com

Infinity Medical Systems Inc.
15996 Grey Stone Road
Poway, CA 92064
800-631-1467
www.infinitydoc.com

JMJ Technologies, Inc.
2155 Post Oak Tritt Road, Suite 540
Marietta, GA 30062
770-509-5653
www.jmjtech.com

Logos Systems, Inc.
8303 Southwest Freeway, Suite 500
Houston, TX 77074
800-722-4534
www.logossytems.com

M2 Information Systems Inc.
144 Railroad Avenue, Suite 100
Edmonds, WA 98020
800-598-6647
www.m2is.com

The Magic Corporation
26 Lafayette Street
Norwich, CT 06360
860-886-2860
www.dreco.com

Med4th Systems Ltd.
2701 University Avenue, Suite 418
Madison, WI 53705
608-833-1985
www.med4th.com

MedCom Information Systems, Inc.
2117 Stonington Avenue
Hoffman Estates, IL 60195
800-213-2161
http://idt.net/~medcom19

Medic Computer Systems
8601 Six Forks Road, Suite 300
Raleigh, NC 27415
800-334-8534
www.medcmp.com

Medical Information Management Systems, Inc.
511 Union Street
Suite 1800
Nashville, TN 37219
615-777-6467
www.mimscorp.com

Medical Information Systems, Inc.
1150 First Avenue
Suite 620
King of Prussia, PA 19406
800-487-9135
www.chartmaker.com

Medical Information Technology
One Meditech Circle
Westwood, MA 02090
781-821-3000
www.meditech.com

MedicaLogic, Inc.
20500 NW Evergreen Parkway
Hillsboro, OR 97124
800-322-5538
www.medicalogic.com

Medicomp Systems
14500 Avion Parkway
Suite 175
Chantilly, VA 20151
703-803-8080
www.medicomp.com

MediMouse Systems
107 Lakefront Drive
Hunt Valley, MD 21030
410-771-0301
www.penta.com/medimouse

MedPlus Inc.
8805 Governors Hill Drive
Cincinnati, OH 45249
800-444-6235
www.medplus.com

Medware Computer Solutions
1055 North Dixie Freeway
Suite 2
New Smyrna Beach, FL 32168
800-316-4786
www.medware.com

Mountainside Software Inc.
780 Keezletown Road
Weyers Cave, VA 24486
800-868-8423
www.mtnsdsoft.com

Oacis Healthcare Systems
1101 Fifth Avenue
San Rafael, CA 94901
415-482-4400
www.oacis.com

Oceania, Inc.
3145 Porter Drive
Suite 103
Palo Alto, CA 94304
888-462-3264
www.oceania.com

Patient Medical Records Inc.
901 Tahoka Road
Brownfield, TX 79316
800-285-7627
www.pmrinc.com

PDA Medical
PO Box 471659
San Francisco, CA 94147
415-447-0504
www.pdamed.com

Per-Se Technologies
2840 Mount Wilkinson Parkway
Atlanta, GA 30326
770-444-4000
www.per-se.com

Physician Micro Systems, Inc.
2033 Sixth Avenue, #707
Seattle, WA 98121
206-441-8490
www.pmsi.com

Physician's Computer Company
15 Pinecrest Drive
Essex Junction, VT 05452
800-722-7708
www.pcc.com

Physix, Inc.
Two Greenway Plaza, Suite 610
Houston, TX 77046
800-749-2585
www.physix.com

PowerMed Corporation
PO Box 128
Medina, NY 14103
888-621-5565
www.PowerMed.Com

PrimeCare Systems Inc.
610 Thimble Shoals Boulevard
Suite 402-A
Newport News, VA 23606
757-591-0323
www.pcare.com

Purkinje Inc.
The Forum 8000
Interstate Highway 10 West, Suite 600
San Antonio, TX 78230
210-476-0030
www.purkinje.com

Quick Notes, Inc.
11346 State Road 84
Fort Lauderdale, FL 33325
800-899-2468
www.qnotes.com

Sirius Technologies America
2100 Habersham Marina Road, #201B
Atlanta, GA 30131
770-889-2351
www.siriustech.com

SMS
51 Valley Stream Parkway
Malvern, PA 19355
610-219-6300
www.smed.com

SpectraSoft Inc.
6100 South Maple Avenue, #118
Tempe, AZ 85283
800-889-0450
www.ssoft.com

3M Health Information Systems
575 West Murray Boulevard
Murray, UT 841123
800-367-2447
www.3Mhis.com

Turbo-Doc Medical Record Systems, Inc.
771 Buschmann Road
Suite G
Paradise, CA 95969
800-977-4868
www.turbodoc.com

VersaForm Systems Corporation
591 West Hamilton Avenue, #201
Campbell, CA 95008
800-678-1111
www.versaform.com

Wang Healthcare
Concord Road Corporate Center
300 Concord Road, 3rd Floor
Billerica, MA 01821
888-813-7575
www.whis.com

Journals and Web Sites

Magazines and Web sites are good sources of information on health care computing. Trade journals often contain interesting and useful observations on issues related to EMR systems. Web sites can also be an aid: *e-MD* is a site aimed at health care providers and is a very good source of useful information; *The Informatics Review* (the e-journal of the Association of Medical Directors of Information Systems) is a site with information on current issues in medical informatics as well as links to a number of useful sites; and *ComputingforClinicians.com* is maintained by the editor of this book who welcomes your questions and comments.

Trade Journals

Advance for Health Information Executives
www.advanceforhie.com

Healthcare Informatics
www.healthcare-informatics.com

Health Data Management
http://HDM.Faulknergray.com

MD Computing
www.mdcomputing.com

Web Sites

ComputingforClinicians.com
www.computingforclinicians.com

e-MD
http://www.edotmd.com/

The Informatics Review
www.informatics-review.com

Organizations and Standards Groups

American Medical Informatics
    Association
4915 St. Elmo Avenue, #401
Bethesda, MD 20814
301-657-1291
www.amia.org

Computer-Based Patient Record
    Institute
4915 St. Elmo Avenue, #401
Bethesda, MD 20814
301-657-1291
www.cpri.org

Medical Records Institute
567 Walnut Street
PO Box 600770
Newton, MA 02460
617-964-3923
www.medrecinst.com

Standards Groups

ASTM	www.astm.org
CPT	www.ama-assn.org/med-sci/cpt/cpt.htm
DICOM	www.nema.org
HL-7	www.HL7.org
ICD-10	www.vaccines.ch/whosis/icd10/index.html
LOINC	www.regenstrief.org/loinc/loinc_information.html
MEDCIN	www.medicomp.com
NDC	www.fda.gov/cder/ndc/
READ Codes	www.schin.ncl.ac.uk/mig/terms.htm
SNOMED	www.snomed.org/

Hardware and Technology

Below are sites which provide timely information on the latest technology trends and reviews of products. *Infoworld* and *PC Week* are weekly technology newsletters. Both offer in-depth reviews and analysis of trends and issues. They also offer searchable archives of past reviews and articles. Both Web sites offer access to a wealth of additional, mostly free, resources including full-text articles and product reviews. Ziff-Davis Publishing offers a number of consumer-oriented computer publications (including excellent Macintosh coverage) and all are available on-line; *PC Week* is one of its publications (Web site: *www.zdnet.com*).

Infoworld: www.infoworld.com

PC Week: www.zdnet.com/pcweek

For those who would like buying books, nothing beats the *For Dummies...* series for price, quality, or range of topics covered:

For Dummies Books: www.dummies.com

APPENDIX C
Using the EMR
Evaluation Form

Jerome H. Carter

The sample EMR evaluation form reproduced in this Appendix may be found useful in creating a Request for Proposal or evaluation materials for site visits and demonstrations. Of course, it should be altered to fit your particular situation. Opposite the list of features are three columns. The first, "Present/Absent", provides a simple means for noting which features are available in the product. This is a good way to do a "first cut" of the product candidates. Next, determine which features are essential (i.e., which features, if absent, automatically remove the product from further consideration). Comparing the "Present/Absent" column to the "Essential?" column provides a quick way of assessing the potential value of the products under consideration. This makes it easy for those who did not complete the form (e.g., other committee members) to rapidly review products and assess their relative suitability. The final column, "Point Value", is used to record the quality of the implementation of a feature. For example, if the feature under consideration is "Allergy List", then a product that provides for easy list updates in two steps and alerts the user during prescription writing may be deemed superior to one that requires a four-step list update process and that requires the user to remember to look up the patient's allergy history. The former product may be given, for example, a score of 1 (maximum usefulness) for "Allergy List", whereas the latter may be given a score of only 0.7. Using this approach, fine differences between close competitors can be made more objective and analyzable. Of course, the rules for assigning points to various feature components must be determined by those performing the evaluation. Ideally, point assignments are made based upon information gleaned from process analyses.

Product Name:_____

Company:_____

Evaluation Date:_____

Product features deemed essential are in roman type; "wish list" items appear in italic.

	Present/ Absent	Essential?	Point Value (Quality If Present)
CHART FEATURES			
Medication Features			
Medication list			
Long-term			
Per episode			
Active/inactive			
Failed after trial			
Allergy list			
Automatic allergy warning			
Prescription writer			
E-mail or fax to pharmacy			
Maintains prescription history			
Maintains formulary information			
By insurance plan			
Drug interactions			
Multiple drug-drug			
Practitioner-specific medication list			
Drug information			
Side effects			
Adverse reactions			
Overdose			
Dosages			
Forms supplied			
Reports by			
Patient			
Medication			
Provider			

Checklist of EMR Features

	Present/ Absent	Essential?	Point Value (Quality If Present)
Laboratory/X-ray/Pathology Features			
Maintains test history			
By patient			
By provider			
Permits automatic data download from outside facilities			
Permits uploading of orders to other facilities (e.g., lab orders)			
Maintains profile of available tests and indications			
Flags abnormal results			
Permits tracking of abnormal lab followup			
Permits creation of panels			
Disease specific			
Patient specific			
Population specific			
Alerts for redundant testing			
Guideline-aware order entry			
Reports by			
Patient			
Test			
Provider			
Telephone Call Features			
Maintains call history			
Patient			
Site			
Provider			
Number called from			
Automatic dialing			
Captures call reason and action taken			
Provides alerts and reminders for required followup			

Checklist of EMR Features (*continued*)

	Present/ Absent	Essential?	Point Value (Quality If Present)
Report by			
Patient			
Provider			
Call reason			
Call action			
Diagnosis Features			
Problem list			
Long-term			
Per episode			
Guideline-based advice			
Access to knowledge resources			
Internet			
Practice guidelines			
Report by			
Patient			
Provider			
Diagnosis			
Referral Features			
Maintains list of referral sites and providers by			
Specialty			
Reason for referral			
Location			
Maintains referral history			
Patient			
Provider			
Site			
Reason/diagnosis			
Maintains list of approved providers/sites by			
Insurance plan			
Provider preference			

Checklist of EMR Features (continued)

	Present/ Absent	Essential?	Point Value (Quality If Present)
Report by			
Patient			
Provider			
Reason/diagnosis			
Referral site/provider			
Reports by e-mail			
Store and forward images			
Preventive Medicine Features			
Maintains patient intervention history			
Permits design of intervention protocols by			
Sex			
Age			
Disease state			
Insurance plan			
Permits guideline-based protocols			
Provides user-defined alerts			
Report by			
Patient population			
Patient			
Provider			
Diagnosis			
Protocol			
Health status			
SF-36			

Checklist of EMR Features (continued)

	Present/ Absent	Essential?	Point Value (Quality If Present)
Clinical Encounter Features			
Progress note			
Plain text			
Encoded and searchable			
Vital signs			
Clinical findings			
E&M templates			
Defined by end-user			
Specialty specific			
Disease-based guidelines/protocols			
Defined by end-user			
Specialty specific			
Patient Education Features			
User definable			
Preloaded			
Updated regularly (quarterly)			
Web access to educational materials			
ANALYSIS AND MANAGED CARE			
Managed Care Features			
Provider profiles			
Medications			
Labs			
Referrals			
Preventive health			
Site profiles			
Medications			
Labs			
Referrals			
Preventive health			

Checklist of EMR Features (*continued*)

	Present/ Absent	Essential?	Point Value (Quality If Present)
Outcomes by			
Guideline/protocol			
Provider			
Disease			
Site			
Pre-defined reports			
HEDIS			
JCAHO			
Cost analysis			
Labs			
Disease			
Protocols			
Referral			
Patient			
Provider			
COMMUNICATIONS AND INFRASTRUCTURE			
Communications			
Remote access			
Fax support or linkage			
Word processor support or linkage			
Spreadsheet support or linkage			
Provides e-mail support or linkage			
Internet			
Web-enabled version			
Decision Support			
Statistical analysis (internal)			
Knowledge resources (access from within EMR)			
MEDLINE			
Internet resources			
Electronic textbooks			

Checklist of EMR Features (*continued*)

	Present/ Absent	Essential?	Point Value (Quality If Present)
Data Storage and File Formats			
Permits data export			
ASCII			
Support for clinical data repository			
Data warehouse			
Statistical analysis packages			
Permits data import			
ASCII			
Relational database files			
Application programming interface			
Supports varied data formats			
Sound			
Video			
Graphics			
File formats supported			
Proprietary			
Commercial standard (Oracle, Sybase, etc.)			
ASCII			
Standards Supported			
HL-7			
CORBA			
SNOMED			
ICD			
CPT			
MEDCIN			
READ codes			
LOINC for lab data			

Checklist of EMR Features (*continued*)

	Present/ Absent	Essential?	Point Value (Quality If Present)
Interface Options			
Pen			
Voice			
Keyboard			
Graphics			
User modifiable			
Security Features			
Audit trail			
Permits audit trail analysis			
Automatic activation			
Passwords			
Text numeric			
Biometric			
Face			
Voice			
Fingerprints			
Multiple levels by user type			
Data validation			
Back-up process			
Encryption			
Operating Systems			
Unix			
Macintosh			
Windows 95/98			
Windows NT			
Novell			
Internet based			
Client/server			
Number of tiers			

Checklist of EMR Features (*continued*)

	Present/ Absent	Essential?	Point Value (Quality If Present)
Technology			
Database			
Relational			
Object			
Multi-dimensional			
SQL support			

Total Desired Features Present: _____

Total Number of Essential Features: _____

Total Quality Points: _____

Evaluation Computation Suggestion:

Step 1: Narrow product field to no more than four packages.

Step 2: Add up "Total Desired Features Present". Eliminate low ranking products.

Step 3: Add up "Total Number of Essential Features". Eliminate low ranking products.

Step 4: For all remaining products determine the quality of implementation for all features of each product. The winning products will be candidates for more in-depth demonstrations and site visits.

Checklist of EMR Features (*continued*)

Appendix D
Sample Request for Proposal

Sarah T. Corley

Section I: Practice and Company Information

Practice Information (Supplied by Practice)

- Main contact at the practice: Name, Title, Address, Telephone, Fax, and E-mail.

- Person (if not the main contact) who will negotiate terms of the relationship: Name, Title, Address, Telephone, Fax, and E-mail.

- Total number of physicians, advanced practice providers, nurses, and administrative staff.

- Total number of exam rooms and workstations.

- Details of software that will need interfaces designed.

- Name and contact person for outside lab(s) information system.

Company Information

- Main contact for this proposal: Name, Title, Address, Telephone, Fax, and E-mail.

- Person (if not the main contact) who will negotiate terms of relationship: Name, Title, Address, Telephone, Fax, and E-mail.

- Address of company headquarters and main telephone number if different from the contact address and telephone.

- Provide the name, address, and phone number of your parent organization and any specific division or subsidiary company completing this proposal. Provide the name of and résumé for the President/CEO, Development Director, Marketing Director, Maintenance Director, Installation Manager, and Support Manager.

- Provide the total number of employees within your organization that are directly and exclusively associated with the EMR product. Provide the number and average tenure of employees in Marketing and Sales, Research and Development, Maintenance, Quality Control/Quality Assurance, Technical Support, Client Services,/ Installation, Field Service, and End-User Support.

- Provide information concerning your organization's annual research-and-development plans in the area of EMR systems. Indicate current and projected (3 year) expenditures for research-and-development activity in both absolute terms and as a percent of gross revenues.

- Describe the major releases planned for the proposed platform we would use, with the release and implementation time frames.

- Describe your progress and plans to incorporate the following items into your products: speech (voice) recognition, graphics- or icon-based interfaces, touch screens, light pens, decision support, Internet, and wireless transmission.

- Give a brief description and history of your company.

- Provide copies of audited financial statements for the last three years and a banking reference.

- Provide the number of clients in practices of a similar size and composition to ours and three references including name, address, and telephone number.

- Provide the total number of software licenses sold each year over the last three years.

- Provide the total number of software licenses installed each year over the last three years.

- Provide the name, address, and telephone number of clients representing your ten most recent sales.

- Provide the name, address, and telephone number of clients representing your ten most recent installations.

- Describe your three *most successful* and three *least successful* installations for the proposed system within the past two years. Highlight those practices that are similar in size and scope to ours. Include the following information:

    ✔ Client name, address, telephone number, and contact person

    ✔ Number of users

    ✔ Date of contract commencement

    ✔ Brief hardware configuration, including the number and type of workstations, scanners, printers, and other system components

- Submit a complete list of all clients using your system: name, address, telephone number, date purchased, and date of first productive use.

- Describe any litigation your company is involved in.

- List all technology and/or distribution partnerships and alliances including partner-name, address, telephone number, and a brief description of the nature of the relationship.

- Is your company's software HL-7 compliant? What data interchange standards does your company adhere to?

- Have any objective studies of your system's benefits been reported in journals? If so, please include a copy.

- Do you have a users group? How often does it meet? Do you have a regular client newsletter? How often is it published? Include all copies for the past year.

Section II: Functional Requirements

For each numbered area below please indicate the status of the feature as follows:

C = Current feature supported in a commercially available release
P = Planned feature for a future release (include the expected month/year of the commercially available release)
N = Not planned
O = Other product. The feature is available in another product either from your company or from another company with which you have a distribution relationship. Include any relevant cost or future date information.

Write a narrative description that describes the capabilities of your product in each area. You may include additional information in the Appendix.

1. **Chart Summary**
   Status: _____ Date/Other Info: _____
   Narrative Description:

2. Links Between Chart Elements
Status: _____ Date/Other Info: _____
Narrative Description:

3. Flexible Data Collection
Status: _____ Date/Other Info: _____
Narrative Description:

4. Results Display
Status: _____ Date/Other Info: _____
Narrative Description:

5. Health Maintenance
Status: _____ Date/Other Info: _____
Narrative Description:

6. Intuitive Interaction Model
Status: _____ Date/Other Info: _____
Narrative Description:

7. Standards-Based Encoding
Status: _____ Date/Other Info: _____
Narrative Description:

8. Scheduling
Status: _____ Date/Other Info: _____
Narrative Description:

9. Intraoffice Messaging
Status: _____ Date/Other Info: _____
Narrative Description:

10. To-Do Lists
Status: _____ Date/Other Info: _____
Narrative Description:

11. Rapid User Interaction Model
Status: _____ Date/Other Info: _____
Narrative Description:

12. Referral Management
Status: _____ Date/Other Info: _____
Narrative Description:

13. Order Entry
Status: _____ Date/Other Info: _____
Narrative Description:

14. Client–Server
Status: _____ Date/Other Info: _____
Narrative Description:

15. Oracle, Sybase, Informix (for larger practices)
Status: _____ Date/Other Info: _____
Narrative Description:

16. Communications Manager
Status: _____ Date/Other Info: _____
Narrative Description:

17. Scalability
Status: _____ Date/Other Info: _____
Narrative Description:

18. System and Data Security
Status: _____ Date/Other Info: _____
Narrative Description:

Section III: Support and Services

- How are new releases handled? Be specific about costs and time frames.

- How is routine technical support handled? Be specific about costs and time frames.

- Provide address and telephone numbers for support locations nationally and the closest support available for our practice.

- Attach a standard contract and describe any exclusions.

- List any procedures expected from clients to ensure smooth system operation.

- Describe all hardware and software maintenance options.

- Describe any additional services offered if hardware is purchased as part of the transaction.

- Describe your approach to providing appropriate clinical content and knowledge bases for the specialties in our practice.

- List all third-party products to which your system has been interfaced.

- Describe your problem escalation policies in general and specifically for software errors, hardware errors, and disasters.

Section IV: Costs

- Detail the proposed hardware including manufacturer, model numbers, unit prices, quantities, and total cost.

- Detail the proposed software including module name, unit prices, quantities, and total cost.

- Detail the proposed implementation and training services including costs per day, number of FTEs from your organization, number of FTEs recommended from our practice, number of service days, number of calendar days, and total services cost.

- Detail the proposed hardware maintenance services including costs.

- Detail the proposed software maintenance services and technical support including costs.

- Describe the fee structure for help/questions, troubleshooting, general-release enhancements (upgrading, debugging), system performance fine-tuning, training (at vendor and on-site), and custom development/modifications.

Section V: Appendix

Please supply any additional material that you consider relevant to your proposal.

INDEX